D1790428

RED ROCKS COMMUNITY COLLEGE
U18960 042 983 6

RD 31 .G4 1985

General surgery

DATE DUE

NOV 8 '93			

DEMCO 25-380

CURRENT OPERATIVE SURGERY

General Surgery

Other volumes in the Current Operative Surgery series

Vascular Surgery (Ed.) C. W. Jamieson

Forthcoming volumes

Orthopaedics and Trauma (Ed.) S. P. F. Hughes

Plastic and Reconstructive Surgery (Ed.) I. F. K. Muir

Urology (Ed.) A. R. Mundy

CURRENT OPERATIVE SURGERY

General Surgery

Edited by

A. Cuschieri, MD, ChM, FRCS, FRCS (Ed)

Professor, Department of Surgery, Ninewells Hospital and Medical School, Dundee

and

T. P. J. Hennessy, MA, MCh, FRCS, FRCSI

Professor, Department of Clinical Surgery, University of Dublin

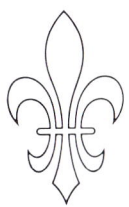

Baillière Tindall London Philadelphia Toronto
Mexico City Rio de Janeiro Sydney Tokyo Hong Kong

Baillière Tindall 1 St Anne's Road
W. B. Saunders   Eastbourne, East Sussex BN21 3UN, England

West Washington Square
Philadelphia, PA 19105, USA

1 Goldthorne Avenue
Toronto, Ontario M8Z 5T9, Canada

Apartado 26370—Cedro 512
Mexico 4, DF Mexico

Rua Evaristo da Viega 55, 20° andar
Rio de Janeiro—RJ, Brazil

ABP Australia Ltd, 44–50 Waterloo Road
North Ryde, NSW 2113, Australia

Ichibancho Central Building, 22–1 Ichibancho
Chiyoda-ku, Tokyo 102, Japan

10/fl, Inter-Continental Plaza, 94 Granville Road
Tsim Sha Tsui East, Kowloon, Hong Kong

© 1985 Baillière Tindall

All rights reserved. No part of this publication may be reproduced, stored in a retrieval system or transmitted, in any form or by any means, electronic, mechanical, photocopying or otherwise, without the prior permission of Baillière Tindall, 1 St Anne's Road, Eastbourne, East Sussex BN21 3UN, England.

First published 1985

Typeset and printed in Great Britain by Butler and Tanner Ltd, Frome and London

British Library Cataloguing in Publication Data

General surgery.—(Current operative surgery)
 1. Surgery
 I. Cuschieri, A. II. Hennessy, T. P. J. III. Series
 617 RD31
ISBN 0–7020–1072–3

List of Contributors

Henri Bismuth MD, Professeur à la Faculté, Chirurgie Hépato-Biliaire et Digestive, Hôpital Paul-Brousse, 14 Avenue P. V. Couturier, 94800 Villejuif, France.

F. C. Campbell MD, FRCS, Lecturer, Department of Surgery, Ninewells Hospital and Medical School, Dundee DD1 9SY, Scotland.

Denis Castaing MD, Hôpital Paul-Brousse, 14 Avenue P.V. Couturier, 94800 Villejuif, France.

A. Cuschieri MD, ChM, FRCS(Ed), Professor and Head, Department of Surgery, Ninewells Hospital and Medical School, Dundee DD1 9SY, Scotland; Senior Honorary Consultant Surgeon, Ninewells Hospital and Tayside Health Board.

Robert J. Freeark MD, Professor and Chairman, Department of Surgery, Stritch School of Medicine, Loyola University, 2160 South First Avenue, Maywood, IL 60153, USA; Surgeon-in-chief, Foster G. McGaw Hospital of Loyola University; Consultant, Hines Veterans' Administration Hospital, Maywood.

T. P. J. Hennessy MA, MCh, FRCS, FRCSI, Regius Professor of Surgery, Trinity College, University of Dublin; Consultant Surgeon, St James's Hospital, James's Street, Dublin 8, Republic of Ireland, and Royal City of Dublin Hospital.

M. Hobsley MChir, PhD, FRCS, Professor of Surgery, Department of Surgical Studies, The Middlesex Hospital Medical School, London W1N 8AA; Honorary Surgeon, The Middlesex Hospital.

George W. Johnston MCh, FRCS, FRCSI, Honorary Senior Lecturer in Surgery, Queen's University, Belfast; Consultant Surgeon, Royal Victoria Hospital, Grosvenor Road, Belfast BT12 6BA, Northern Ireland.

Leon Morgenstern MD, FACS, Clinical Professor of Surgery, UCLA School of Medicine; Director of Surgery, Cedars-Sinai Medical Center, 8700 Beverly Boulevard, Los Angeles, CA 90048, USA.

Contents

	Preface	ix
1	Conservative and Reconstructive Surgery of the Breast F. C. Campbell & A. Cuschieri	1
2	Gun Transection for Oesophageal Varices G. W. Johnston	27
3	Pyloric Reconstruction M. Hobsley	42
4	Reconstruction of the Gastric Reservoir A. Cuschieri	62
5	Conservative Surgery of the Spleen L. Morgenstern	74
6	Segmentectomy 4 H. Bismuth & D. Castaing	93
7	Peritoneovenous Shunting for Intractable Ascites A. Cuschieri	106
8	Surgery for Morbid Obesity R. J. Freeark	123
9	Injection Sclerotherapy for Oesophageal Varices T. P. J. Hennessy	141
	Index	145

Preface

In producing this volume, the editors had to select a number of procedures which have emerged within general surgical practice over the past 10 to 15 years. The selection was not an easy one and was influenced to some extent by the editors' clinical interests, but incorporated those procedures which are topical and which constitute a significant change from the orthodox scene.

Some of the operations included are, as of right, newer forms of surgical treatment which are as yet not in general use but remain under study in a number of centres and still require long-term evaluation within prospective clinical trials. The history of general surgery is characterized by operations which appeared *ab initio* as logical and useful but subsequently were observed to be attended by long-term consequences which precluded their continued usage. Rather cryptically, Heneage Ogilvie remarked that 'a gastric operation is always good ... until it is found out'. On average it takes 10 to 20 years (at times a whole generation of surgeons) to confirm the benefit of or alternatively to discredit an operation.

Other procedures in current usage indicate a different approach to orthodox surgical practice, consequent on the realization that traditional therapy is either too ablative or attended by a substantial morbidity. Often these alternative approaches concern more conservative surgery such as splenic preservation for trauma, and lumpectomy with postoperative radiotherapy for the primary local control of breast cancer.

The third category of the newer surgical procedures constitutes a resurgence of well-established but previously unpopular operations. Often the change follows the emergence of new technology which allows a more effective and safer use of these procedures, as in sclerotherapy and gun transection for oesophageal varices.

In this volume we have chosen examples of the above categories of 'newer operations' and trust that we have achieved the right balance and breadth of interest. The entire artwork for this volume has been ably undertaken by Mr M. J. Courtney. Aside from a uniform style throughout, the volume has been enriched by excellent line drawings of the various operative procedures.

We are greatly indebted to our fellow authors for their cooperation and for the excellence of their contributions. In this respect our editorial work has been an easy task. We would like to express our appreciation for the advice and help obtained from our publishers during the preparation of this volume. In particular, we are grateful to Dr G. Smaldon who was receptive to the idea for the *Current Operative Surgery* series, and kept us on course and strove valiantly to keep us on schedule. Finally, we would like to thank our secretaries, Mrs Joyce MacKenzie and Mrs Bernadette Kelly, for their assistance and excellent typing.

A. Cuschieri
T. P. J. Hennessy

1

Conservative and Reconstructive Surgery of the Breast

F.C. Campbell
A. Cuschieri

CONSERVATIVE SURGERY OF THE BREAST

Prior to the advent of effective diagnostic techniques, the surgery of all breast disease was dominated by the fear of cancer. Benign disorders could only be reliably distinguished from cancer by histology after excision and the natural inclination for all diagnostic biopsies, duct removals, etc. was to carry out wide local excision, together with a large surrounding margin of healthy breast tissue. Failure to do so risked transection of a cancerous lump and spillage of cancer cells, which in theory had drastic consequences. Little consideration was given to any breast deformity. This approach persists in the present day to some extent, despite the widespread availability of good preoperative diagnostic facilities, such as mammography, aspiration cytology and needle biopsy.

For established breast cancer, the surgeon's primary consideration was the achievement of 'adequate tumour clearance' which required excision of the whole breast with tumour, all draining lymphatic channels, any structures which they crossed and all accessible nodes. To this end, breast cancer was treated by radical mastectomy,[1] extended radical mastectomy[2,3] and eventually super radical mastectomy[4,5] The breast itself was considered an inessential organ and cosmetic results seemed unimportant. However, numerous well-conducted clinical trials have conclusively shown that radical breast excision and wide lymph node dissection, however extreme, failed to improve the survival of women with breast cancer.[6-12] Recent evidence suggests that the biological aggressiveness of the cancer which can be assessed after surgery, is a much more important determinant of prognosis than physical factors, such as the choice of operation or spillage of cancer cells.[13]

Another development which has changed our approach to breast surgery is the recognition of the psychiatric morbidity associated with the loss of a breast.[14] Approximately half of all women undergoing mastectomy react adversely to this procedure and are dissatisfied with their resulting scars. Profound social withdrawal occurs in 10–15%[15] but fortunately, many of those persistently distressed can respond well to breast reconstruction. Most surgeons, therefore, have become concerned to minimize breast deformity, and in the case of cancers, have begun a search for acceptable methods of breast conservation which would allow optimum local cancer control.

The modern surgical treatment of women with operable breast cancer entails a preliminary explanation by the surgeon to the patient of the available surgical options, with their advantages and disadvantages. With some guidance, the intelligent patient makes the final decision herself. In general, breast conservation is requested by the younger premenopausal patients although exceptions are encountered and breast awareness seems to be an important factor at all age groups.

This chapter includes a description of the modern approach to the common clinical problems of women with breast disease and thereafter deals with conservative surgery for breast cancer, namely subcutaneous mastectomy and reconstructive surgery after mastectomy.

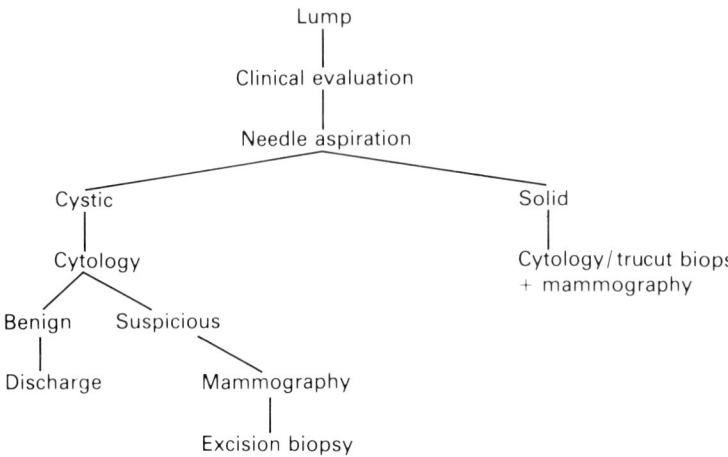

Figure 1.1 *Management of a breast lump.*

Assessment of patients

The pathological classification of breast disease is complex. The clinical spectrum is narrow however, and the patient commonly presents to the surgeon with one of the following:

1. Breast lump
2. Breast lumpiness
3. Nipple discharge
4. Nipple excoriation
5. Breast pain

The approach to any of these problems is dominated by 2 questions:

Does the patient have breast cancer?
Does the patient have a benign condition for which there is an effective treatment?

These questions can be answered in the majority of women before recourse to surgery by clinical evaluation, mammography, aspiration cytology or trucut biopsy. Each problem is managed in a slightly different manner:

1. **Lump** (Figure 1.1). Needle aspiration is indicated for all breast lumps to determine whether they are solid or cystic. Aside from confirming the diagnosis, aspiration of a cyst is therapeutic and obviates the need for excision in the first instance. Aspiration of a cyst should always be followed by repalpation of the area. Excision biopsy is advisable in the presence of a residual lump after aspiration or when the cyst fluid is blood-stained or mucoid or its cytology is suspicious. In practice malignant cystic lesions are very rare.

All solid lumps should have aspiration cytology or trucut needle biopsy. The former is less painful for the patient and it is possible to carry it out for *all* breast lumps, whereas trucut biopsy is rarely successful with fibroadenomas since the large needle cannot penetrate their tough rubbery substance. Mammography is indicated for all solid lumps to help ascertain the nature of the lesion and for complete examination of the opposite breast. A confident diagnosis can be made preoperatively in the majority of patients.

2. **Lumpiness** (Figure 1.2). The clinical recognition of a discrete lump in a breast which is nodular is often difficult. Nonetheless a carcinoma may arise just as frequently in a lumpy breast as in one with a smooth consistency. A careful examination is extremely important in this very common condition, and in the absence of suspicious features such as localized nodularity or oedema, a young woman aged under 35 years may be reassured and discharged. Mammography has a poor yield in young women but it is recommended for women over 35 years and for all patients with suspicious clinical features. A marker biopsy is indicated in the presence of suspicious mammographic abnormalities (subclinical lumps, areas of disordered architecture, vascularity or microcalcification).

3. **Nipple discharge** (Figure 1.3). A blood-stained nipple discharge is associated with a duct papilloma or carcinoma, but it is not generally realized that a serous discharge from a single duct also has an appreciable risk.[16] The first step in clinical evaluation therefore is to ascertain whether the

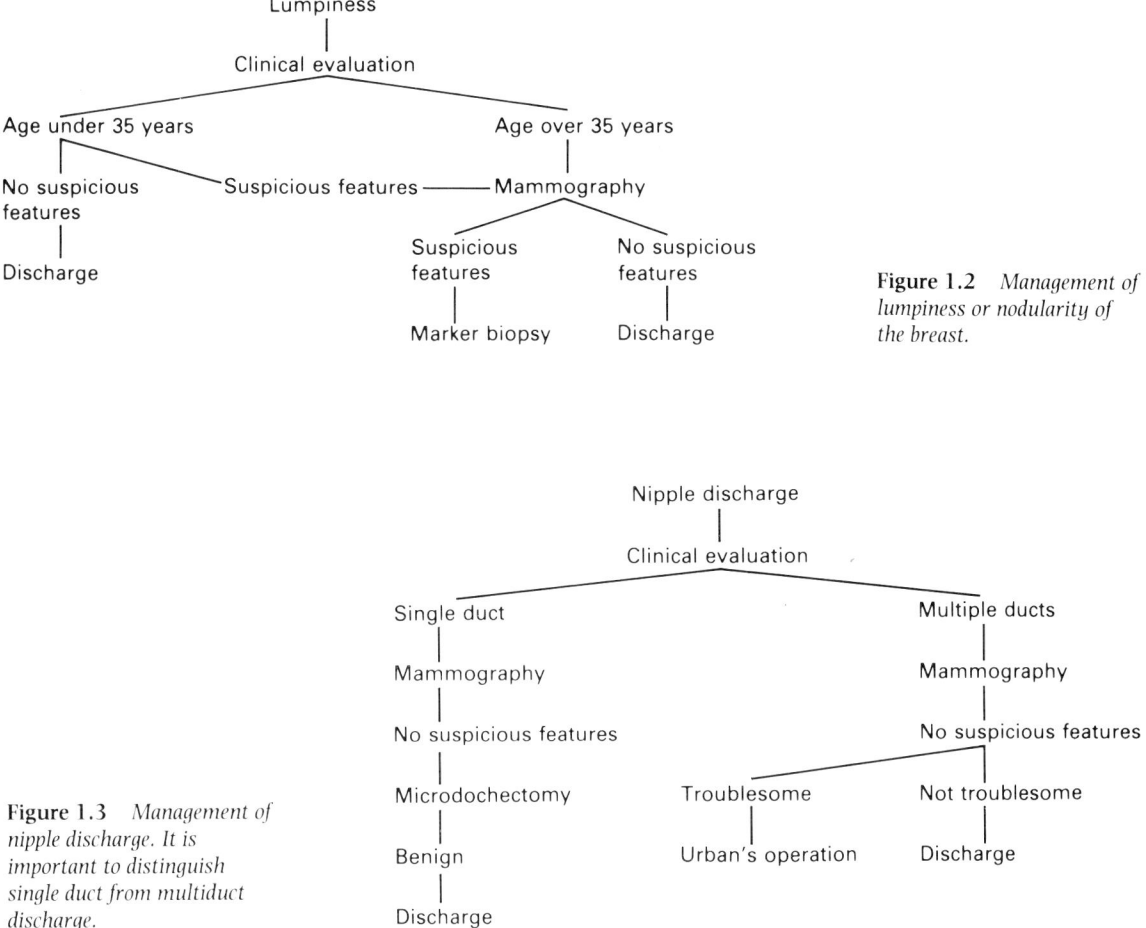

Figure 1.2 *Management of lumpiness or nodularity of the breast.*

Figure 1.3 *Management of nipple discharge. It is important to distinguish single duct from multiduct discharge.*

discharge emanates from a single duct or from multiple ducts. A careful examination is imperative and each breast should be gently compressed around the periphery of the areola. Multiduct discharge is usually serous or white, often affects both breasts, but is rarely associated with carcinoma. Mammography is indicated and in the absence of suspicious features, the patient can be reassured. If the discharge is troublesome then the patient would be best advised to have surgery (Urban's subareolar excision of lactiferous ducts) since there is no effective drug therapy. Surgery is always indicated in single duct discharge to exclude intraduct carcinoma. A microdochectomy will reveal the cause of the discharge and is also therapeutic.

4. **Nipple excoriation** (Figure 1.4). Paget's disease of the nipple is the commonest cause of excoriation. Paget's disease may be diagnosed, after careful clinical examination and mammography, by nipple biopsy which can be carried out under local anaesthesia at the outpatient clinic.

Sir James Paget described a disease of the mammary areola which preceded the development of clinical cancer[17] and which is nowadays considered to be an epidermotropic carcinoma of nipple ducts. However, patients frequently present with Paget's change in the nipple, which is accompanied by clinical or mammographic evidence of an underlying carcinoma. When this is the case, then treatment appropriate for the carcinoma

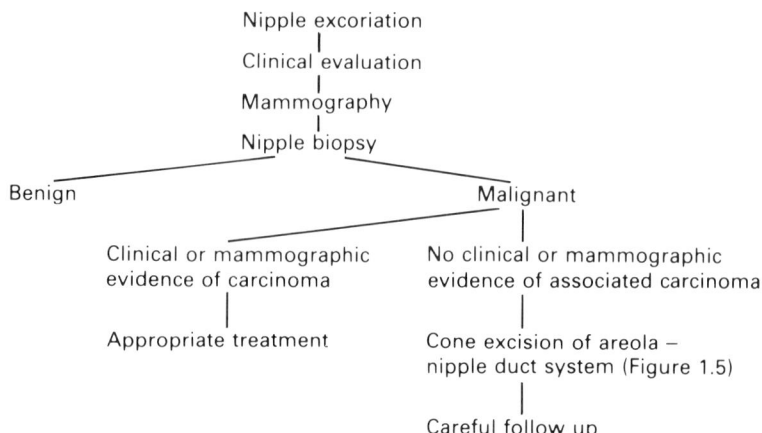

Figure 1.4 *Management of nipple excoriation.*

should be carried out. With increasing surveillance for breast cancer, true Paget's disease of the nipple is diagnosed more frequently. These patients show no evidence of a palpable mass or mammographic abnormality and may be treated with conservative surgery, i.e. with a cone excision of the areola and nipple duct system to a depth of 5 cm (Figure 1.5). In a recent study, women treated in such a manner showed no evidence of recurrence at 50 months of follow up.[18]

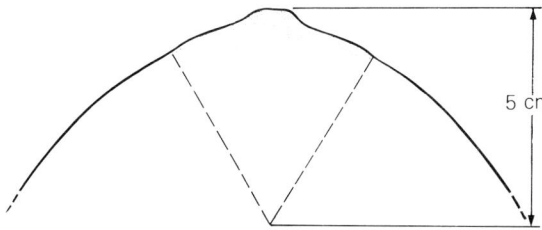

Figure 1.5 *Diagrammatic scheme of cone excision of nipple for Paget's disease. Primary closure after excision preserves the breast mound with an acceptable cosmetic appearance.*

5. **Breast pain** (Figure 1.6). Breast pain is rarely associated with carcinoma but it is the commonest symptom which brings a woman to the Breast Clinic. A careful and detailed history is necessary to distinguish two definite categories of pain, namely cyclical mastalgia where a strong relationship to the menstrual cycle is evident and non-cyclical mastalgia where no such relationship exists. Clinical examination will reveal areas of local tenderness which should be noted on representative drawings. Mammography is indicated for all women over 35 years or for younger women with suspicious clinical features.

Irrespective of whether pain is cyclical or non-cyclical, most women will require only firm reassurance, the recommendation of a good supporting bra and the occasional simple analgesic. It is when symptoms have failed to respond to this regime that the distinction of cyclical from non-cyclical mastalgia becomes important. The former may respond well to specific agents which can alter the hormonal environment of the breast whereas the latter is unlikely to benefit. Three drugs are effective in relieving the tenderness of cyclical mastalgia. Evening Primrose Oil (Efamol) is the richest natural source of essential fatty acids which are important cofactors for prolactin metabolism. This drug is virtually free from side-effects, and has been shown in a placebo-controlled trial to improve cyclical mastalgia.[19] It is given in a dose of 500 mg six times daily, together with ascorbic acid 200 mg three times daily. Bromocriptine, a dopamine agonist, is also effective, but is associated with nausea, vomiting and headache. Side-effects can be minimized by starting with a low dose of 1.25 mg daily, gradually increasing to 2.5 mg twice daily. Adequate contraceptive methods should be used during therapy. Danazol has a place in treatment of cyclical mastalgia but is associated with weight gain and amenorrhoea.

Reliance is placed on conventional analgesics for non-cyclical mastalgia. Excision of 'trigger spots',

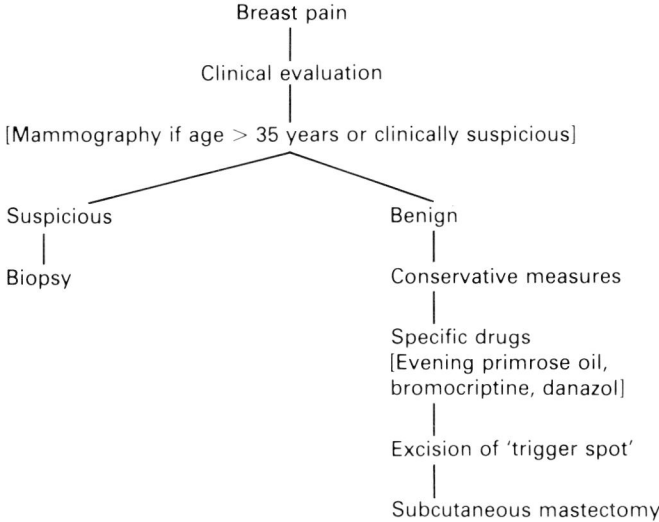

Figure 1.6 *Clinical approach to breast pain. The majority of women require only simple supportive measures and reassurance.*

i.e. localized areas of maximum tenderness, may also be helpful. Subcutaneous mastectomy should be considered in the last resort for refractory pain, either cyclical or non-cyclical, which makes the patient's life a misery. A good cosmetic and symptomatic result is often achieved in such circumstances.[20]

Diagnostic procedures

Fine needle aspiration cytology

An accurate preoperative diagnosis avoids the traditional, but unpleasant approach whereby the patient must proceed to theatre for a frozen section biopsy, not knowing whether she will awaken with a diagnosis of cancer. Most centres use a trucut needle biopsy to obtain a tissue diagnosis preoperatively, but fine needle aspiration cytology which requires skilled expertise, and a trained cytologist, has a higher diagnostic yield, is less traumatic for the patient and can provide an immediate answer at first attendance.

Technique. The equipment is simple and inexpensive. A 10 ml syringe fitted with a fine disposable hypodermic needle and containing 0.2 ml heparin (5000 u/ml) is mounted into an aspiration gun (Figure 1.7).

The breast is gently swabbed with an antiseptic solution, while the lump is raised into prominence by the opposite hand. With continuous suction applied to the gun, multiple rapid 'runs' are made into the lump in a slightly tangential direction so as to avoid puncturing the chest wall (Figure 1.8). Within 15–30 seconds the operator will see aspirate material appearing in the bottom of the syringe. The needle is withdrawn maintaining a reduced suction. The cellular aspirate is emptied forcibly onto a slide and smears are prepared. The haematological 'Diff Quick' stain is used. This allows the cytologist to issue a report within a few minutes of the aspiration (Figure 1.9).[21] If no duct cells are found on the smears the aspirate is regarded as unsatisfactory and the procedure should be repeated. The final report is issued after staining with Giemsa or Papanicolaou.

Breast cytology smears are graded on the 1–5 Papanicolaou scale (Table 1.1). Grades 1 and 2 are benign and if there is no discrepancy between the cytological report and the clinical or mammographic findings, these lesions do not require removal. In our experience 90% of grade 4 and 98% of grade 5 are malignant and thus all of these require urgent attention. Grade 3 is either an active benign cellular lesion or an invasive cancer and since the two cannot be reliably differentiated by cytology, our policy has been to biopsy all these lesions irrespective of clinical and mammographic findings.

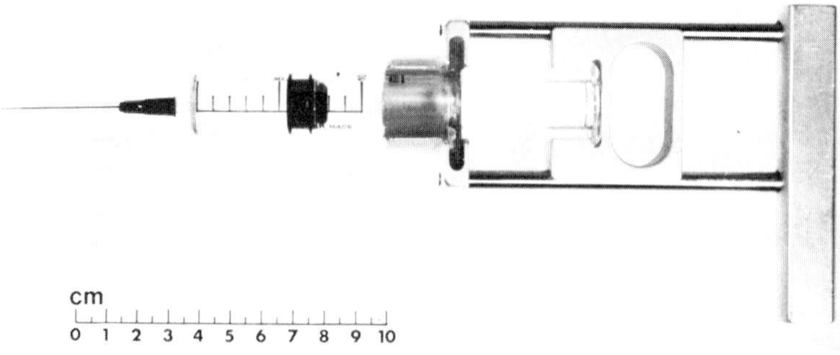

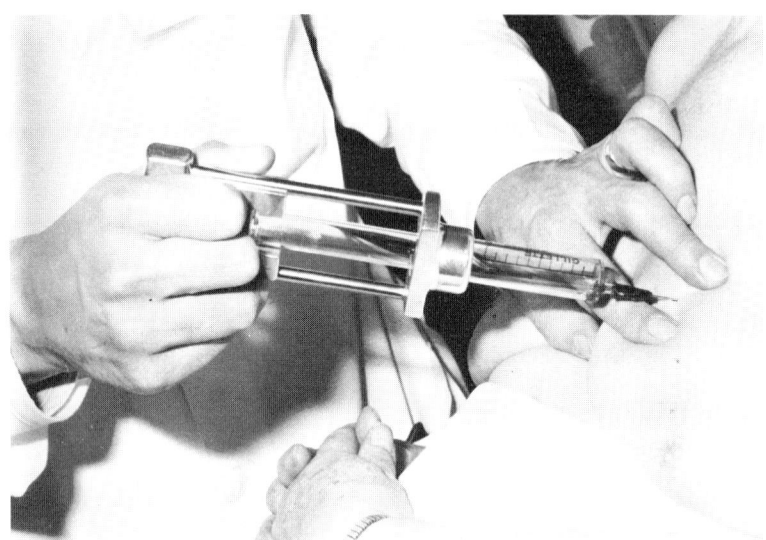

Figure 1.7 *Fine needle aspiration gun used at the Ninewells Breast Clinic. It accommodates a 10 ml Gillette syringe.*

Figure 1.8 *Fine needle aspiration gun in use. The left hand is used to steady the lump. Several runs are made through the lump while maintaining suction with the right hand.*

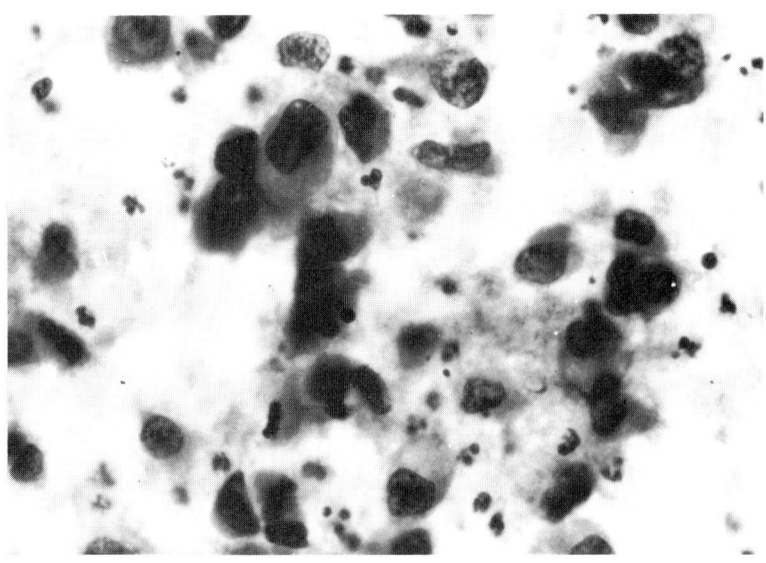

Figure 1.9 *Cytology smear using 'Diff Quick'.*

Table 1.1 Cytological grading of breast smears.

Grade	Definition
1	Normal
2	Hyperplastic duct cells
3	Irregularly proliferating cells
4	Cells highly suspicious of malignancy
5	Conclusive evidence of malignancy

Marker biopsy

Mammography is a useful tool for the early diagnosis of breast cancer, and may show features suggestive of malignancy in a clinically normal breast. Approximately half of these radiologically suspicious lesions are malignant and therefore accurate localization with complete excision of the radiological abnormality but with minimal removal of normal breast tissue is mandatory.

Technique. X-ray localization is carried out on the morning of surgery, using a needle or radio-opaque dye. The radiologist passes a needle or injects 0.5 ml of a mixture of 25% Hypaque and methylene blue (this latter stain allows recognition at surgery) into the centre of the suspect area. Mammograms taken in two planes confirm the localization.

The needle or dye is exposed through a circumferential incision and with reference to the mammograms, the suspect area is excised. The specimen is returned to the x-ray department while the patient remains anaesthetized. If specimen radiology confirms that the suspect area has been removed, the wound is closed and the patient returns to the ward. Urgent paraffin histology is more reliable than frozen section histology, particularly in the case of subclinical lesions where the histological differentiation between proliferative benign lesions, dysplasia, in situ or early invasive cancer can be difficult, even to an experienced pathologist.

Excision biopsy

This is indicated as a diagnostic procedure for all clinically suspicious lumps irrespective of negative preoperative investigations. Some surgeons still prefer frozen section histology, with immediate mastectomy on finding a positive result. Our own preference, however, is for urgent paraffin histology so that the diagnosis can be explained to the patient in advance of her definitive operation and the most appropriate procedure can be chosen.

Circumareolar and circumferential incisions for central and lateral lumps respectively are recommended because they confer better cosmetic results than radially disposed incisions.

Breast conservation in the primary treatment of breast cancer

This method of treatment has been in use since 1954,[22] and is currently being reassessed by two clinical trials in the UK. The first prospective randomized trial comparing local excision and postoperative radiotherapy with radical mastectomy was conducted at Guy's Hospital.[23] Although results were similar between the two groups in stage 1 disease, patients with stage 2 cancer randomized to the local excision arm, fared substantially worse with an unacceptably high incidence of loco–regional recurrence. The most important criticism levelled against this trial concerns the dose of radiotherapy administered which is universally considered to be too low and certainly inadequate to sterilize residual tumour tissue within the breast and axilla. A more recent trial comparing radical mastectomy versus quadrantectomy with axillary dissection and radiotherapy has not shown any differences in loco–regional recurrence, disease-free interval or survival to date.[12] Other studies have also suggested that local excision followed by radiotherapy to the breast, axilla and neck is as effective as conventional mastectomy in achieving adequate local control of the disease.[24,25]

Indications

Although these have been clearly defined and universally accepted, most surgeons practising this approach limit the procedure to mobile tumours not exceeding 3.0 cm in diameter. Skin fixation wide of tumour and deep tethering are contraindications to the procedure.

Procedure and nomenclature

The treatment consists of wide local excision through non-involved breast tissue with axillary sampling or lower axillary clearance. Postoperative radiotherapy is commenced two to three weeks postoperatively. A total of 45–50 Gy are administered in 20 fractions to the breast, ipsilateral axilla and supraclavicular nodes. Irradiation of the breast alone is performed in some centres when the axillary nodes are found to be not involved by histological examination.

Several names have been used to describe wide local excision of breast cancer: lumpectomy, tylectomy, quadrantectomy and segmentectomy. Aside from the different and rather confusing terminology, the surgical principle is the same. The tumour is excised with a minimum of 1 cm margin of apparently non-involved breast tissue. In small to medium breasts this approximates to removal of the affected quadrant. The term tylectomy is of Greek derivation and correctly describes excision of a lump but does not qualify its removal with normal surrounding breast tissue. Segmentectomy is an inaccurate term for the procedure and is best avoided.

Our practice has been wide local excision through curved transverse incisions which should not exceed 5 cm in length and lower axillary clearance.

Lower axillary clearance

1. Incision. The skin incision which is approximately 5.0 cm long is placed along the axillary tail of the breast and the anterior axillary fold (Figure 1.10). It is deepened to expose the lateral margin of the pectoralis major (Figure 1.11).

2. Exposure of pectoralis minor. The pectoralis major is retracted medially to expose the pectoralis minor down to its origin from the chest wall. The pectoral fascia is then incised along the lateral margin of the muscle (Figure 1.12) which is then mobilized and retracted medially. A few pectoral vessels require ligature and division at this stage.

3. Exposure of the axilla. The retraction of the mobilized pectoralis minor opens the axilla. The axillary contents are cleared from the level of the axillary vein downwards and between the latissimus dorsi and the chest wall down to and including the axillary tail of the breast (Figure 1.13). The subcapsular vessels and nerve are preserved. The clearance achieved by this technique is equivalent to that obtained by Patey mastectomy.

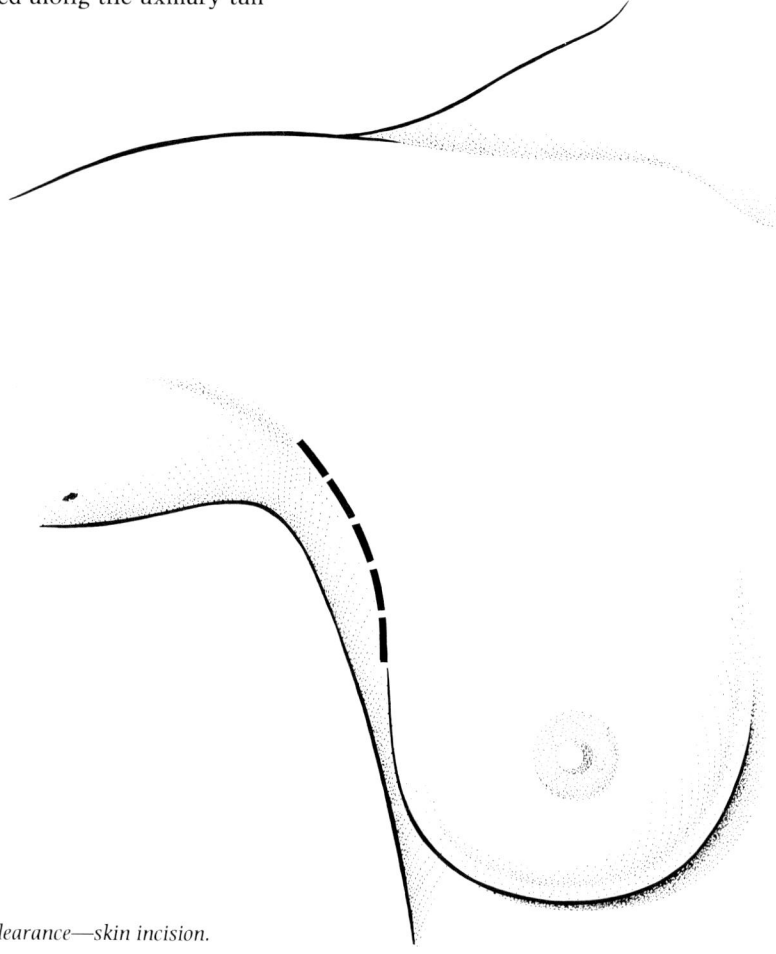

Figure 1.10 *Lower axillary clearance—skin incision.*

CONSERVATIVE AND RECONSTRUCTIVE SURGERY OF THE BREAST 9

Figure 1.11 *Lower axillary clearance—exposure of pectoralis major.*

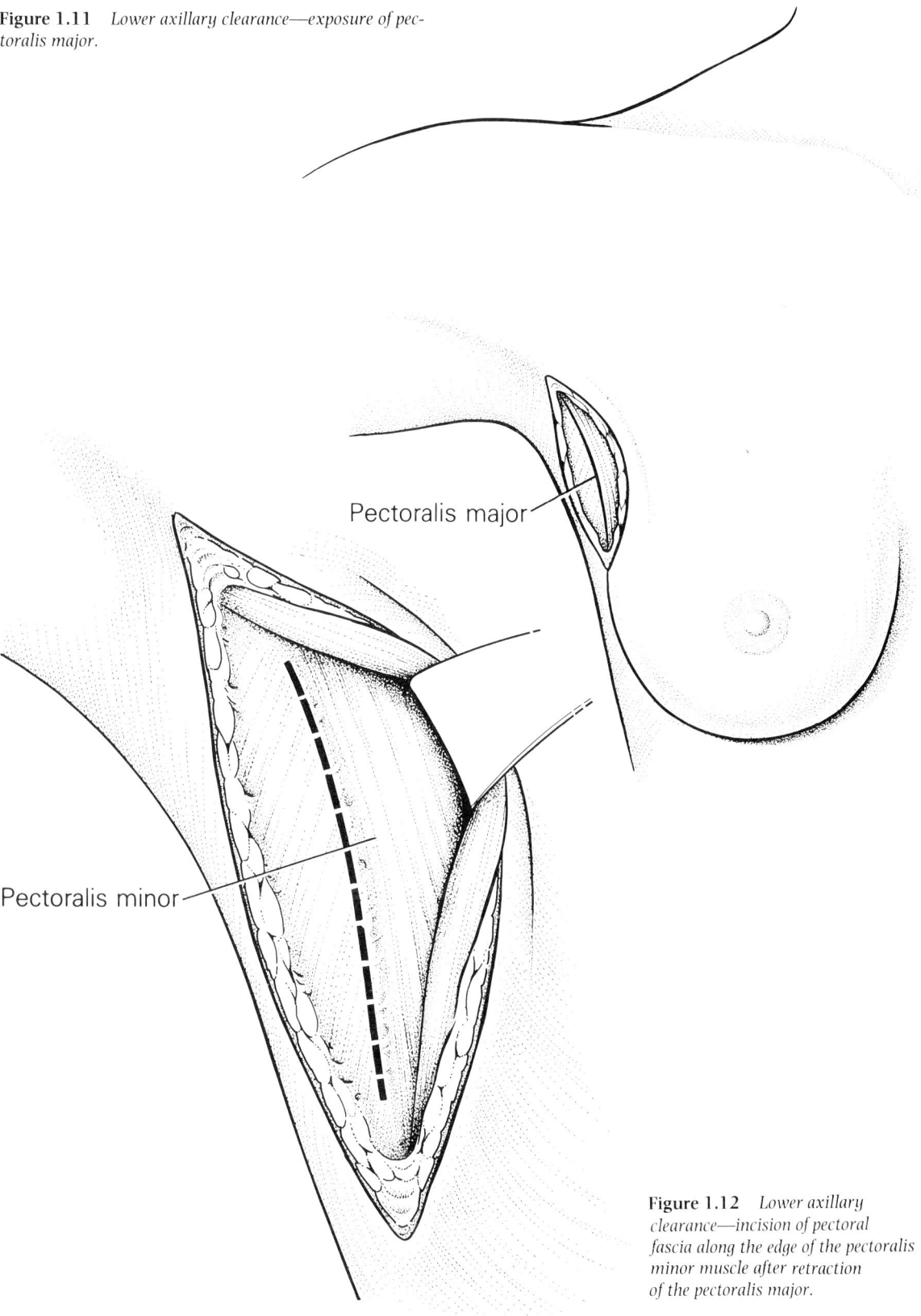

Figure 1.12 *Lower axillary clearance—incision of pectoral fascia along the edge of the pectoralis minor muscle after retraction of the pectoralis major.*

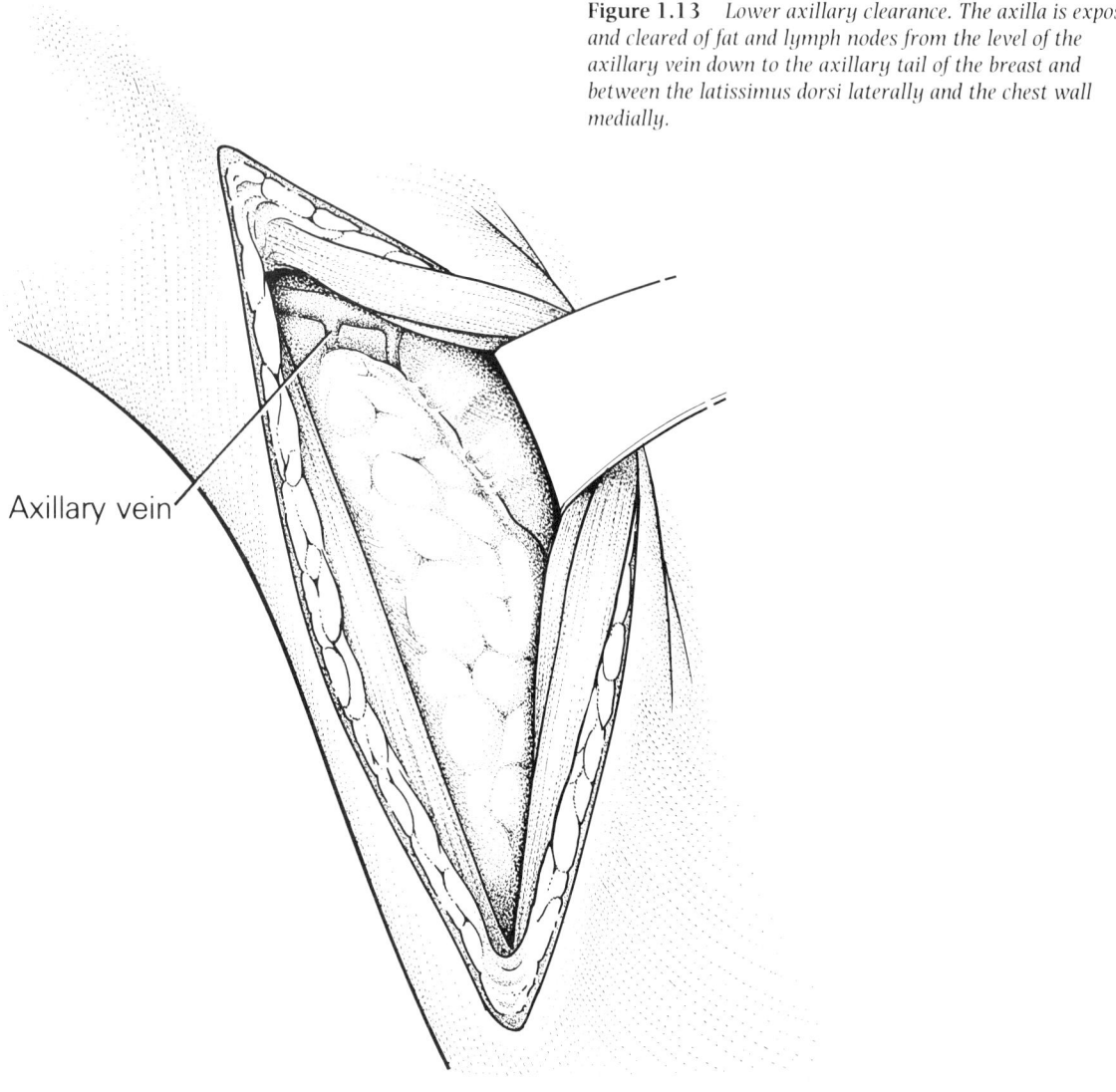

Figure 1.13 *Lower axillary clearance. The axilla is exposed and cleared of fat and lymph nodes from the level of the axillary vein down to the axillary tail of the breast and between the latissimus dorsi laterally and the chest wall medially.*

Subcutaneous mastectomy

In this operation, the breast parenchyma is removed from underneath the skin and immediate or delayed reconstruction is carried out, usually with a silicone prosthesis. Cosmetic results are poorer in fat women because skin and subcutaneous tissues are stretched as prostheses are larger and cause greater tension on suture lines. Thus healing is poorer.

Indications in benign breast disease

Intractable breast pain. The operation is often successful in women with intractable breast pain which has been resistant to any other treatment. It is important to emphasize that all causes of referred pain from other sites should be excluded and that conservative methods should be given a fair trial.

Premalignant breast disease. Epithelial hyperplasia, particularly in the presence of cellular *atypia*, carries an increased risk of malignancy.[26] Women with this condition are usually managed by prolonged follow up, and repeat clinical and mammographic assessment, with surgical intervention as indicated. However, a minority of women will develop a cancerophobia and will request a prophylactic mastectomy. We have also treated patients having painful fibrocystic disease involving frequent recurrence of macrocyst formation with subcutaneous mastectomy. In addition to their severe symptoms, these patients have a higher risk of breast cancer.[20]

Indications in malignant disease

Subcutaneous mastectomy is the procedure of choice in patients with non-invasive breast cancer. A bilateral procedure is advisable for patients with lobular carcinoma in situ. There is some evidence that subcutaneous mastectomy is an acceptable alternative to simple mastectomy in the treatment of operable invasive breast cancer. Two studies failed to find any significant differences in survival or disease-free interval in patients treated by total or subcutaneous mastectomy.[27,28] Subcutaneous mastectomy is suitable for mobile breast cancers (T1–2) either without or with minimal (<1.0 cm) skin dimpling. It is however less favoured than wide local excision and radiotherapy by surgeons practising conservation breast surgery. The procedure is unsuitable for centrally placed tumours.

Operative technique

1. **Position of the patient.** The operation is performed with the patient placed symmetrically on the table having both arms abducted. Routine skin preparation is carried out on both sides, including the axillae, and towels are sutured to the skin leaving both breasts exposed.

2. **Incision.** The infralateral submammary incision gives a good cosmetic result and is the incision of choice in patients with small breasts. It allows access for axillary node sampling in patients with cancer but is inadequate for axillary clearance. The submammary approach is difficult in patients with medium to large breasts and is attended by forceful retraction of the skin flap during the procedure. The risk of both operative damage to the flaps and subsequent ischaemic necrosis is enhanced in these patients. The circumareolar lateral incision is safer in these patients and facilitates the mastectomy. Furthermore it permits axillary clearance in patients with cancer. The incision skirts the lower half of the areolar margin and is then extended along the lateral radius to the periphery of the breast mound (Figure 1.14).

Whenever subcutaneous mastectomy is performed for a carcinoma with slight skin dimpling (<1.0 cm), the affected area of skin is excised as a separate transverse ellipse and the edges approximated by interrupted sutures. However, the exposure is not altered and this added step does not usually jeopardize the blood supply to the breast skin flaps.

The assistant holds the breast under tension and the skin incision is made starting at the areolar end. It is deepened to the plane of separation between the breast parenchyma and the subcutaneous fat. This plane is easily identified as it lies underneath a plexus of veins which covers the large fat globules of the breast tissue (Figure 1.15).

3. **Demarcation and preservation of the nipple disc.** The vascular integrity of the areola and nipple is ensured by the preservation of a disc of breast tissue including the terminal lactiferous ducts about 0.5–1.0 cm in thickness depending on the size of the breast. The diameter of this disc corresponds to that of the areola and is outlined by sharp knife dissection to separate it from the remaining breast tissue. The upper (alveolar) skin edge is lifted up with skin hooks and the breast tissue is divided by scalpel parallel to the areolar skin and nipple (Figure 1.16). Thereafter the periphery of the disc is incised down to the subcutaneous fat corresponding with the areolar margin on the outside (Figure 1.17).

4. **Elevation of the inferior flap.** This is facilitated by traction on the skin edges using skin hooks. The plane is identified and dissection is carried out deep to the venous plexus and should be relatively avascular consisting of loose areolar tissue between the breast fat and the venous plexus. Elevation of the inferior skin flap is completed when the lower half of the breast is separated from the overlying skin and subcutaneous fat and the rectus sheath is exposed at the periphery of the breast (Figure 1.18).

5. **Detachment of the breast tissue from pectoralis major.** The fascia along the lower edge of the exposed breast tissue is divided and the edge of the breast is then grasped in tissue-holding forceps. The breast is thereafter detached from the pectoral muscle (Figure 1.19). Diathermy coagulation of the perforating pectoral vessels is necessary during this step. The mobilization of the breast tissue from the underlying muscle is otherwise easy and consists of both blunt and sharp dissection as necessary. It should extend medially to the sternal edge and superiorly to the clavicle and pectoralis major tendon.

Figure 1.14 *Subcutaneous mastectomy—the circumareolar/lateral incision used for medium to large breasts.*

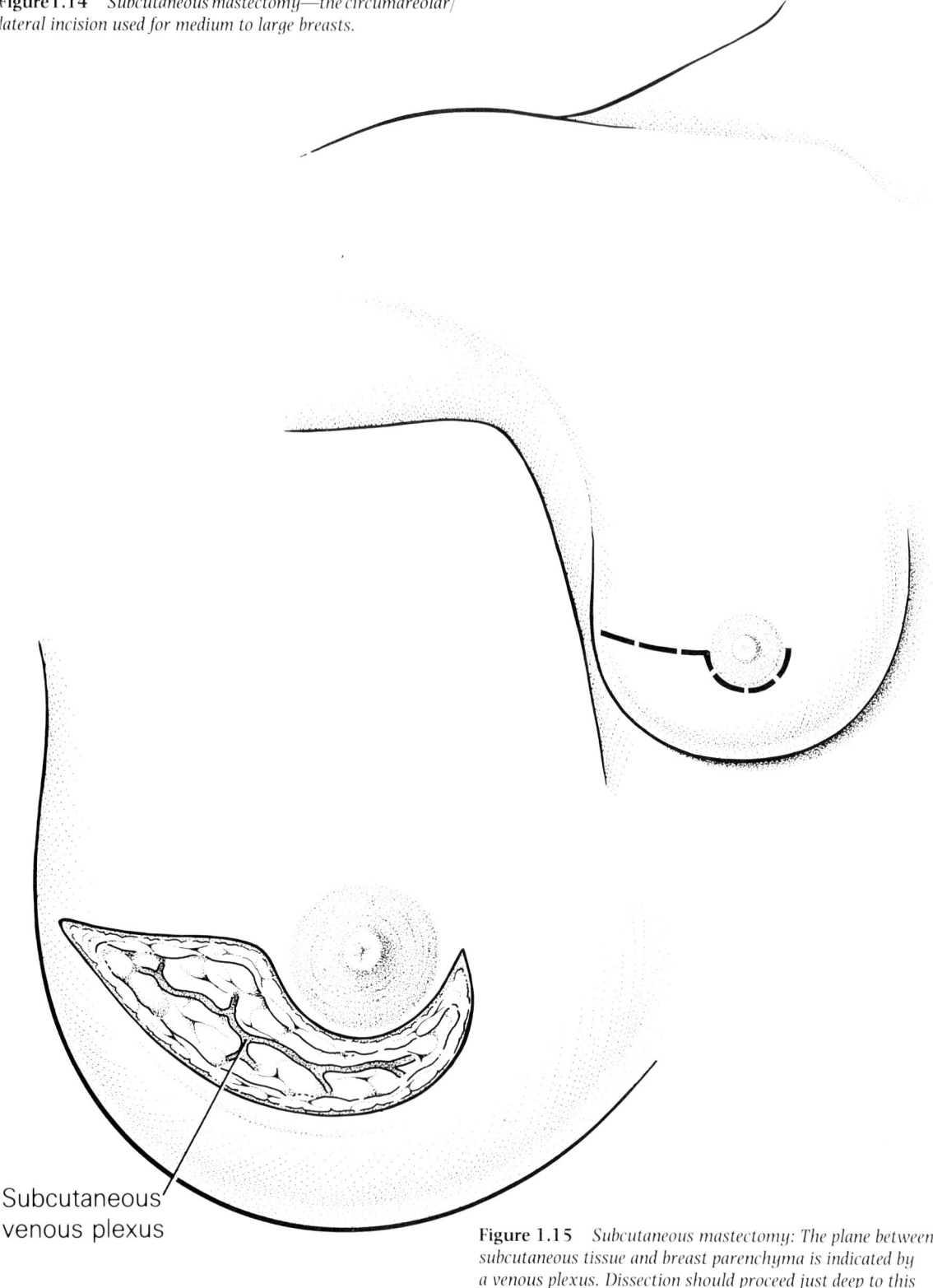

Subcutaneous venous plexus

Figure 1.15 *Subcutaneous mastectomy: The plane between subcutaneous tissue and breast parenchyma is indicated by a venous plexus. Dissection should proceed just deep to this venous plexus.*

CONSERVATIVE AND RECONSTRUCTIVE SURGERY OF THE BREAST

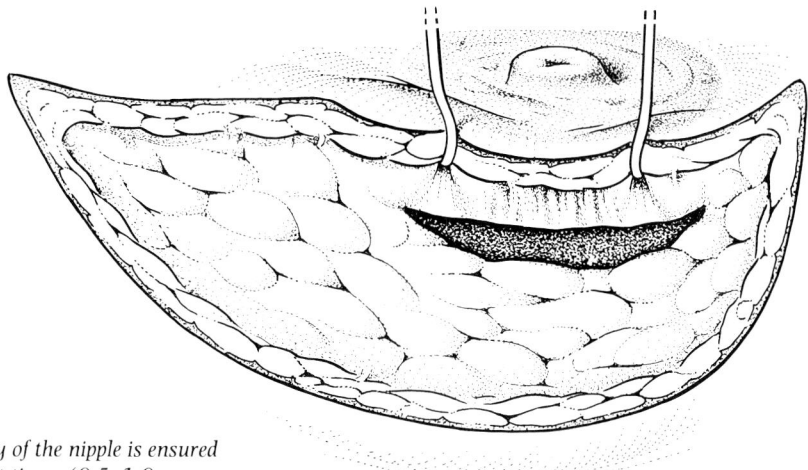

Figure 1.16 *The vascular integrity of the nipple is ensured by the preservation of a disc of breast tissue (0.5–1.0 cm thick) corresponding to the nipple–areola extent. The upper areola skin edge is elevated by skin hooks and the breast tissue is divided by scalpel parallel to the areolar skin.*

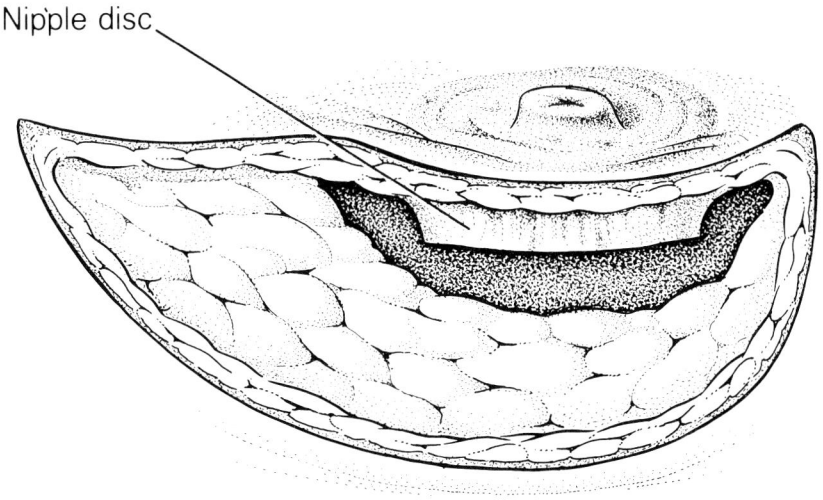

Figure 1.17 *The periphery of the disc is incised down to the subcutaneous fat corresponding with the areolar margin.*

Figure 1.18 *The inferior flap has been elevated and is retracted downwards to expose the periphery of the breast lying on the rectus sheath. The loose fascia tethering the breast to the rectus sheath is divided.*

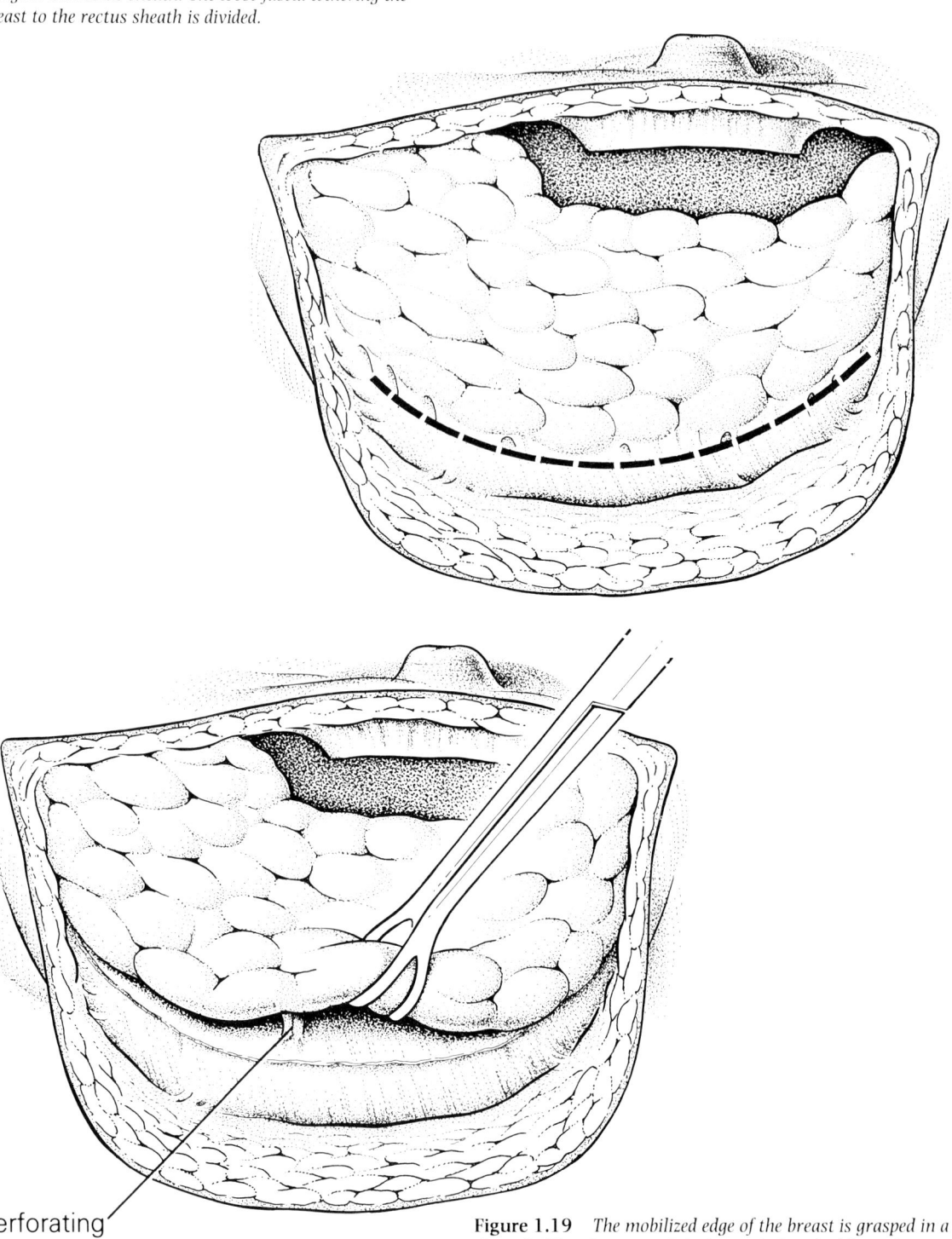

Perforating pectoral vessels

Figure 1.19 *The mobilized edge of the breast is grasped in a tissue holding forceps and the breast is detached from the underlying pectoral muscle. Diathermy coagulation of the perforating pectoral vessels is required during this step.*

CONSERVATIVE AND RECONSTRUCTIVE SURGERY OF THE BREAST 15

6. **Elevation of the superior flap.** Prior mobilization of the deep surface of the breast facilitates this step and minimizes blood loss. The same technique is used as with the inferior flap, with fine scissor dissection deep to the venous plexus. The breast tissue is then detached medially and superiorly and wrapped in gauze, and is held in the operator's left hand.

7. **Dissection of the axillary tail.** A refractor is placed at the lateral extremity of the upper flap and the axillary tail dissected off the pectoralis major tendon and the floor of the axilla (Figure 1.20). If axillary nodal clearance is considered necessary, the dissection is carried medially to expose the pectoralis minor which is then retracted together with the pectoralis major tendon. A clearance of the axillary contents from the level of the axillary vein downwards is feasible with this approach but may require an upward extension of the lateral extremity of the wound. The breast is removed. The sites of the areolar disc and the axillary tail are marked with non-absorbable sutures for orientation and the excised breast is then weighed. The breast weight in grams is the best guide to the size of the implant necessary.

8. **Choice of implant.** Nowadays silicone gel or combined gel–saline prostheses are used. The latter are said to cause less encapsulation. The tear-drop shaped variety approximates more closely to the natural shape than the circular one. In practice the difference is marginal with regard to the cosmetic outcome. The disadvantage of the tear drop prosthesis is that accurate orientation is crucial which is not a problem with the circular variety. The size of the implant in millilitres should approximate to the weight of the breast in grams, although with large breasts a discrepancy of up to 60 ml is acceptable.

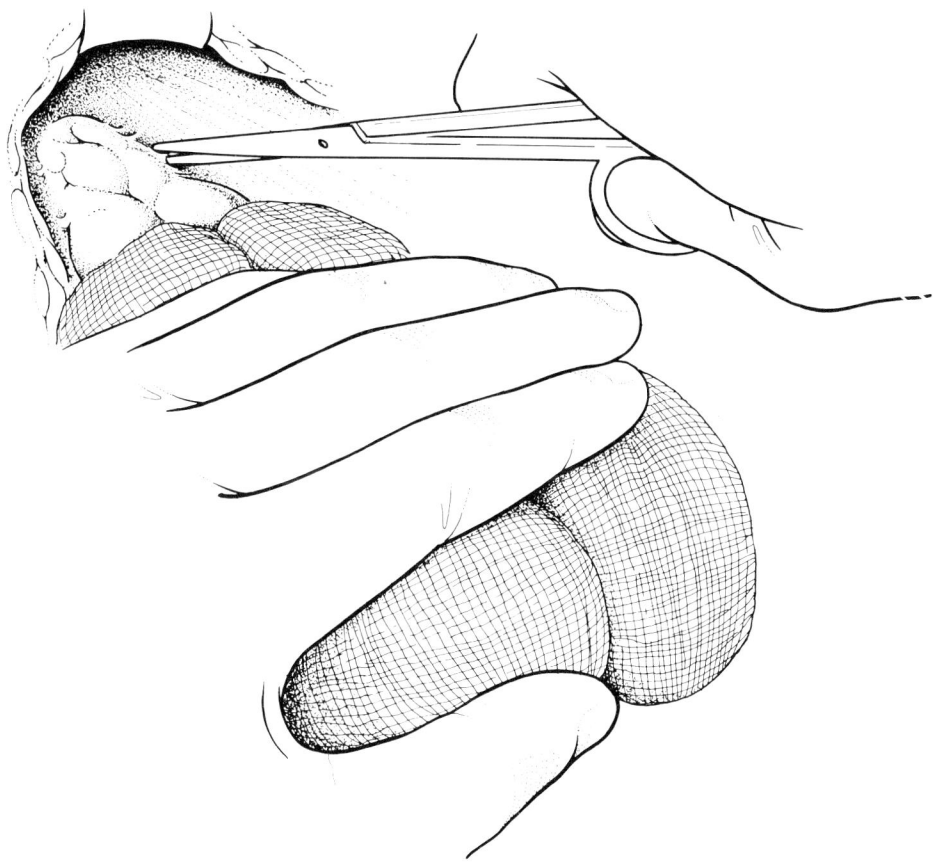

Figure 1.20 *The mobilized breast has been wrapped in gauze and is held in the surgeon's left hand. A retractor is placed at the lateral extremity of the upper flap and the axillary tail is dissected off the pectoralis major tendon and the floor of the axilla.*

The prosthesis can be placed either superficial or deep to the pectoralis major. A better immediate profile is obtained when the superficial plane is employed but the risk of early wound complications is higher and encapsulation, when it occurs, is more noticeable. For these reasons we favour the subpectoral approach. The subpectoral pouch has been modified to accommodate larger prostheses and to avoid the lateral flattened appearance which results when the edge of the pectoralis major is sutured to the chest wall over the implant.

9. **Extended subpectoral pouch.** An incision is made through the muscle layer down to the rib cage, along the digitations of the serratus anterior curving downwards and medially to the rectus sheath and dividing the origin of the pectoralis minor from the chest wall (Figure 1.21). By a mixture of blunt and scissor dissection the lower and medial digitations of the pectoralis major are divided and this muscle is elevated from the underlying rib cage taking care not to perforate its substance and leaving its lower and medial margins attached to the chest wall.

The pouch is extended laterally by elevating with sharp scissor dissection the lower digitations of the serratus anterior and rectus abdominis over a depth of 2.5–5.0 cm depending on the size of the implant necessary (Figure 1.22). After haemostasis is ensured, a suction drain is inserted and tunnelled well away from the pouch emerging

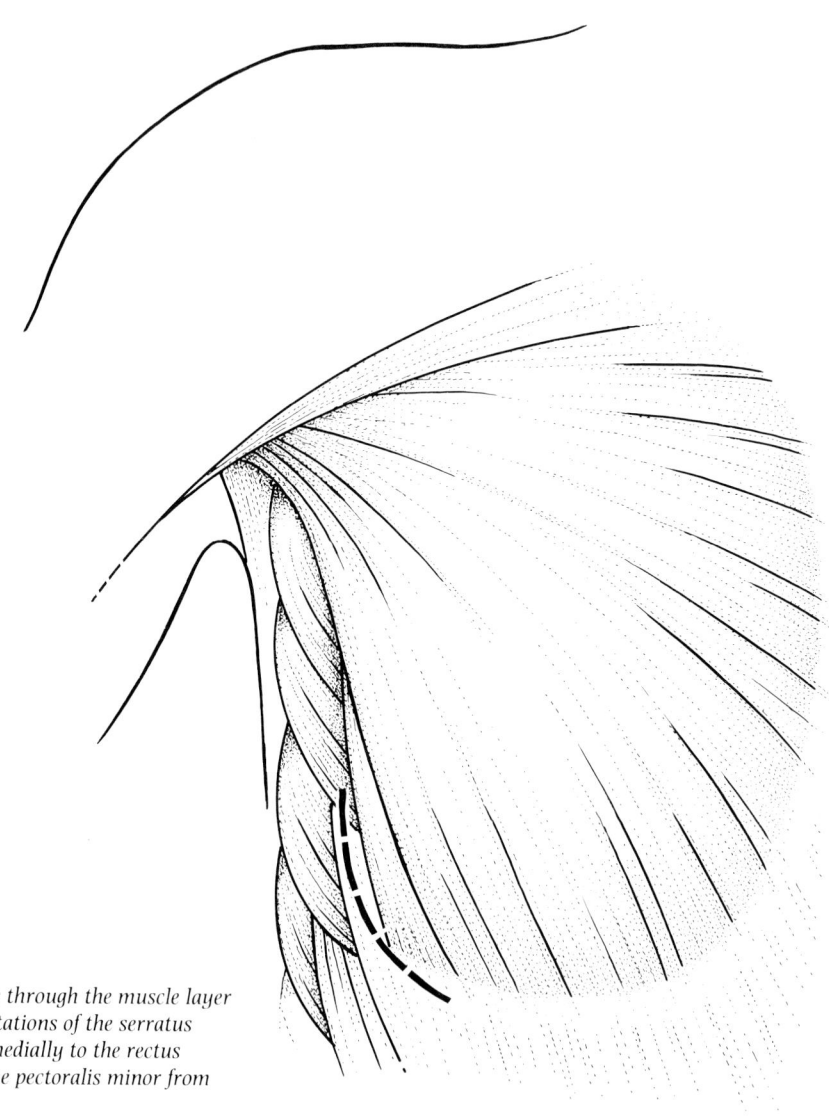

Figure 1.21 *An incision is made through the muscle layer down to the rib cage along the digitations of the serratus anterior curving downwards and medially to the rectus sheath and dividing the origin of the pectoralis minor from the chest wall.*

CONSERVATIVE AND RECONSTRUCTIVE SURGERY OF THE BREAST 17

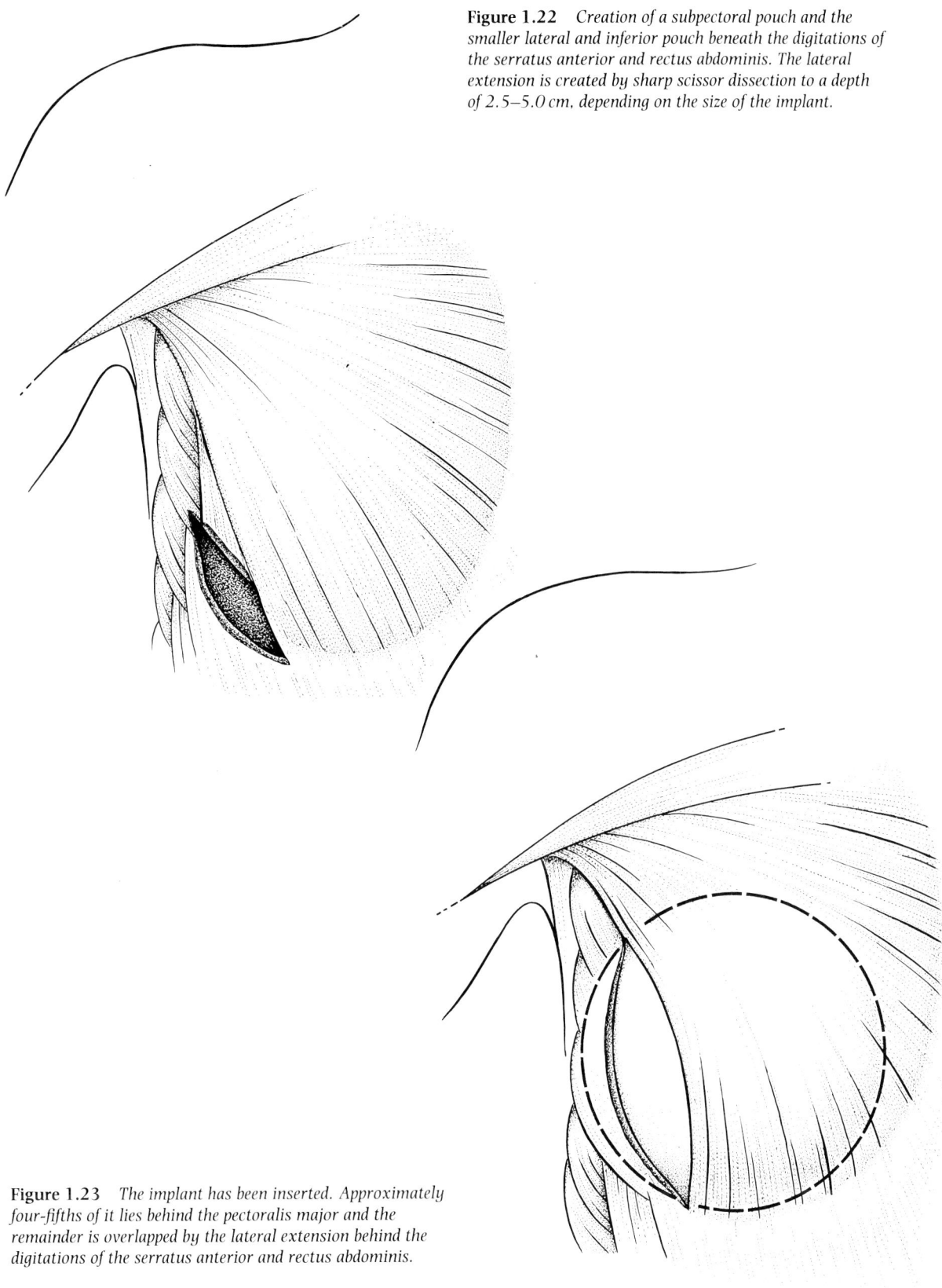

Figure 1.22 *Creation of a subpectoral pouch and the smaller lateral and inferior pouch beneath the digitations of the serratus anterior and rectus abdominis. The lateral extension is created by sharp scissor dissection to a depth of 2.5–5.0 cm, depending on the size of the implant.*

Figure 1.23 *The implant has been inserted. Approximately four-fifths of it lies behind the pectoralis major and the remainder is overlapped by the lateral extension behind the digitations of the serratus anterior and rectus abdominis.*

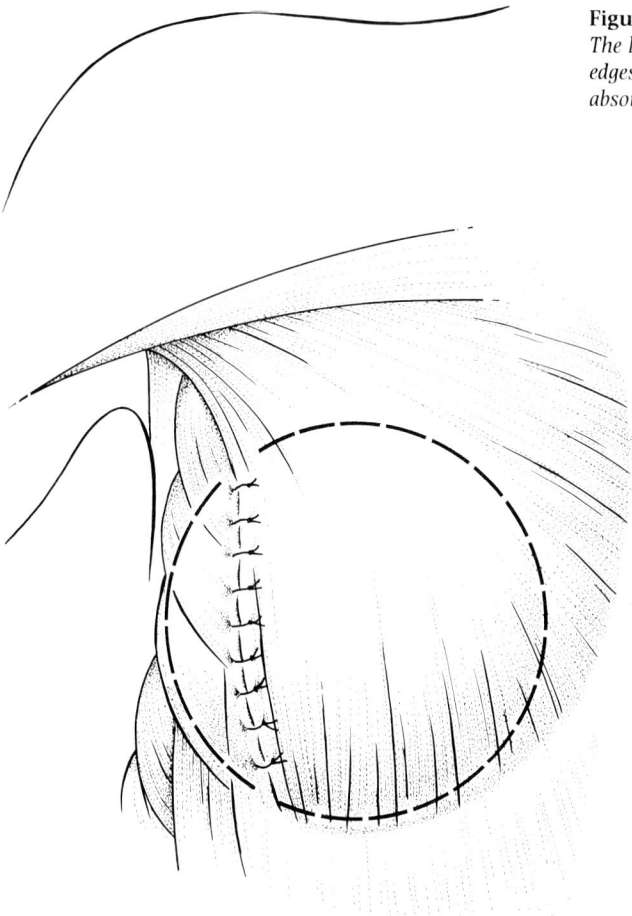

Figure 1.24 *Closure of the extended subpectoral pouch. The lateral edge of the pectoralis major is sutured to the cut edges of the serratus anterior of rectus digitations with absorbable 2/0 material.*

through the skin of the epigastrium. The implant is then inserted. Approximately four-fifths of it lies behind the pectoralis major and the remainder is overlapped by the digitations of the serratus anterior and rectus abdominis (Figure 1.23). The lateral edge of the pectoralis major is then sutured to the cut edges of the serratus anterior/rectus digitations using interrupted absorbable 2/0 sutures (Figure 1.24). Care must be taken to avoid puncture of the silicone implant during this step and a protective spatula should be placed over the implant during insertion of the sutures.

10. **Wound closure.** The wound is closed by fine (3/0 prolene) interrupted mattress sutures starting medially at the areola. Wound dressings are applied and then padded with cotton wool before the application of circumferential crêpe bandaging.

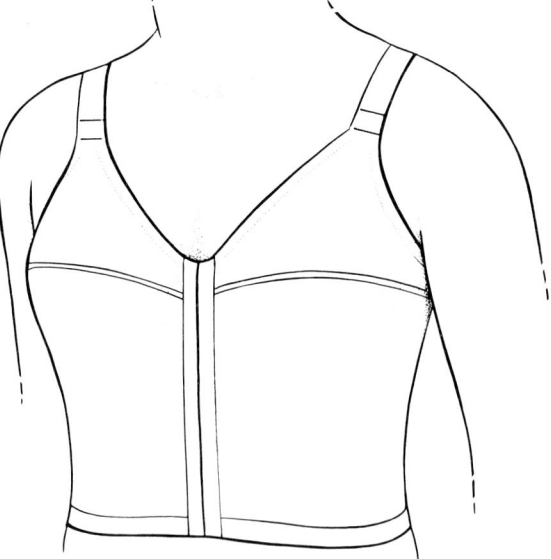

Figure 1.25 *Elasticated bodice-bra used for the first fortnight after subcutaneous mastectomy.*

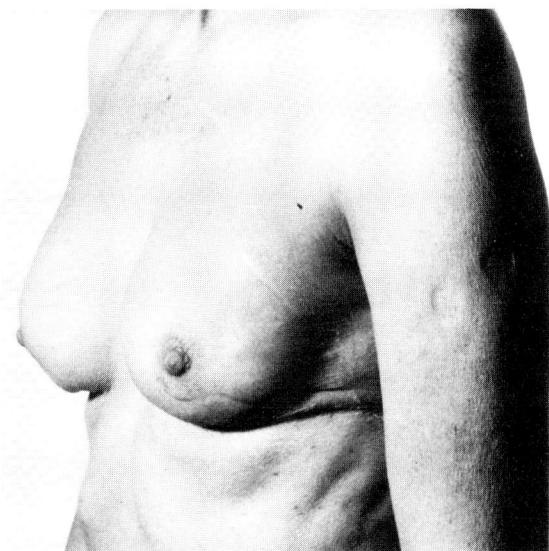

Figure 1.26 *Subcutaneous mastectomy. Twelve months after surgery.*

Postoperative care

The dressings are taken down after 24 hours and the wounds and skin inspected. Fresh gauze dressings are then applied and the patient wears an elasticated bodice-bra with a front zip for the next fortnight (Figure 1.25). Thereafter she reverts to wearing an ordinary well-supported full cup bra. The patient is instructed to massage her implants daily after the fourth week. This practice reduces the incidence and severity of encapsulation of the implants. Cosmetic results are usually excellent (Figure 1.26).

Complications

Skin necrosis. This results from impairment of the blood supply to the skin during the operation and is more prone to occur in patients who have had previous excision biopsies. The area most at risk is the areola and nipple. This complication is best avoided by ensuring that dissection is carried out in the appropriate plane (deep to the venous plexus), by avoidance of metal retractors on the skin flaps and by the preservation of a nipple disc of breast tissue. Superficial (epidermal) necrosis is of little consequence. This commonly affects the nipple/areolar skin and is always followed by rapid regeneration of the epidermis. Small areas of full-thickness necrosis can be excised and the fresh edges sutured. In the presence of extensive necrosis (>2.5 cm) it is best to remove the implant and achieve healing of the skin. Reinsertion of the implant is then undertaken two to three months later. In the meantime the patient is instructed to massage the skin and scar daily to prevent contracture and adhesions to the chest wall.

Conversion to simple mastectomy has not been necessary in the authors' experience. The adoption of the circumareolar–lateral approach in favour of the submammary one in all patients has resulted in the avoidance of skin necrosis in the last 32 consecutive subcutaneous mastectomies.

Accumulation of serous/blood-stained fluid. This has occurred in three out of 53 subcutaneous mastectomies. The fluid accumulates between the skin flaps and the underlying muscles and results in a tense congested breast. Evacuation is possible by aspiration with the needle held parallel to the skin to avoid puncture of the muscle layer and implant. Accumulation of solid blood clot requires open evacuation, control of any bleeding vessel and re-suture of the wound edges.

Infection. This has been observed in two out of 53 patients and this incidence is similar to that reported in another series.[27] In the absence of wound dehiscence, it is treated conservatively with antibiotics. Otherwise it requires open drainage and removal of the implant with reinsertion a few months later. It has not been our practice to use prophylactic perioperative antibiotic therapy in patients undergoing subcutaneous mastectomy.

Capsule formation. Encapsulation (Figure 1.27) is invariable and, when gross, results in a rounded tense breast mound with tenderness and pain. Severe symptomatic encapsulation has been encountered in one-third of our patients at three to six months after the operation. The incidence of this complication can be reduced but not abolished by regular massage of the implants. It is best treated by closed capsular disruption. The procedure entails forcible squeezing of the breast mound until the capsule is felt to split. If encapsulation is severe, the procedure is best carried out under general anaesthesia. Closed capsulotomy fails in about 5% of patients and then open capsulotomy is required. In practice this often necessitates replacement of the implant since the original one is invariably damaged during the operation. The object of open capsulotomy is to divide the capsule from inside down to the subcutaneous fat around its perimeter. It thus necessitates prior removal of

The most commonly used technique of breast reconstruction entails the insertion of a subpectoral implant to restore a breast mound. This is the method used in the presence of an intact pectoralis major and adequate chest wall skin. The technique of insertion of the implant is identical to that described for subcutaneous mastectomy (see p 10). The other commonly used technique which is especially useful in patients with inadequate skin/muscle is the latissimus–dorsi myocutaneous flap. Other techniques include the use of rectus abdom-

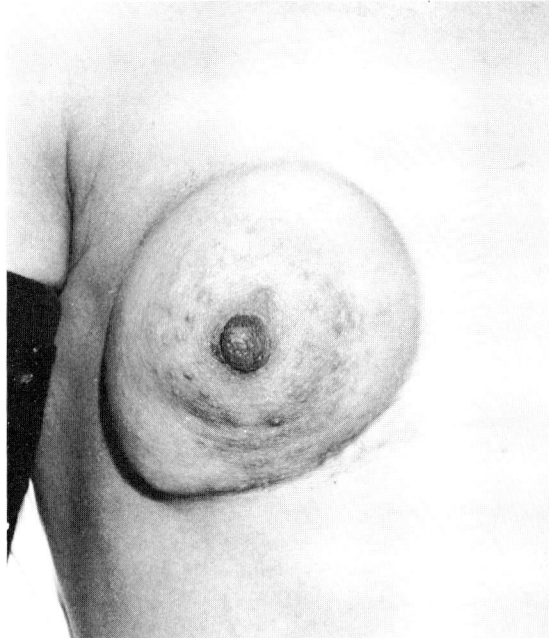

Figure 1.27 *Severe encapsulation of silicone implant, six months after subcutaneous mastectomy performed through the inferolateral approach.*

the implant which is reinserted after capsular division is completed.

RECONSTRUCTION OF THE BREAST AFTER TOTAL MASTECTOMY

This can be performed at the time of mastectomy (immediate) or delayed for varying periods thereafter. Increasingly, immediate reconstruction is gaining preference since it avoids a second operation and the psychological trauma (albeit temporary) of mutilation. The argument for delayed reconstruction cannot however be ignored. Many patients undergoing mastectomy are subject to stress to an extent that precludes valid decision-making with regard to the option for or against reconstruction. In practice many change their minds after mastectomy with some requesting reconstruction despite refusing it initially and vice versa. The fear that primary reconstruction may result in a high local recurrence rate has not materialized.[29]

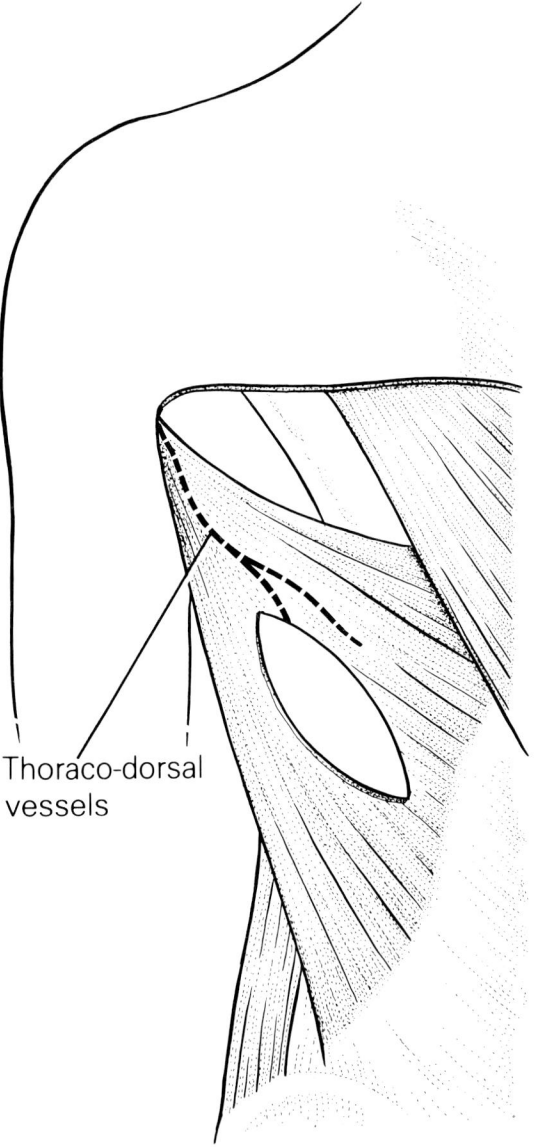

Figure 1.28 *Latissimus dorsi myocutaneous flap. The muscle and skin island are nourished by the thoracodorsal vessels.*

inis flaps and omental graft which is covered with split skin grafts.

Latissimus dorsi myocutaneous flap

This safe and reliable flap was introduced by Olivari[30] and popularized for breast reconstruction by Bostwick.[31] It is particularly indicated when the anterior chest skin is tight, scarred or damaged by previous radiotherapy and/or when the pectoralis major muscle has been removed. Either the latissimus dorsi muscle alone (to provide bulk and replace a pectoralis major defect) or the muscle together with an oval skin island of up to 30 × 10 cm can be transposed to provide skin and muscle cover usually over a silicone implant.

The latissimus dorsi myocutaneous flap is shown in Figure 1.28. The muscle derives its major blood supply from the thoracodorsal subcapsular vessels and this stresses the need for the preservation of these vessels during the axillary dissection in the course of mastectomy for breast cancer. The skin blood flow is maintained via perforating vessels passing through the muscle to the dermis. The muscle arises from the spines of the lower six thoracic, the lumbar and the sacral vertebrae, from the edge of the iliac crest (posterior third) and lower three ribs. Attachment of the latissimus dorsi to the lumbosacral spine and iliac crest is via the posterior layer of the lumbar fascia. However the origin from the thoracic spinous processes is direct and is overlapped by the trapezius muscle.

1. **Position and mapping of skin incision.** The patient is placed in the full lateral position as for a thoracotomy with the arm on a rest. The margins of the latissimus dorsi muscle and skin ellipse are outlined with a skin marker. The size of the skin island depends on the extent of the skin cover required. The incision outlines an ellipse with an oblique longitudinal axis running downwards and medially in line with the posterior axillary fold (Figure 1.29).

2. **Exposure of latissimus dorsi.** The skin edges on either side of the ellipse are elevated to expose the muscle (Figure 1.29). Considerable undermining is necessary and facilitates primary closure of the wound following transfer. The muscle is detached from the lower ribs after retraction of the trapezius from the lower thoracic spine. Several bleeding vessels are encountered and require ligation. The muscle is then detached at its junction with the lumbar fascia and iliac crest.

3. **Transposition of the myocutaneous flap.** The skin of the posterior axillary fold is dissected away from the latissimus dorsi and this muscle with its cutaneous island is then transposed to the anterior chest wall. The lower margin of the muscle is sutured to the serratus anterior and rectus sheath beneath the lower skin flap with interrupted 2/0 absorbable sutures. Similarly the transposed latissimus dorsi is sutured medially to the sternal edge (Figure 1.30). A silicone implant of suitable size is then inserted underneath the transposed latissimus

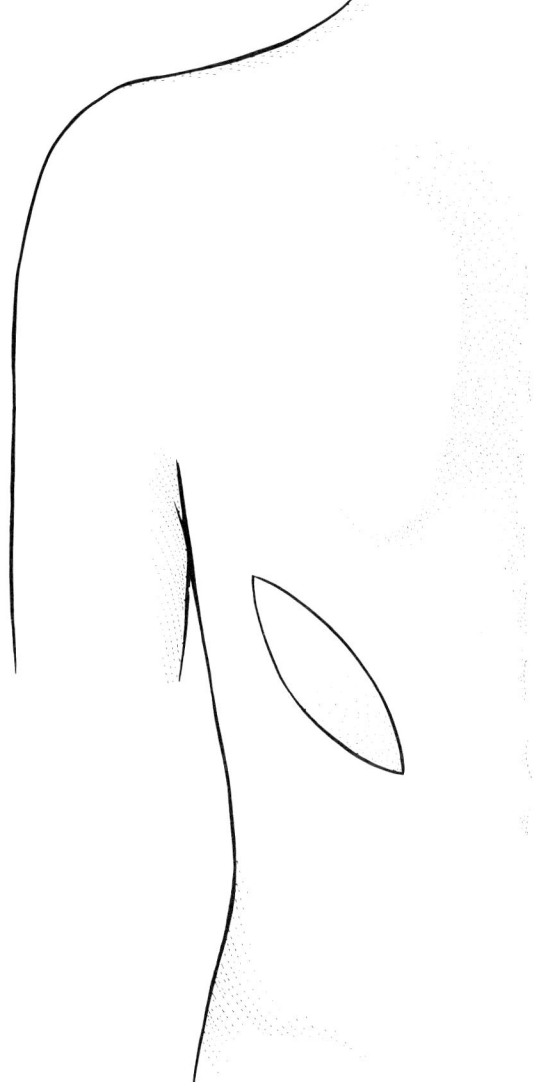

Figure 1.29 *Skin incision outlining the skin ellipse. The oval cutaneous island can measure up to 30 × 10 cm. Usually a 14 × 5 cm suffices but exact measurements are dictated by the size of the skin defect. The skin edges on either side of the ellipse are elevated to expose the latissimus dorsi muscle.*

22 GENERAL SURGERY

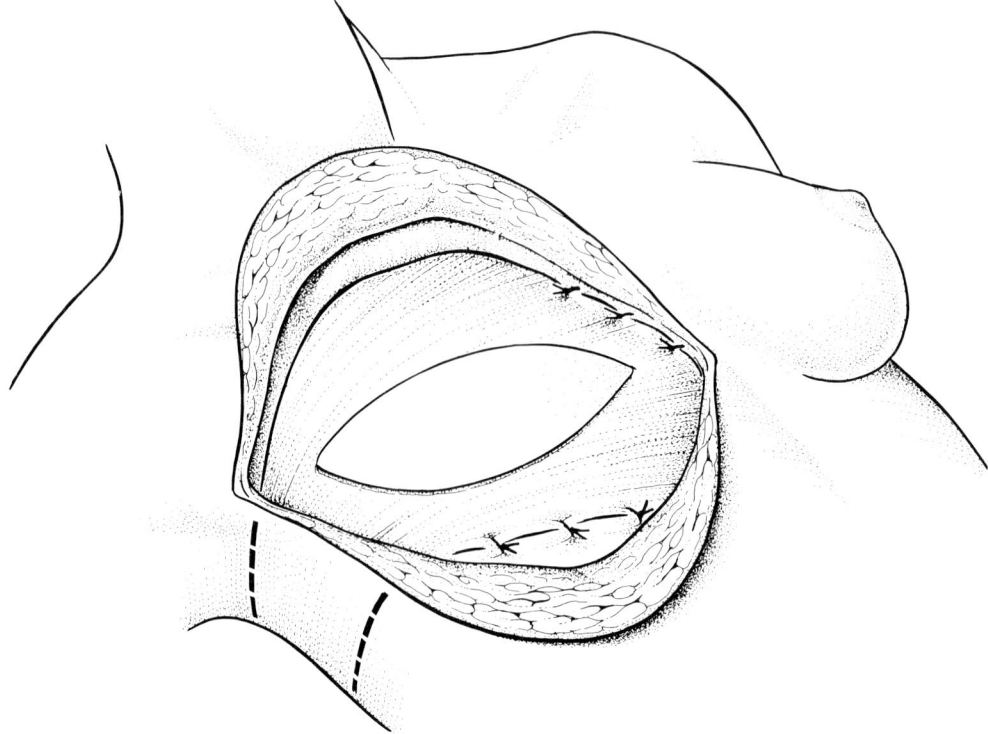

Figure 1.30 *The mobilized myocutaneous flap has been transposed to the pectoral region. The edges of the muscle are sutured to the serratus anterior and rectus sheath inferiorly and the sternal edge medially.*

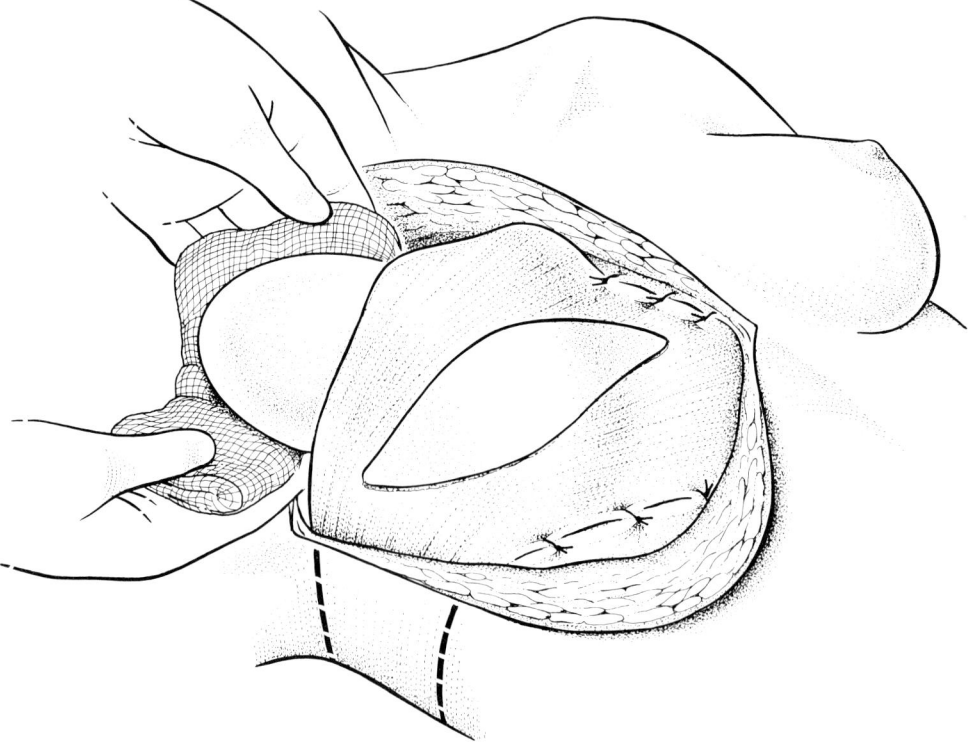

Figure 1.31 *A silicone implant of appropriate size is then inserted beneath the transposed latissimus dorsi and its upper margin is sutured to the medial third of the clavicle.*

CONSERVATIVE AND RECONSTRUCTIVE SURGERY OF THE BREAST 23

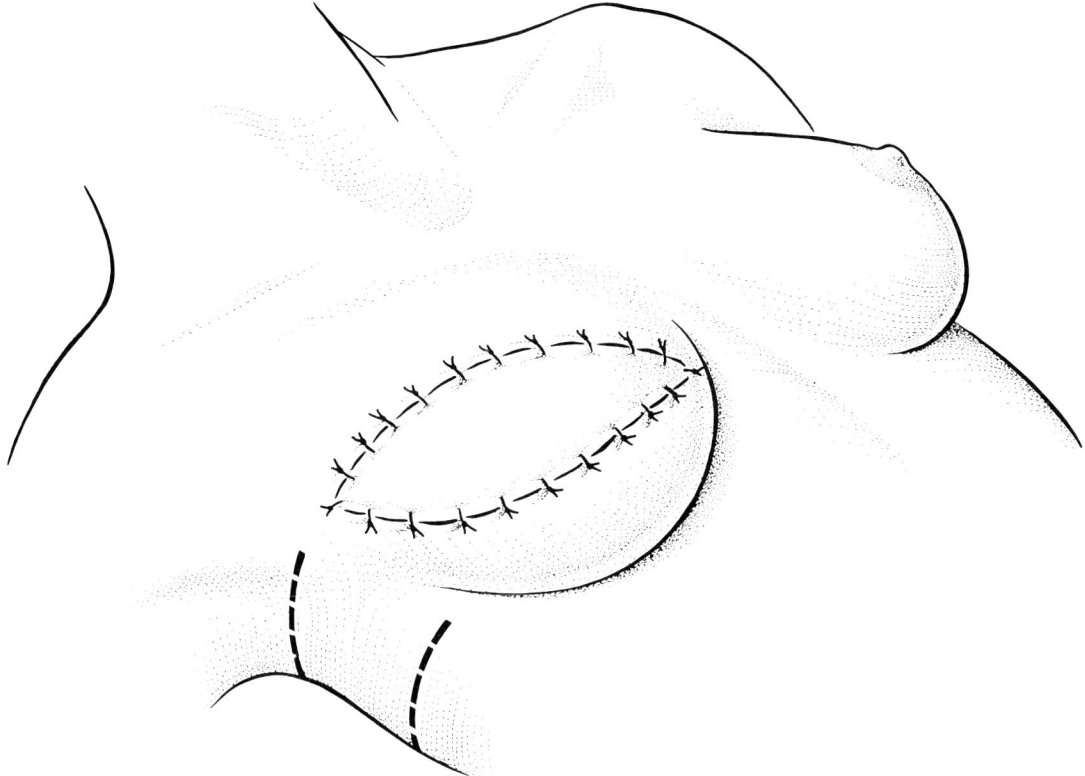

Figure 1.32 *The edges of the skin ellipse of the myocutaneous flap are sutured to the skin flaps with fine (3/0) monofilament sutures.*

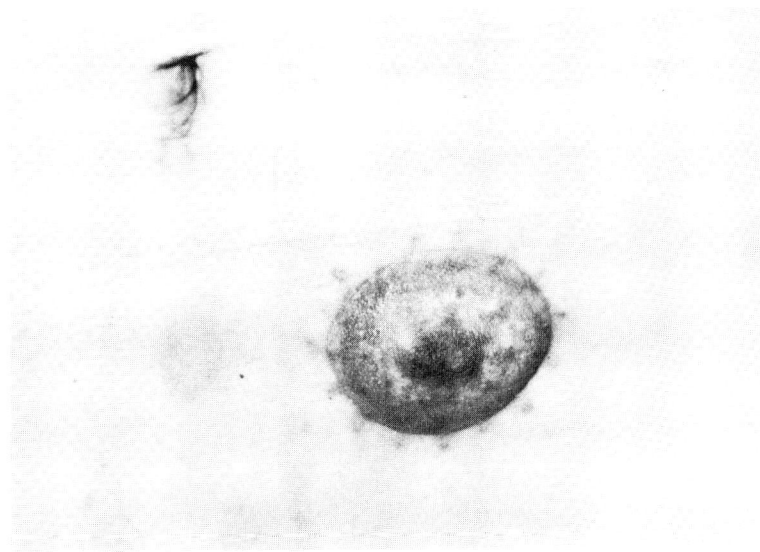

Figure 1.33 *Nipple–areola transfer to the left groin. The patient had reconstruction 12 months later when the nipple–areola complex was regrafted on the newly fashioned breast mound.*

dorsi, the upper margin of which is sutured to the medial third of the clavicle (Figure 1.31).

4. **Closure of donor site wound.** Provided sufficient undermining has been carried out, the edges of the skin can be approximated with interrupted sutures. The resulting scar should lie mainly in the bra line.

5. **Suture of chest skin to cutaneous island.** Some trimming may be necessary. If so it is best to trim the chest wall skin rather than the transposed ellipse since elevation of this from the muscle might jeopardize its blood supply. The suturing of the ellipse to the chest wall skin is performed with loose fine (3/0 prolene) interrupted sutures (Figure 1.32).

Complications

These are uncommon since this is a safe well-vascularized flap. Areas of skin necrosis can occur but are usually limited to the medial corner of the ellipse. These are best left for demarcation and are then excised and the edges sutured or the area is skin grafted depending on the size of the defect.

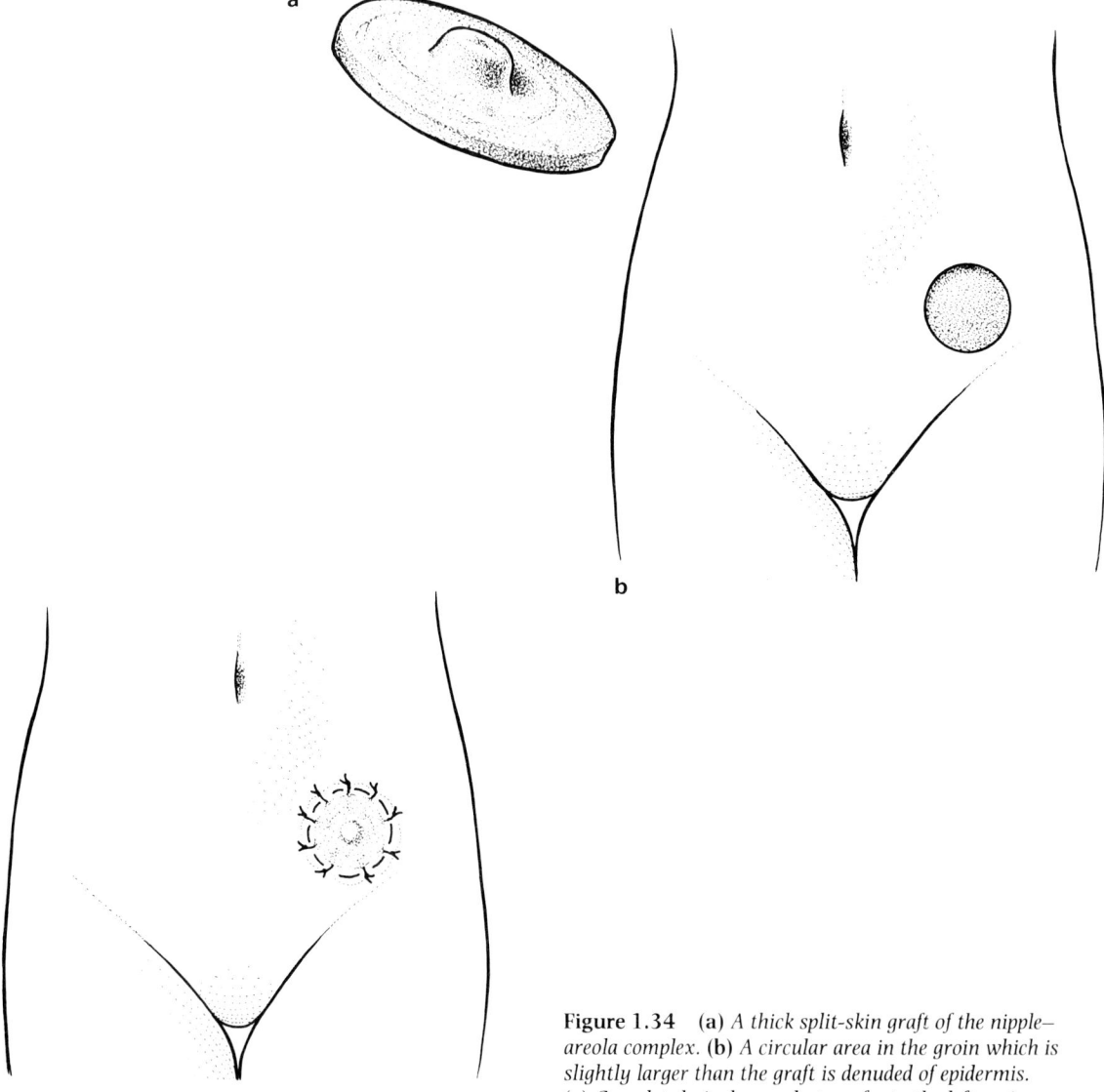

Figure 1.34 (a) *A thick split-skin graft of the nipple–areola complex.* (b) *A circular area in the groin which is slightly larger than the graft is denuded of epidermis.* (c) *Completed nipple–areola transfer to the left groin.*

Nipple–areola grafting

There is no substitute for the patient's own nipple and areola. Primary grafting of a thick split-skin graft onto the dermis of the skin of a myocutaneous flap can be performed when reconstruction is carried out at the time of mastectomy.

We have found transfer of the nipple–areola complex to the groin very useful when reconstruction is delayed after mastectomy (Figure 1.33). Histological confirmation of the absence of cancer infiltration by frozen section is necessary before obtaining a thick split-skin graft which is preferable to a full thickness one since the latter tends towards depigmentation to a greater extent. A circular area in the groin of slightly larger size than the graft is denuded of epidermis to create a dermal bed for the transposed nipple–areola complex (Figure 1.34).

Nipple–areola reconstruction

The procedures available include sharing from the opposite nipple–areola using a concentric spiral technique or reconstruction from auricular tissue or labia minor. The latter carries the disadvantage of subsequent hyperpigmentation which tends to contrast rather unfavourably with the opposite areola.

REFERENCES

1. Halsted WS (1895) The results of operations for the cure of cancer of the breast performed at the Johns Hopkins Hospital, from June 1889–January 1894. *Johns Hopkins Hospital Reports* **4**: 297–305.
2. Urban JA (1956) Radical mastectomy with en bloc in continuity resection of the internal mammary lymph node chain. *Surgical Clinics of North America* **36**: 1065–1082.
3. Dahl Ivensen E & Tobiassen T (1963) Radical mastectomy with parasternal and supraclavicular dissection for mammary carcinoma. *Annals of Surgery* **157**: 170–175.
4. Wangensteen OH (1949) Remarks upon a more radical operation for breast cancer. *Annals of Surgery* **130**: 315–316.
5. Wangensteen OH, Lewis FJ & Arhelger SW (1956) The extended or super-radical mastectomy for carcinoma of the breast. *Surgical Clinics of North America* **36**: 1051–1063.
6. Lacour J, Bucalossi P, Cacares E, Jacobelli I, Koszarowski T, Le H, Veronesi U & Rumeau Rouquette C (1976) Radical mastectomy versus radical mastectomy plus internal mammary dissection. *Cancer* **37**: 206–214.
7. Patey DH & Dyson WH (1948) The prognosis of carcinoma of the breast in relation to the type of operation performed. *British Journal of Cancer* **2**: 7–13.
8. Kaae S & Johansen H (1962) Breast cancer: five year results. Two random series of simple mastectomy with postoperative irradiation versus extended radical mastectomy. *American Journal of Roentgenology* **87**: 82–88.
9. Brinkley D & Haybittle JL (1966) Treatment of stage II carcinoma of the female breast. *Lancet* **ii**: 291–295.
10. Roberts MM, Blumgart LH, Davies M, Henk JM, Forrest APM, Campbell H, Gleave EN, Kunkler PB, Shields R, Hulbert M, Jamieson CW & Sellwood RA (1973) Simple versus radical mastectomy. *Lancet* **i**: 1073–1076.
11. Den Besten & Ziffren SE (1965) Simple and radical mastectomy, a comparison of survival. *Archives of Surgery* **90**: 755–759.
12. Veronesi U, Saccozzi R, Del Vecchio M, Bane A, Clemente C, De Lena M, Gallus G, Greco M, Luini A, Marubini E, Muscolino G, Rilke F, Salvadori B, Zecchin A & Zucali R (1981). Comparing radical mastectomy with quadrantectomy, axillary dissection and radiotherapy in patients with small cancers of the breast. *New England Journal of Medicine* **305** (1): 6–11.
13. Haybittle JL, Blamey RW, Elston CW, Johnson J, Doyle PJ, Campbell FC, Nicholson RJ & Griffiths K (1982) A prognostic index in primary breast cancer. *British Journal of Cancer* **45**: 361–366.
14. Maguire P, Brooke M, Tait A, Thomas C & Sellwood R (1984) The effect of counselling on physical disability and social recovery after mastectomy. *Clinical Oncology* **9**: 319–324.
15. Maguire P, Tait A, Brooke M, Thomas C & Sellwood R (1980) Effect of counselling on the psychiatric morbidity associated with mastectomy. *British Medical Journal* **281**: 1454–1456.
16. Seltzer MH, Perloff LJ, Kelley RL & Fittis WT (1970) The significance of age in patients with nipple discharge. *Surgery, Gynecology & Obstetrics* **131**: 519–522.
17. Paget J (1874) On disease of the mammary areola preceding cancer of the mammary gland. *St Bartholomew's Hospital Report* **10**: 87–89.
18. Lagios MD, Westdahl PR, Rose MR & Concannon S (1984) Paget's disease of the nipple: alternative management in cases without or with minimal extent of underlying breast carcinoma. *Cancer* **54**: 545–551.
19. Pashby NL, Nansel RE, Hughes LE & Preece PE (1983) A clinical trial of evening primrose oil in mastalgia. *British Journal of Surgery* **68**: 801.
20. Cuschieri A (1980) The results of subcutaneous mastectomy for severe diffuse and symptomatic be-

nign disease of the breast. *British Journal of Surgery* **67**: 827.
21 Duguid HL, Wood RAB, Irving AD, Preece PE & Cuschieri A (1979) Needle aspiration of the breast with immediate reporting of material. *British Medical Journal* **ii**: 185–187.
22 Mustakallio S (1954) Treatment of breast cancer by tumour extirpation and roentgen therapy instead of radical operation. *Journal of the Faculty of Radiologists* **6**: 23–26.
23 Atkins H, Hayward JL, Klugman DL & Wayte AB (1972) Treatment of breast cancer: a report after 10 years of a clinical trial. *British Medical Journal* **ii**: 423–424.
24 Levene MB, Harris JR, Hellman S (1977) Treatment of carcinoma of the breast by radiation therapy. *Cancer* **39**: 2840–2845.
25 Calle R, Pilleron JP, Schlenger P & Vilcoa JR (1978) Conservative management of operable breast cancer: ten years experience at the Foundation Curie. *Cancer* **42**: 2045–2053.
26 Black MM, Barclay THC, Cutler SJ, Henkey BF & Asire A (1972) Association of atypical characterization of benign breast lesions with subsequent risk of breast cancer. *Cancer* **29**: 338–346.
27 Hinton CP, Doyle PJ, Blamey RW, Davies CJ, Holliday HW & Elston CW (1984) Subcutaneous mastectomy for primary operable breast cancer. *British Journal of Surgery* **71**: 469–472.
28 Ward DC & Edwards MH (1983) Early results of subcutaneous mastectomy with immediate silicone prosthetic implant for carcinoma of the breast. *British Journal of Surgery* **70**: 651–653.
29 Goldwyn RM (1975) Reconstruction after mastectomy. *Archives of Surgery* **110** (3): 246.
30 Olivari N (1976) Latissimus flap. *British Journal of Plastic Surgery* **29**: 126–128.
31 Bostwick J, Vasionez LD & Jurkiewicz JH (1978) Breast reconstruction after a radical mastectomy. *Plastic and Reconstructive Surgery* **61**: 682–683.

2
Gun Transection for Oesophageal Varices

George W. Johnston

Oesophageal varices result from persistent elevation of the portal venous pressure most commonly secondary to intrahepatic disease. However the mere presence of varices does not necessarily mean that treatment is indicated. Indeed because of the poor life expectancy in cirrhotic patients, half of those with demonstrable varices will never bleed. Although portal hypertension does not require treatment, active therapy is essential for the patient who experiences an episode of haemorrhage, not only for control of the acute bleeding but also to try to prevent recurrent haemorrhage. The patient who survives an episode of bleeding from oesophageal varices is almost certain to bleed again, the majority within the next six to 12 months. There is no general agreement as to which method of treatment is best for either the acute bleeding episode or indeed for the more long-term prevention of recurrent bleeding. It is difficult to ascertain from the literature what constitutes an ideal programme because of the variety of operations carried out on vastly differing populations with many different aetiologies of portal hypertension. Ideally the management of each individual patient should be tailored according to the medical fitness of the patient. However the line of treatment followed will depend to a large extent on the medical facilities available in the area. Where no local expertise is available, patients should, where possible, be transferred to a neighbouring centre with a special interest in the field of portal hypertension.

PATHOPHYSIOLOGY OF BLEEDING OESOPHAGEAL VARICES

Although there are many sites of portal systemic anastomoses, the only clinically significant one is at the lower end of the oesophagus. Some considered that this area was vulnerable because of the possibility of acid reflux and oesophagitis with the erosion of the mucosa overlying the varices. However it is now clear from many studies that 'erosion from without' is not a major factor. The other theory, 'explosion from within', requires further probing. Certainly increased portal pressure is essential for the development of varices, but the raised hydrostatic pressure alone cannot be the sole factor since there is poor correlation between the height of portal pressure and the risk of bleeding.[1] In portal hypertension the increase in portal pressure extends throughout the portal venous system and so one has to try and explain why it is rare to find major haemorrhage from the haemorrhoidal portal systemic anastomoses, while bleeding is common in the lower oesophagus. Of course the oesophagus within the chest is subjected to negative intrathoracic pressure, which, when added to the high venous pressure, throws a very large strain on the thin-walled oesophageal varices. Inspiration against a closed glottis markedly increases the pressure within the varices. However these pressure changes should obtain throughout the whole intrathoracic oesophagus, yet bleeding occurs almost exclusively at the lower end. We feel that it is a difference in the venous anatomy of this segment of the oesophagus which accounts for the prevalence of bleeding at this site. Using a

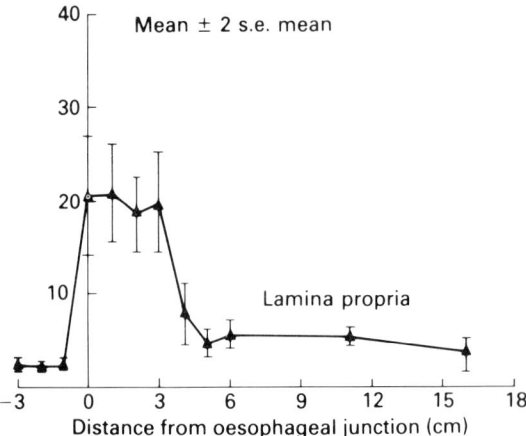

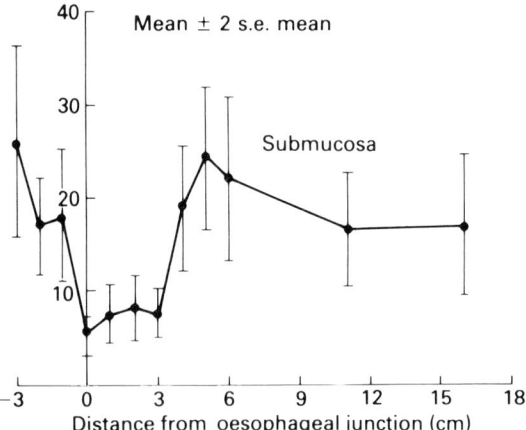

Figure 2.1 *Graph showing percentage area occupied by the veins in the lamina propria (above) and in the submucosa (below) in the normal oesophagus.*

computer image analysis system to study the venous anatomy of the stomach and oesophagus one notes an abrupt change in the vessel pattern at the oesophagogastric junction. In the normal individual the veins of the lowest three to five centimetres of the oesophagus lie mainly in the lamina propria, i.e. between the muscularis mucosa and the basement membrane of the epithelium. In the stomach, however, and in the more proximal oesophagus, the veins lie mainly in the submucosa, i.e. deep to the muscularis mucosa.[2] There is a sevenfold increase in the area occupied by veins in the lamina propria of the lower oesophagus compared to the corresponding area of the stomach (Figure 2.1). In portal hypertension it is these vessels in the lamina propria of the lowest 3–5 cm of the oesophagus which become varicose, while in the stomach and proximal oesophagus it is mainly the vessels in the submucosa which undergo dilatation. Thus, although oesophageal varices often extend throughout the length of the oesophagus and into the stomach, it is only in this lowest few centimetres of the oesophagus that the veins lie close to the oesophageal lumen. In addition large intraepithelial channels develop and these are often separated from the oesophageal lumen by only a few desquamating epithelial cells (Figure 2.2). It is likely that these intraepithelial channels seen microscopically correspond to the cherry red spots viewed endoscopically. Although these intraepithelial channels are relatively very small, serial sections demonstrate that they do communicate with the larger vessels in the lamina propria and may well be the source of bleeding (Figure 2.3). It is considered that blue or red varices exhibiting these cherry red spots are more liable to haemorrhage than white varices without them. Although haemorrhage from varices is often described as torrential, there is a sense in which it is the vomiting of accumulated blood which is torrential. Even when varices are known to be the source of upper gastrointestinal bleeding, radiologists usually find it difficult to demonstrate any leak into the oesophageal lumen on angiography. Similarly, using the flexible endoscope, one often fails to demonstrate a bleeding point on a varix, though if one follows flexible endoscopy with rigid oesophagoscopy, the obturator effect of the larger instrument distends the varices and this mechanism sometimes delineates the site of haemorrhage. When the venous pressure is elevated it does not take a large opening to allow a significant loss of blood in a short time; through a pinhole opening, the size of the lumen of a 21 SWG needle, one can lose over a litre of blood in one hour at the level of pressure one experiences in portal hypertension.

If it is true that bleeding occurs from a very small opening in a very limited area of the oesophagus, perhaps more attention should be directed towards this localized danger area. Hence there has been a recent upsurge in interest in both sclerotherapy and oesophageal transection–devascularization operations which attack this vulnerable area.

CLINICAL FEATURES

History

In the British Isles probably only about 10% of the patients admitted with upper gastrointestinal

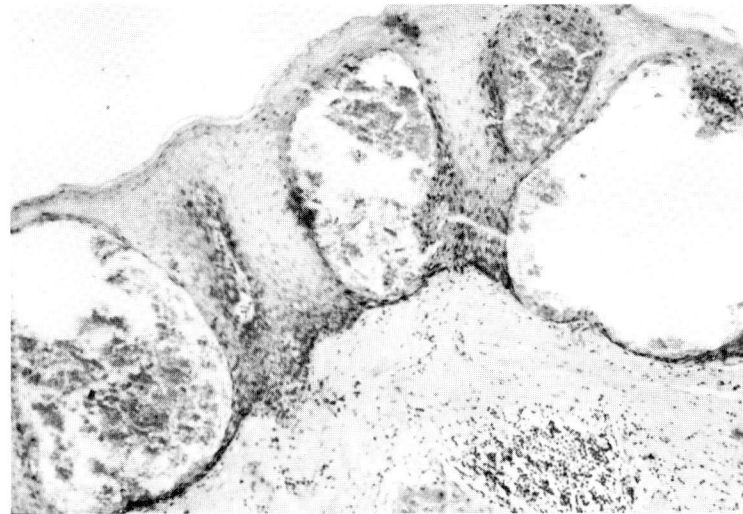

Figure 2.2 *Photomicrograph demonstrating the large intraepithelial channels in the lower oesophagus in portal hypertension.*

bleeding will be bleeding from oesophageal varices and yet it is vital to recognize this group. A good history and careful physical examination of the patient will alert the clinician to the majority of these patients. Many will have had the diagnosis of cirrhosis, portal hypertension and oesophageal varices already established during previous hospitalization. If such patients with known varices are admitted with serious upper gastrointestinal haemorrhage, there is an 80–90% chance that the varices are the source of bleeding. For other patients presenting at hospital for the very first time, other pointers should be sought. For example, a past history of jaundice or previous residence in an area where hepatitis B or schistosomiasis is endemic should put one on alert. History of alcohol abuse is important though one must realize that initially most alcoholics tend to minimize the quantity of alcohol they admit to consuming. Even if they do admit to excess drinking, bleeding could be coming from alcoholic gastritis or a Mallory–Weiss ulceration subsequent to alcoholic vomiting bouts. Although the ingestion of anti-inflammatory agents is not an important cause of variceal bleeding, it is worth checking on this aspect of the history. In children a recent upper respiratory tract with spasms of coughing may be significant since inspiration against a closed glottis markedly increases portal pressure and hence the strain on any thin-walled varices. Also one should enquire about symptoms suggestive of hiatus hernia, peptic ulceration, gastric neoplasm, etc.

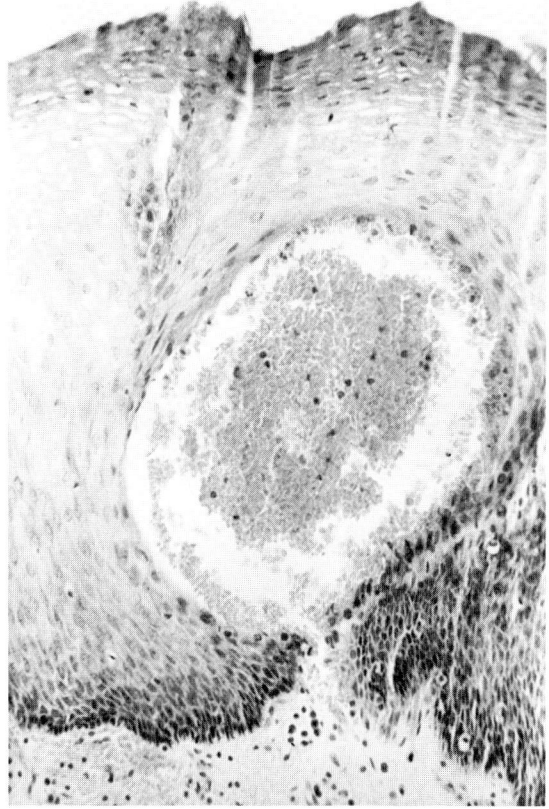

Figure 2.3 *Photomicrograph showing the communication between the intraepithelial channels and the lamina propria veins.*

It is worthwhile trying to get some idea of the extent of blood loss by enquiring about the frequency and quantity of vomiting, the presence of abdominal colic and the frequency, size and colour of any stools passed. It should be remembered that blood loss arising in the oesophagus can produce stools which are red in colour rather than black, if the transit time through the bowel is less than 10 hours; this indicates major and rapid blood loss. With less major episodes of bleeding the patient may only have melaena.

Physical examination

Hepatic cirrhosis is the commonest cause of portal hypertension and therefore any stigmata of chronic liver disease should be sought. In the hands one can look for palmar erythema, finger clubbing, vascular spiders, Dupuytren's contracture and flapping tremor. The head and neck is the best area to see skin telangiectasia, vascular spiders, xanthelasma and of course jaundice. In the trunk one should look for gynaecomastia, ascites, prominent periumbilical and anterior abdominal wall veins, and loss of pubic hair and testicular atrophy in the male. The liver may or may not be enlarged depending on the stage of cirrhosis, but if the portal hypertension is intrahepatic in origin, the liver texture will be abnormally firm. In the vast majority of patients with portal hypertension the spleen will be enlarged although not invariably so. It has, of course, to be at least twice its normal size before it is palpable below the costal margin. However percussion may pick up splenic enlargement before it is large enough to be palpated. Percussion along a line from the umbilicus to the lower margin of the posterior axillary fold is normally resonant due to the presence of gas in the colon, stomach and lung. Dullness to percussion in the upper part of this line may represent early splenomegaly, provided dullness due to ascites has been excluded. In children with bleeding oesophageal varices due to portal vein obstruction the spleen is invariably palpable in our experience.

EARLY MANAGEMENT OF THE PATIENT

Resuscitation

About 90% of the patients admitted with variceal haemorrhage are suffering from some form of hepatic cirrhosis and many have severely compromised liver function. The acute loss of blood and resulting hypotension is a further insult to the already sick liver. In addition the large protein load from the blood in the lumen of the gut may precipitate portal systemic encephalopathy. Ideally a central line should be established for blood transfusion and, if required, vasopressin infusion. Measures should be taken to try and reduce the risk of hepatic coma; the bacterial flora of the large intestine can be reduced by a combination of neomycin and metronidazole orally or via the gastric limb of a Sengstaken tube, should this be in place. Lactulose given orally in a dosage of 10–30 ml three times daily also reduces the absorption of ammonia by lowering faecal pH and by stimulating bowel evacuation.

Endoscopy

Obviously, early control of bleeding is necessary for efficient resuscitation and it is therefore necessary to confirm the exact source of bleeding as soon as is practical. However, where a patient is still vomiting blood, emergency endoscopy is fraught with difficulties and probably does not reduce morbidity or mortality. In these circumstances, if one is fairly certain that the patient is bleeding from varices, it is justifiable to institute oesophageal tamponade, as both a diagnostic and therapeutic tool. Of course even in patients with proven oesophageal varices, haemorrhage can occur from a different source, although in the past the incidence of non-variceal bleeding has been over-emphasized, merely because an active bleeding point on a varix was not demonstrated endoscopically. Prior to endoscopy one should spend some hours getting the patient into a stable condition, the bleeding controlled by either vasopressin or oesophageal tamponade, and the stomach evacuated of blood, preferably with the help of 10–20 mg of metoclopramide given intravenously. Even if there is some blood in the stomach at the time of endoscopy it is usually possible to get a fairly adequate examination of the common sites of upper gastrointestinal bleeding from all causes. Thus with the patient in the left lateral position, any remaining blood pools in the fundus of the stomach and it is usually possible to inspect the oesophagus, the lesser curvature of the stomach, the gastric antrum and the duodenum. Diagnostic endoscopy can be converted to therapeutic endoscopy if one's scheme of things includes injection sclerotherapy.

Control of the acute bleeding episode

In a number of patients, particularly the good-risk patients, haemorrhage often stops spontaneously and no emergency intervention is indicated. Time is available for a more thorough investigation of these patients prior to any definitive procedure. In the majority of the remaining patients bleeding can be controlled initially by vasopressin or tamponade. Vasopressin is particularly useful in children where the block is extrahepatic and where bleeding usually stops on conservative treatment thus avoiding the use of the rather terrifying Sengstaken–Blakemore tube if at all possible. Vasopressin is also useful in the adult with a relatively small haemorrhage; however in the presence of massive bleeding it is probably wiser to proceed straight to oesophageal tamponade, thereby minimizing blood loss. Bolus injection of 20 units of vasopressin in 100 ml of 5% dextrose given over a 20 minute period can be effective. Continual infusion at a rate of 0.4 u/min may be more efficient but if given into a peripheral vein it can precipitate cutaneous gangrene adjacent to the superficial vein.[3]

Although oesophageal tamponade is unpleasant for the patient it can be life-saving. The dangers attributed to the technique are almost all the result of misuse of the method. The use of the four lumen tubes with a pharyngeal aspirator reduces the risk of aspiration into the trachea. Traction should generally be avoided since this increases the patient's discomfort and also the risk of ulceration to the nares. There should be no problem of acute airway obstruction if the patient is kept under constant observation during the time the oesophageal balloon is distended. Ulceration of the lower oesophagus occurs only after unduly prolonged tamponade or if the wrong pressures are used. After 12–24 hours tamponade, at a time convenient to the staff, the oesophageal balloon is deflated while the gastric balloon position is maintained. The patient may now be allowed to drink and constant nursing supervision is no longer necessary. Test aspiration is performed to check for recurrent bleeding, and frequent monitoring of the patient's vital signs is continued. Should bleeding recur, the oesophageal balloon is reinflated after careful repositioning of the gastric balloon snugly at the cardia. Arrangements are then made for such patients to go to the operating theatre for more definitive treatment within the next 24 hours. Patients who do not bleed in the day following deflation of the oesophageal balloon can have the gastric balloon released and the tube removed.

Whether patients stop bleeding spontaneously, or stop with the use of vasopressin or tamponade, or rebleed after these conservative measures, all require more definitive treatment to try to prevent recurrent haemorrhage. The plan of management we employ is shown in Figure 2.4.

PREOPERATIVE ASSESSMENT AND PATIENT SELECTION

A discussion of all the various investigations available for patient assessment is outside the scope of this chapter. I have therefore confined myself to those tests considered most helpful in selecting the procedure best suited to the individual patient. Ideally one would like to be able to offer the patient an operation which would eliminate the risk of further variceal bleeding but not all patients are fit for major surgery. For example, doing an emergency shunt on the Child's Grade C patient with

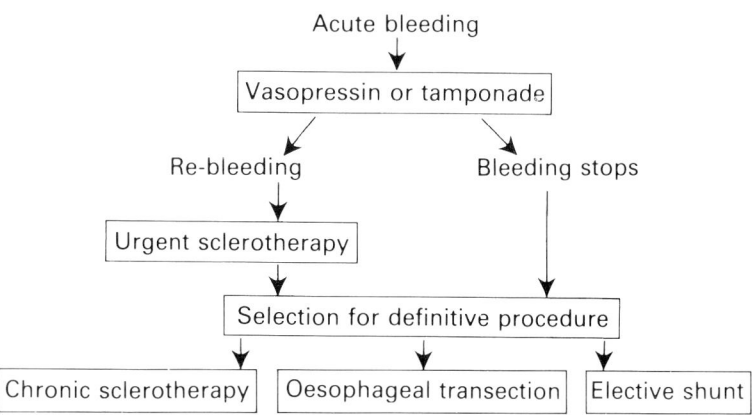

Figure 2.4 *Flow diagram for management of patients with bleeding oesophageal varices.*

ascites and encephalopathy is pointless; the few patients who would survive would be crippled with postoperative encephalopathy. It is therefore essential to get at least some basic assessment before deciding the best line of treatment for each patient. Clinical assessment is vital but the old adage, 'The patient who looks well, and feels well, does well', can be fallacious. Although the deeply jaundiced patient with primary biliary cirrhosis often withstands surgery well, the combination of significant jaundice, ascites and encephalopathy in the cirrhotic patient are usually contraindications to major surgery. A full haematological and biochemical profile is essential and coagulation studies are also necessary since most of the clotting factors are made in the liver; the platelet count will also demonstrate if there is any hypersplenism.

It is also useful to have documented evidence of the varices on barium studies of the oesophagus, although confident diagnosis can usually be made at endoscopy. The non-invasive dynamic isotope liver scan provides a reliable measure of liver and splenic size and also a good estimate of hepatic blood flow. The serum albumen and the liver size are two of the best indicators of prognosis. Liver biopsy is useful to establish the exact diagnosis and also to exclude active hepatitis which would discourage major surgery. However if one has proven the presence of varices as the source of bleeding, and if one is going to operate in any case, it may be justifiable to defer biopsy until the actual time of surgery. If shunt surgery is contemplated venographic studies are essential, but where injection sclerotherapy or a transection–devascularization procedure is envisaged, it is doubtful whether such invasive investigations are justified. With the clinical and biochemical data, one can establish the Child's classification of the patient or some modification of it. Perhaps division into good- and poor-risk patients is all that is necessary, surgical intervention being avoided in the latter group. Those patients who fail to stop bleeding, or rebleed on cessation of vasopressin therapy, or oesophageal tamponade, require emergency intervention. I feel that for these patients the best form of initial treatment is injection sclerotherapy. In the 25-year period since 1958 we have treated 264 patients with a total of 445 injections during 369 admissions for acute bleeding. We reported a control rate of 91.4% and an admission mortality of 14.9%.[4] It is doubtful if we could achieve these figures with any other form of emergency intervention. Of course patients who survive emergency injection sclerotherapy still have to go on to some other form of treatment at a later date to try to prevent recurrent haemorrhage. This may mean chronic injection sclerotherapy, oesophageal transection or some form of shunt surgery.

How do we decide which patients to choose for which procedure? I think it is easiest if we start with the very good-risk patients. In spite of the bad press received by shunt surgery, I feel that there is still a place for portal decompression in perhaps 10–20% of patients; where definitive shunt surgery is used, the evidence suggests that the Warren shunt gives less postoperative morbidity. Certainly the risk of post-shunt encephalopathy can be reduced if one avoids shunt surgery in patients with Child's Grade C liver disease, those with diabetes, patients over the age of 50 years and in those patients where portal hypertension is secondary to schistosomiasis. This leaves about 80–90% of the patients in the 'shunt reject' pool. For these patients we have tended to use chronic injection sclerotherapy for the poorer risk ones and reserve oesophageal transection for those considered better risk. The trouble with chronic injection sclerotherapy is that repeated visits to hospital are required and so our policy has been to reserve this method for the patients we feel would not tolerate laparotomy, e.g. patients with marked jaundice, gross ascites, small liver size and poor liver function. At present about half of our patients in the shunt reject pool are treated with injection sclerotherapy and the remainder by oesophageal transection. We are now embarking on a controlled trial of chronic injection sclerotherapy versus oesophageal transection for prevention of recurrent haemorrhage.

THE TECHNIQUE OF GUN TRANSECTION—DEVASCULARIZATION

Boerema[5] and Crile[6] pioneered transoesophageal ligation of varices and subsequently many modifications have been devised and widely practised. Walker's modification[7] used a vertical incision for the muscle layers and a transverse cut for the submucosa and mucosa thereby reducing the risk of suture line leakage. Hassab[8] introduced the concept of transabdominal gastro-oesophageal decongestion together with splenectomy for bleeding oesophageal varices in bilharzial cirrhosis; his technique did not include oesophageal or gastric transection. Japanese surgeons, disillusioned by the results of shunt surgery, devised an extensive transthoracic para-oesophageal devascularization operation together with oesophageal transection.[9] An abdominal component of the operation adds

GUN TRANSECTION FOR OESOPHAGEAL VARICES 33

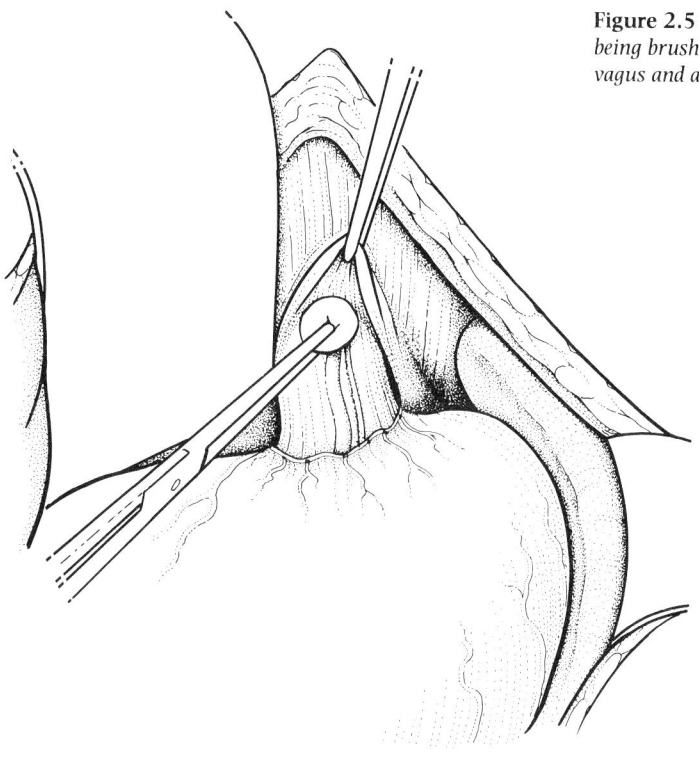

Figure 2.5 *Diagram showing the phreno-oesophageal fold being brushed upwards to expose the underlying anterior vagus and accompanying veins.*

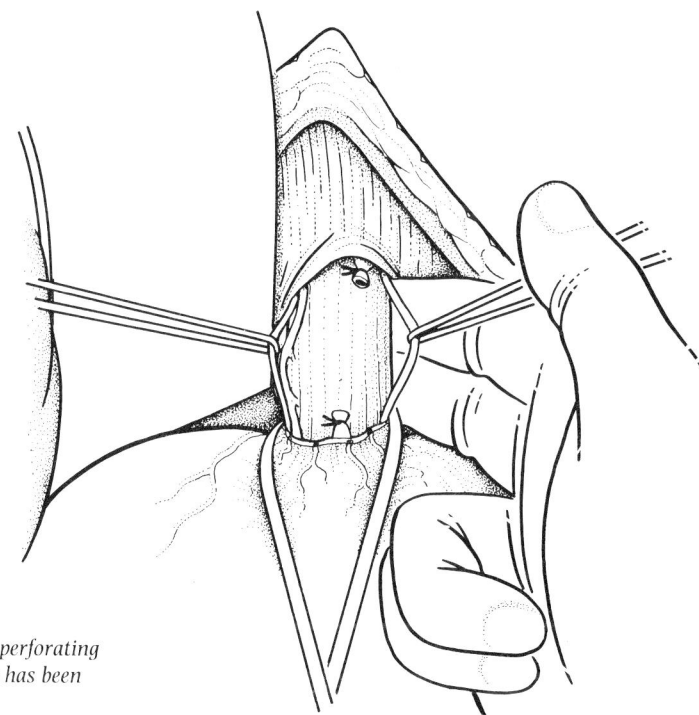

Figure 2.6 *Diagram illustrating the posterior perforating veins which need to be divided. The anterior vein has been divided.*

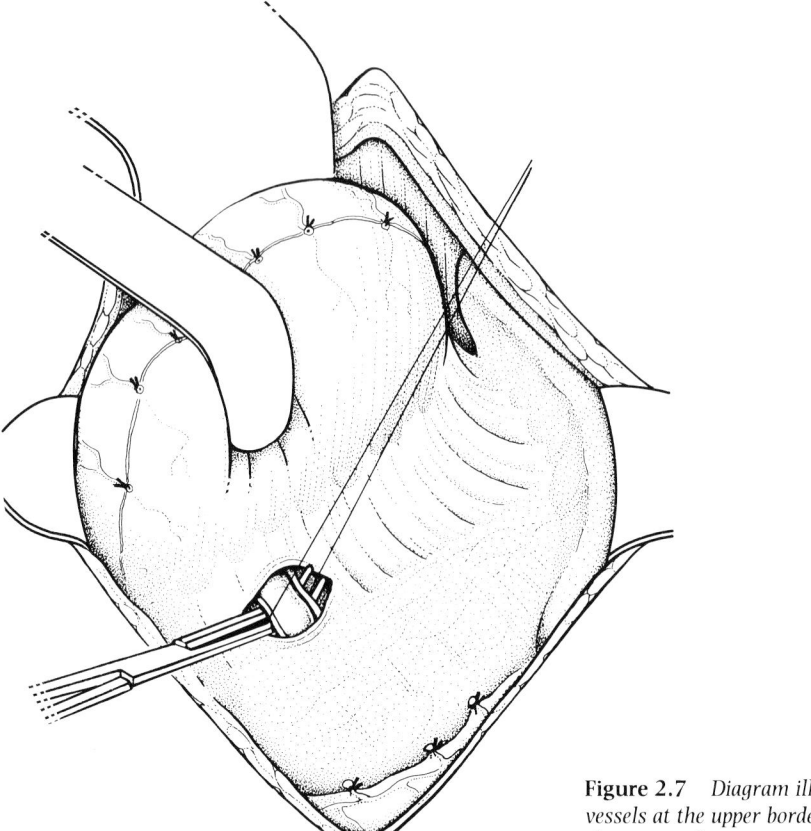

Figure 2.7 *Diagram illustrating ligation of the left gastric vessels at the upper border of the pancreas via a window in the gastrocolic omentum.*

splenectomy and devascularization of the upper stomach together with vagotomy and pyloroplasty. This extensive procedure is not well tolerated by the poor-risk cirrhotic patients encountered in Western society and has not, as yet, become popular outside Japan. The advent of circular stapling guns made the oesophageal transection simpler and safer and was first reported by Vankemmel.[10] The advantage of gun transection is that it gives a full thickness division of the oesophagus via the abdominal approach and at the same time allows sub-diaphragmatic devascularization. Encouraged by the results reported by Vankemmel in 1974 we began using the technique in January 1976 and now have experience of 110 transections. There have been some minor modifications to the method initially described for the Russian SPTU gun.[11]

Technique

The patient lies supine on the operating table; a slight head-up tilt can be helpful. A midline incision from the umbilicus to the xiphisternum usually gives adequate exposure. If splenectomy is indicated because of hypersplenism the left subcostal approach is preferable. Preliminary exploration of the abdomen should confirm the diagnosis and exclude the presence of a hepatoma or any other serious pathology. The position of the oesophagus is palpated and the transverse white line indicating the lower border of the phreno-oesophageal ligament identified. There are usually multiple dilated vessels in the peritoneal layer and these should be diathermied prior to division of the pre-oesophageal peritoneum at the level of the phreno-oesophageal ligament. Using a gauze dissector the ligament is brushed upwards to expose the underlying oesophagus and bring into view the large peri-oesophageal collateral veins which run with the anterior vagus nerve (Figure 2.5). These can usually be separated off from the nerve without difficulty, but if not, the anterior vagus can be sacrificed, providing one ensures that the posterior vagus is preserved. The oesophagus is mobilized at

Figure 2.8 *With the vagi retracted, the oesophagus, freed of its venous connections, is encircled by a stout ligature.*

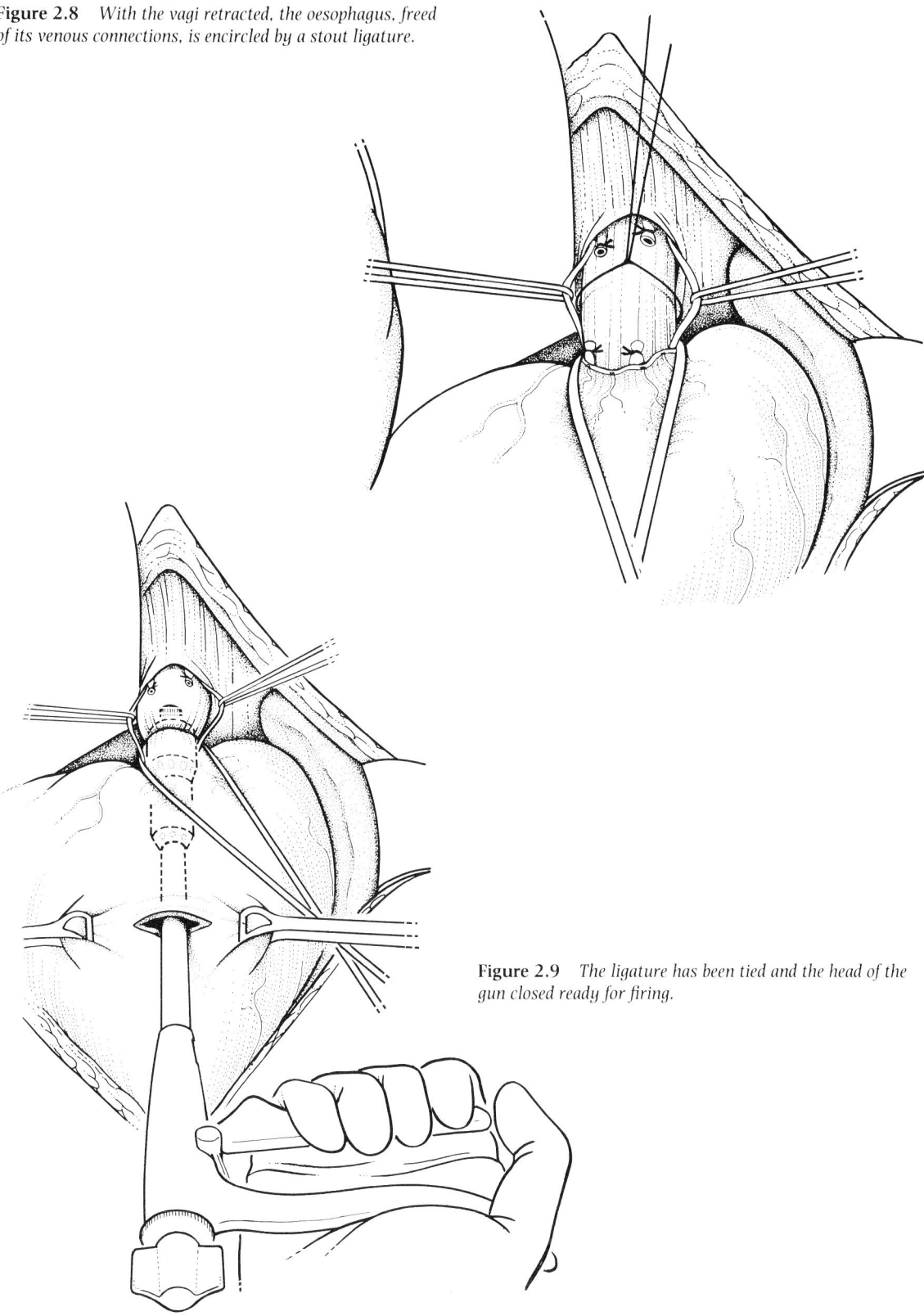

Figure 2.9 *The ligature has been tied and the head of the gun closed ready for firing.*

the sides and posteriorly using a gauze dissector. This brings into prominence the collateral vessels running with the posterior vagus; these are usually larger than those at the front of the oesophagus. These vessels are freed from the posterior vagus and the nerve protected by a silastic sling. A rubber sling is passed round the mobilized oesophagus which is now held forward to allow division of the many perforating oesophageal veins under direct vision (Figure 2.6). Usually there are only one to three perforators coming off the anterior vessel but there are three to six from the lowest 5 or 6 cm of the oesophagus to the posterior veins. The significance of these perforating veins in portal hypertension has been demonstrated recently using Doppler flow studies and intravariceal injection radiography.[1,2] It is essential that this vulnerable area of the oesophagus, namely the lowest 5 cm, is freed of all these extrinsic venous connections. It is often stated that dissection around the hiatus carries a serious risk of haemorrhage in patients with portal hypertension, but this has not been our experience. Peri-oesophagitis secondary to hiatus hernia, or previous injection sclerotherapy, however, make mobilization of the oesophagus more difficult and tedious. At this stage of the operation a loose wipe is placed down at the area of dissection and attention is turned to the left gastric vessels. This leash of vessels can be approached either through the gastrohepatic omentum or via a window in the gastrocolic omentum (Figure 2.7); we generally use the latter route since this gives excellent access to the lesser sac and also the splenic artery, should one wish to do splenic artery ligation. The left gastric pedicle is identified at the upper border of the pancreas and mass ligature of all the vessels is carried out in continuity; usually about three ligatures are applied and we also put on the largest size of metal ligaclip since this can be a useful marker should subsequent venography be required. If hypersplenism is present splenic artery ligation may be carried out. Where the spleen is not being removed some surgeons like to ligate and divide the uppermost short gastric vessels for more adequate devascularization.

Attention is now redirected to the lower oesophagus. With the vagi freed from the oesophagus a stout linen ligature is passed around the oesophagus and loosely tied (Figure 2.8). A small gastrotomy is made in the anterior wall of the stomach and an obturator-sizer is passed into the oesophagus to determine the largest size of gun head which can be slipped into the oesophagus safely. It is important to make sure that neither the linen ligature nor the rubber sling around the oesophagus cause any obstruction posteriorly, when the gun head is being guided into the lower oesophagus. When the closed gun has been advanced into the lower third of the oesophagus the head is opened up to give a gap of about 3 cm. The gun is then withdrawn down the oesophagus until the lowest part of the gap lies immediately above the oesophagogastric junction. It is essential that the assistant maintains this position of the gun until the linen ligature is tightened round the oesophagus just immediately above the cardia (Figure 2.9). The rubber sling should be removed from around the oesophagus before tightening up the head because it can easily intrude into the gap. When the gap in the head of the gun has been reduced to less than 2.5 mm the trigger is pulled; approximately 1 cm of full thickness oesophageal wall is removed. It is necessary to reopen the gap in the head of the gun before withdrawing the instrument through the newly formed anastomosis; a complete 'doughnut' indicates a satisfactory transection. An index finger is inserted through the gastrotomy wound to assess the quality and position of the suture line and to direct a nasogastric tube into the stomach for postoperative decompression. The gastrotomy wound is closed in two layers, liver biopsy performed and the abdomen closed without drainage.

If hypersplenism is a significant problem, splenectomy can be added but for this a left subcostal approach is preferred. Where the patient has a concomitant duodenal ulcer, it is best to place the gastrotomy in the most dependent part of the stomach so that it can be subsequently used for gastrojejunostomy in conjunction with the vagotomy. This step adds very little to the operative time.

Postoperative care

Nasogastric aspiration of the stomach is maintained for 24–48 hours, after which the tube is withdrawn. However all oral fluids are withheld until the fourth or fifth postoperative day. By this stage one can start giving 15–30 ml of water hourly and gradually build up the diet over the next few days. For the first dozen patients in the series we performed routine gastrographin studies of the anastomosis prior to allowing food but we no longer think that this is necessary. It is important to remember that these patients are without oral calories for over a week and therefore require intravenous feeding through a central line until established on an adequate diet. Prior to discharge all patients are warned that they may experience some difficulty initially in swallowing solid food. This dysphagia is usually mild and temporary but if it distresses the patient he is advised to return for barium studies to see if dilatation is necessary.

RESULTS

Since January 1976 we have performed 110 stapled oesophageal transections with sub-diaphragmatic devascularization. All 110 patients were considered unsuitable for any form of portal systemic shunt. In 26 patients this was because of acute bleeding, in 12 because of extrahepatic block and in the others because of advanced years, poor liver function or the presence of diabetes. Ninety-six patients had portal hypertension due to intrahepatic disease and 14 had extrahepatic portal hypertension. There were 50 Child's Grade A patients in the series including the 14 patients with extrahepatic block, 25 Grade B and 35 Grade C (Table 2.1). There were 59 males and 51 females; mean age was 54 years with a range of 14–80 years (21 patients were over 70 years). Twenty-six patients underwent emergency transection and the remainder had their operations electively, sometimes during the same admission and usually within the six weeks following the haemorrhage. In the first 61 patients in the series we used the Russian SPTU gun with either the 26 or 29 mm heads. In the remainder of patients we used the American EEA stapler with either the 28 or 31 mm heads.

Preoperative problems

Thirty-six patients had mild to moderate ascites at the time of surgery; ascites probably increases the risk of operation. Fourteen patients had experienced portal systemic encephalopathy preoperatively but in the majority this was related to episodes of gastrointestinal bleeding. Thirty-three patients had hypersplenism as defined by a platelet count of less than $50\,000/mm^3$. In addition 15 patients were diabetic, eight had duodenal ulceration, seven had cholelithiasis, five had hiatus hernias, four had gastritis and two had gastric ulcers. Malignancies were present in six of the patients at the time of surgery; in three patients primary hepatomas were found only after laparotomy but the other three patients were known to have carcinoma of the lung, carcinoma of the larynx and non-Hodgkin's lymphoma respectively.

In addition to oesophageal transection and sub-diaphragmatic devascularization 24 patients had splenectomy and a further nine had splenic artery ligation. Eight patients had vagotomy and drainage for concomitant peptic ulceration. In another 35 patients the anterior vagus nerve was sacrificed in order to obtain more complete devascularization. Six patients required cholecystectomy, four had herniorrhaphies and one had a partial hepatectomy for a resectable hepatoma.

Table 2.1 *110 Consecutive oesophageal transections, 1976–1984.*

Aetiology	No. of patients	Sex M	Sex F	Age (years)	Child's Class	Mortality Operative	Mortality Late	Rebleeding
Extrahepatic	14	10	4	37 (14–58)	14A	0	0	4
Intrahepatic								
Alcoholic	37							
Cryptogenic	28							
Chronic active hepatitis	16							
Primary biliary	8				36A	5	10	9
Haemochromotosis	1	49	47	57	25B	2	6	8
Granulomatous	1			(15–80)	35C	10	18	6
Cystic fibrosis	1							
Partial nodular transformation	1							
Schistosomiasis	2							
Lupoid hepatitis	1							
TOTAL	110	59	51	54 (14–80)	50A 25B 35C	17	34	27

Complications

Anastomotic leakage

It is with some surprise that we report that no patient in the series developed a leak from the oesophageal suture line. However one patient did develop an oesophageal leak about 2 cm above the transection. We think this was probably due to oesophageal damage following intraoperative dilatation from below, of a pre-existing oesophageal stricture; this patient died subsequently from mediastinitis. A further patient for no apparent reason also developed a leak about 1.5 cm above the anastomosis. This perforation was sub-diaphragmatic; following repair nine days after the initial procedure she made a satisfactory recovery. One further patient who started drinking fluids the evening of the operation leaked from his gastrotomy wound and developed a subphrenic abscess; following drainage of the abscess a temporary fistula resulted but this resolved spontaneously.

Dysphagia

Although many patients experienced some minor temporary dysphagia on commencement of solid food, this resolved spontaneously in the majority. However 14 of the 93 patients who survived to leave hospital required dilatation on at least one occasion. The average number of dilatations was 1.5 with a maximum of five in one patient. In retrospect probably eight of these 14 patients would not have required intervention had we been a little more patient. There was no correlation between the occurrence of dysphagia and previous injection sclerotherapy or the extent of operative peri-oesophageal devascularization. However only two of the last 49 patients, where the EEA stapler was used, have required dilatation. Oesophageal motility and pressure studies in patients with dysphagia have demonstrated some incoordination of swallowing together with impaired sphincter relaxation, resulting in less efficient oesophageal clearing.

Oesophageal reflux and heartburn

Four of our patients were known to have hiatus hernias prior to surgery and repair was not undertaken at the time of transection. However on questioning, some further patients also admitted to reflux and heartburn postoperatively, although this was rarely volunteered spontaneously. Twenty-four hour oesophageal pH monitoring using a radio pill was carried out in 19 patients following oesophageal transection for varices and the results were compared with 14 normal controls. There was no difference in the number of reflux episodes between the two groups. However in the erect position the duration of a pH of less than five was significantly greater in the post-transection group when compared to controls. The duration of a pH of less than four was also greater following transection but this did not reach statistical significance. There was no significant difference between the groups in the supine position.[13]

We also looked at lower oesophageal sphincter pressure and length prior to, and more than one month after, transection in seven patients. The median preoperative pressure was 16.5 mm of mercury compared to a postoperative pressure of 7.1 mm of mercury. The length of the lower oesophageal sphincter dropped from a median of 4.9 cm preoperatively to 2.8 cm postoperatively. However the pH studies have shown that in the majority of patients there is sufficient length and adequate pressure in the remaining sphincter to prevent significant reflux.

Symptoms of heartburn have been controlled well in patients with the use of antacids or one of the alginic acid preparations.

Postoperative encephalopathy

Although 14 patients had had encephalopathy prior to surgery, most of these episodes had been related to a prior haemorrhage. Only six of the 93 patients who survived to leave hospital have had any subsequent encephalopathic episodes. As yet, no patient has developed encephalopathy for the first time subsequent to the operation.

Recurrent haemorrhage

Three patients had recurrent bleeding within the first few days following emergency transection; two bled from an unknown source, possibly the suture line, and one subsequently died. The other patient bled from an acute erosion over a gastric varix and died 19 days after transection from uncontrollable haemorrhage associated with serious coagulation abnormalities. Of the 93 patients who left hospital alive, 27 patients have had recurrent haemorrhage in the follow-up period extending from three months to eight years and three months. There have been 39 bleeding episodes in the 27 patients with seven deaths. Recurrent varices have been shown to be the source of bleeding in 11 of the patients with two deaths. The other sources of bleeding included Mallory–Weiss ulceration in two, oesophagitis in two with one death, gastritis in three with two deaths and peptic ulceration in a further three patients. In six patients the source of bleeding was not known, either because the patients bled outside hospital and were not endoscoped or early endoscopy failed to show the source. There were two deaths in this group, both occurring outside hospital, and both in alcoholic patients who continued to drink heavily. Although at the five-year follow up, 40% of patients have had some further bleeding from the upper gastrointestinal tract (Figure 2.10), this was frequently minor in nature and, more often than not, it occurred from sources other than varices.

MORTALITY

There were 17 deaths in the series, giving a hospital mortality of 15%. Seven of these deaths occurred in the 26 patients undergoing emergency transection, giving an emergency mortality of 27% compared to a 12% mortality in the 84 patients having a more elective procedure. There were no deaths in the extrahepatic group, making the overall mortality in the cirrhotic group 18%. Ten of the deaths occurred in the 35 patients in Child's Grade C group.

SURVIVAL

Yearly cumulative figures were calculated using the statistical package for the Social Services programme and comparisons made between groups using the Lee–Desu statistical method.[14] The overall five-year cumulative survival was 47.2% but if the extrahepatic group are excluded the five-year survival for the cirrhotic group alone drops to 40.1% (Figure 2.11). There was no statistical difference in the five-year survival between the Child's Grade A and B patients (59.3% and 62.4% respectively) but comparison with the Child's Grade C figure of 24% was statistically significant: P = 0.008. Of the 93 patients who survived to leave hospital, 34 have died in the follow-up period; 18 of these patients were Child's Grade C. Causes of death were liver failure in 19, haemorrhage in seven, carcinoma in three, respiratory failure in two, cerebrovascular accident in two and disseminated intravascular coagulopathy in one. This last patient died following insertion of a Denver shunt for intractable ascites three years after transection. Of the 58 patients alive at the time of review, between 85 and 90% are well and free of jaundice, ascites and encephalopathy.

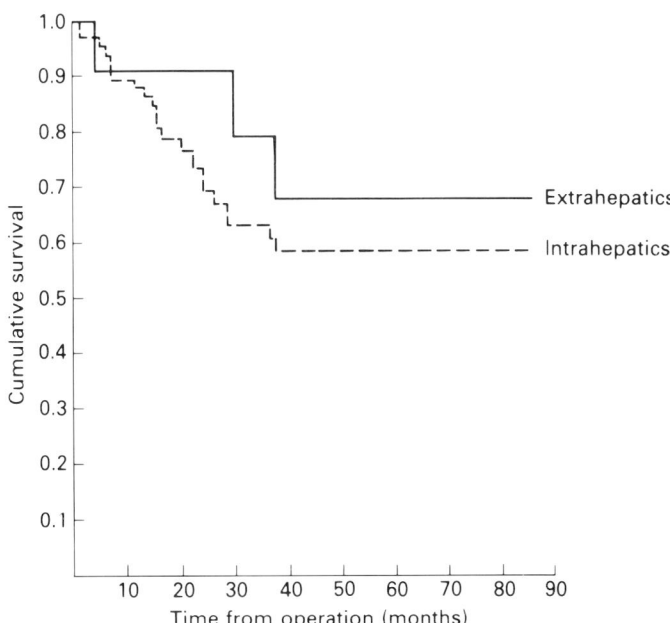

Figure 2.10 Post-transection remission from bleeding.

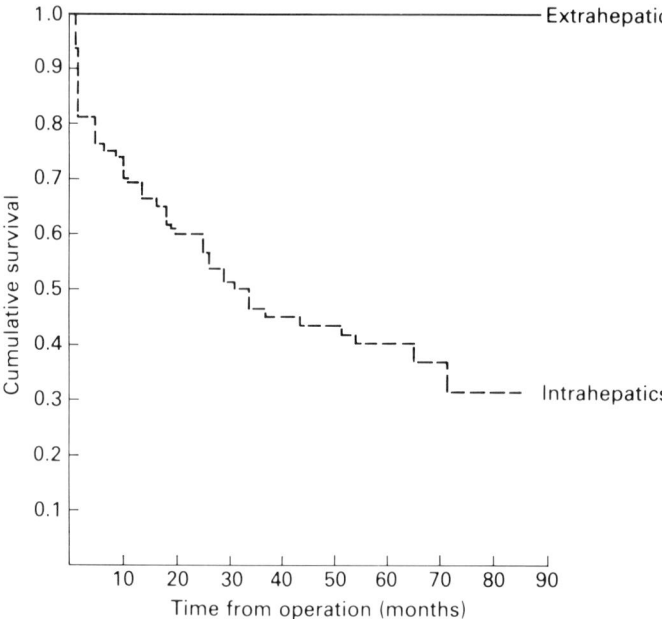

Figure 2.11 *Cumulative survival following transection.*

SUMMARY

Treatment of haemorrhage from oesophageal varices is still controversial. No one disputes the difficulties of management, or the demands on time, effort and resources. However some articles take an unnecessarily depressing attitude forgetting that the five-year survival for these patients is better than for many of the cancers we treat. The best results can be achieved only when patients with portal hypertension and bleeding varices are transferred to units with a special interest in the problem. Early replacement of blood and the minimizing of further blood loss are priorities in good management. If vasopressin or tamponade fail to control acute haemorrhage, urgent sclerotherapy is advised. It is the least invasive and therefore the best tolerated form of emergency intervention. For patients who survive the first haemorrhage early definitive therapy must be planned. This may take the form of chronic injection sclerotherapy, an oesophageal transection–devascularization procedure, or some form of shunt. Only further controlled trials can evaluate the most appropriate treatment. One may prefer to accept a higher risk of rebleeding for a lower risk of encephalopathy or vice versa. Currently we are involved in a three-centre controlled trial of chronic injection sclerotherapy versus transection for the prevention of recurrent bleeding in those patients considered fit for surgery. Even in the patients considered unfit for any form of surgery, injection sclerotherapy has much to offer. Ideally one would like to be able to select the most appropriate procedure for each individual patient on a more scientific basis than is practised at present.

REFERENCES

1. Lebrec D, De Fleury P, Rueff B, Nahum H & Benhamou J-P (1980) Portal hypertension, size of esophageal varices and risk of gastro-intestinal bleeding in alcoholic cirrhotics. *Gastroenterology* **79**: 1139–1144.
2. Spence RAJ (1984) The venous anatomy of the lower oesophagus in normal subjects and in patients with varices: an image analysis study. *British Journal of Surgery* **71**: 739–744.
3. Anderson JR & Johnston GW (1983) Development of cutaneous gangrene during continuous peripheral infusion of vasopressin. *British Medical Journal* **287**: 1657–1658.
4. Spence RAJ, Anderson JR & Johnston GW (1985) Twenty-five years of injection sclerotherapy for bleeding varices. *British Journal of Surgery* **72**: 195–198.
5. Boerema I (1949) Bleeding varices of the oesopha-

gus in cirrhosis of the liver and Banti's disease. *Archivum Chirurgicum Neerlandicum* **1**: 253–269.

6. Crile GS (1950) Transoesophageal ligation of bleeding oesophageal varices: a preliminary report of seven cases. *Archives of Surgery* **61**: 654–660.
7. Walker RM (1964) Esophageal transection for bleeding varices. *Surgery, Gynecology & Obstetrics* **118**: 323–329.
8. Hassab MA (1967) Gastro-oesophageal decongestion and splenectomy in the treatment of oesophageal varices in Bilharzial cirrhosis: further studies with a report on 355 operations. *Surgery* **61**: 169–176.
9. Sugiura M & Futagawa S (1973) A new technique for treating oesophageal varices. *Journal of Thoracic and Cardiovascular Surgery* **66**: 677–685.
10. Vankemmel M (1974) Resection-anastomose de l'oesophage sus-cardial pour rupture de varices oesophagiennes. *Nouvelle Presse Medicale* **5**: 1123–1124.
11. Johnston GW (1977) Treatment of bleeding varices by oesophageal transection with the SPTU gun. *Annals of the Royal College of Surgeons of England* **59**: 404–408.
12. McCormack TT, Rose JD, Smith PM & Johnston AG (1983) Perforating veins and blood flow in oesophageal varices. *Lancet* **ii**: 1442–1444.
13. Spence RAJ, Johnston GW & Parks TG (1984) Prolonged ambulatory pH monitoring in patients following oesophageal transection and control subjects. *British Journal of Surgery* **72**: 99–101.
14. Breslow NE (1970) A generalized Kruskal–Wallis test for comparing K Samples subject to unequal patterns of censorship. *Biometrika* **57**: 579–594.

3
Pyloric Reconstruction

M. Hobsley

When vagotomy was introduced[1] as an alternative to partial gastrectomy as an operation for duodenal ulcer, it was hoped that preserving the reservoir function of the stomach would reduce or abolish the incidence of the postprandial symptoms that were first called the *dumping syndrome* by Mix.[2] Once it had been established that symptoms suggestive of gastric outlet obstruction followed the operation of truncal vagotomy in a significant proportion of patients,[3] it was deemed necessary to add to the vagotomy some procedure at the gastric outlet designed to quicken gastric emptying. Truncal vagotomy with some such 'drainage' procedure thus became standard practice, and in many centres has been so for more than three decades.

It had been hoped that dumping would disappear but perhaps it should have been realized that this was unlikely. Clinicians should have recalled that the classical description of the dumping syndrome—and the first in the English language—was given by Herz[4]; his patient had undergone a simple gastrojejunostomy. In other words, there had been no reduction in the capacity of the patient's stomach so it was unlikely that a gastrectomy had produced the stomach's tendency towards dumping by its reduction in gastric capacity. Similarly, it was unlikely that vagotomy-and-drainage would not produce dumping simply because it does not reduce gastric capacity.

The proof that the incidence of dumping after vagotomy-and-drainage was not significantly less than after partial gastrectomy was provided by the surgeons of Leeds in a well-controlled clinical trial.[5] As a result, the idea that the drainage procedure (the destruction or bypassing of the pylorus) was the factor common to both types of operations that predisposed to the postprandial symptoms gradually became accepted.[6,7]

If the symptoms of the dumping syndrome are related to the drainage procedure, there is a distinct possibility that reversal of the drainage procedure to restore normal anatomy and function might prevent the symptoms. An early communication explicitly stating this idea and giving results of several operations to reconstruct the pylorus after vagotomy and pyloroplasty, originated in Denmark,[8] and since that time there has been a more extensive report from the same group[9] as well as reports from several others.[10–12]

It is important to realize that destruction or bypassing of the pylorus results in two different disturbances: (a) rapid gastric emptying into the duodenum and (b) increased reflux of duodenal contents back into the stomach.[13] While many authorities (e.g. Kelly et al[10]) believe that duodenogastric reflux, particularly of bile, can produce many of the same symptoms as those encountered in the dumping syndrome, there is to date not nearly as much quantitative evidence linking reflux with postprandial symptoms as there is linking rapid gastric emptying with postprandial symptoms. Indeed, a preliminary communication[14] describes poor results in a small group of patients in whom symptoms ascribed to reflux of bile into the stomach failed to respond to reconstruction of the pylorus. On the other hand, there is a clear-cut relationship, recently reviewed,[15] between rapid gastric emptying and the dumping syndrome. The only reliable indication at present for performing reconstruction of the pylorus is in patients with symptoms proven to be consistent with the dumping syndrome and in association with an increased rate of gastric emptying.

SELECTION OF PATIENTS

Good results with this operation are only obtainable if the patients are selected with great care. The aspects requiring consideration are the diagnosis of dumping, the assessment of severity, the timing of the operation, the non-operative management of symptoms and the nature of the previous operation.

Diagnosis of dumping

Clinical features

There is no difficulty in making a clinical diagnosis in a typical case. During or within the first half hour after a meal, the patient experiences abdominal distension, churning sensations in the abdomen, tiredness sometimes amounting to exhaustion, sweating and faintness. The symptoms gradually pass off during a period of half to one hour, and may culminate with watery diarrhoea. There is usually a discernible relationship between the severity of the symptoms and the size of meal, and also with the nature of the food eaten: sweet and stodgy foods such as sugar, jam, cake, bread and pastry are particularly liable to provoke symptoms.

The problem is that a minority of patients have bizarre or borderline symptoms. Meurling[16] drew attention to the large variety of symptoms that have been recorded, and drew particular attention to the fact that they can be separated into two groups (Table 3.1). Some patients present with symptoms virtually confined to one or other group: the author has reviewed the evidence[15] that *bile-vomiting*, the *small stomach syndrome* and *diarrhoea* (as a more or less isolated symptom) are all *formes frustres* of the dumping syndrome.

Add to these facts the consideration that the surgeon is usually trying to make the diagnosis of dumping on the basis of an outpatient interview, and it is obvious that sometimes real difficulty can arise.

Dumping provocation test

The answer to this problem is to attempt to produce the symptoms with the patient under the observation of the clinician. An ordinary meal can be used as the provocation, but there are advantages in standardization. Ever since Roberts et al[17] showed that concentrated glucose solution (50 g/dl) reproduces the symptoms in a patient with a typical history, this has been the stimulus most often used.

The patient attends, having fasted since midnight, at about 9 a.m. He sits on a couch or in a chair, and after a rest for 30 minutes drinks 150 ml of the test meal as rapidly as possible. The clinician notes whether the patient looks unwell, whether he volunteers any symptoms or complains of them on direct enquiry, and especially whether the symptoms mimic those which the patient has been complaining of.

Severity of dumping

There are two reasons for wanting to have a quantitative assessment of the severity of dumping. One is that even after the dumping provocation test has been performed there are still some patients who are difficult to categorize. The other is that without some measurement it is difficult to make an objective assessment of the value of the procedure aimed at alleviating the symptoms. Two such quantitative indices are (a) fall in plasma volume and (b) rate of gastric emptying.

Plasma volume

The fact that the symptoms after a meal of concentrated glucose solution are associated with a fall in

Table 3.1 *Which symptoms constitute the dumping syndrome?*

Abdominal		Systemic
Fullness	Weakness	Nausea
Heaviness	Tiredness	Warmth
Vomiting	Faintness	Palpitations
Discomfort	Dizziness	Dyspnoea
Pain	Headache	Sweating
Diarrhoea		
Churning		

plasma volume was first demonstrated by Roberts et al.[17] The fall reaches its maximum 20–30 minutes after the glucose, and the volume then gradually recovers to the baseline after 40–60 minutes. In Roberts' work the change in plasma volume was measured with Evans blue-labelling of plasma albumin, but Hobsley and Le Quesne[18] showed that the change can be calculated from the change in haematocrit, using the formula:

$$P_2 \text{ (as percentage of } P_1) = \frac{Ht_1}{100 - Ht_1} \times \frac{100 - Ht_2}{Ht_2} \times 100$$

where P_2 and Ht_2 refer respectively to the plasma volume and haematocrit at any time after the meal, and P_1 and Ht_1 refer to the same variables during the baseline period before the meal.

The size of the fall in plasma volume does not divide individuals into two groups, i.e. those without symptoms and those with dumping symptoms. Instead, there is a considerable overlap. Hobsley and Le Quesne also showed that one reason for this overlap is that some patients have a stable circulation that can withstand a temporary fall in circulating volume, whereas others have a labile circulation and experience distress with a relatively small fall in circulating volume. The release of kinins and other vasoactive symptoms in some individuals may explain these differences.[19,20] Nevertheless, in patients without symptoms during the dumping provocation test the fall in plasma volume is in the range 0–12% (median 3.9%), but in patients with symptoms the range is 4–23% (median 12.4%).[21,22]

Gastric emptying rate

Even after the dumping provocation test, and despite observation of the patient's symptoms and measurement of the fall in plasma volume, a small proportion of patients remain difficult to categorize. Since the size of the fall in plasma volume is certainly related to the speed of gastric emptying,[23] measurement of the gastric emptying rate of the same standard glucose meal affords another quantitative criterion which usually resolves the difficulty. If the glucose meal is labelled with a radioactive nuclide (e.g.[113] In) external counting with a gamma camera can detect the rate of disappearance of the meal from the gastric area. Gastric emptying rate can be expressed as the percentage fall in counts per minute, averaged over the first 10 minutes after the meal. In patients in whom the meal does not produce symptoms, this index is in the range 0.1–5.1% (median 1.0%), while in symptomatic patients the corresponding values are 0.5–8.1% (median 4.8%). The measurement of gastric emptying rate and fall in plasma volume can be conducted simultaneously.

Time after operation

There is a strong spontaneous tendency towards the diminution of symptoms after the original operation. The author never undertakes an operative procedure in an attempt to alleviate dumping until one year has passed, and in most patients the author prefers to wait two years. The two important factors bearing on the exact timing of the operation are the results of non-operative treatment in that individual and the nature of the previous operation.

Failure of medical measures

For the first few months after the original operation, the most important therapy is a combination of explanations and reassurance. The fact that the patient's symptoms do not represent anything 'going wrong' but simply one extreme of a range of reactions to the disturbance of physiology necessarily caused by the operation, and reassurance that spontaneous improvement is the rule, are often the only measures needed. In the past such symptoms have often been thought to be psychosomatic, so that the patient was adjured to 'pull his socks up' or 'get a grip of himself', and such an attitude on the part of his surgeon was naturally often resented by the patient. It is particularly important for the surgeon to think of dumping as a possible cause of postprandial symptoms, even if the symptoms seem to be bizarre. The author well remembers one patient who complained of symptoms reasonably compatible with dumping, but only after breakfast: the patient claimed that he could eat other meals with impunity. This problem was only solved by admitting the patient and observing him at all his meals, whereon it soon became clear that his intake of carbohydrate and total calories was far greater at *his* normal breakfast than at any of his other meals.

The symptoms of dumping seem to be due to the shift of liquid from the extracellular space into the bowel, accumulation of liquid in the bowel resulting in the abdominal component and the reduction in circulating volume in the systemic component (see Table 3.1). The mechanism of this shift seems to be the osmotic attraction[24] of foodstuffs that have been delivered too rapidly to the small intestine. Simple measures to combat the tendency to dumping are therefore also advised. The patient should eat small (and therefore frequent) meals, avoiding sugar and all carbohydrates as far as possible, because carbohydrates are broken down more rapidly than fats or proteins into small and therefore osmotically active molecules. He should also try to alter his daily routine to allow for a period of half an hour after a meal when he can sit (or even lie) down and relax.

Should the patient's symptoms still be significant a year after the operation, it may be well worthwhile to try non-operative measures. Insulin is effective in many patients,[25] but requires that the patient inject himself as though he had diabetes, and few patients are prepared to tolerate this regime. Non-insulin hypoglycaemic agents are much less effective. The mechanism of action of insulin is unknown.

More recently attempts have been made to slow the rate of gastric emptying by increasing the viscosity of the meal with additives such as pectin[26] or guar.[27]

If it appears that the original operation is one that can easily be reversed, then there is probably no point in trying the more complicated measures. However, if a reversal operation is likely to be complicated and its results are likely to be uncertain, then such measures should be tried in the hope that either they will succeed or the hoped-for spontaneous resolution will result.

Nature of the previous operation

The nature of the original operation is crucial to the choice of operation meant to relieve dumping symptoms. Reversal of pyloroplasty is only applicable if the original operation was a pyloroplasty of a type in which there was no destruction, merely rearrangement, of the pyloric muscle. The common Heineke–Mikulicz pyloroplasty meets this criterion, and so does the Finney operation, but an anterior pylorectomy does not.

If the original operation was not performed by the present surgeon, no effort should be spared to determine with accuracy what procedure had been performed. It is reasonable to accept written evidence in the form of a photocopy of an original operation note, but not a summary or letter based on the original notes, and certainly not what the patient, or even his general practitioner, says.

In the absence of the original operation note, a barium meal examination is the most reliable investigation, particularly with respect to whether the whole stomach is still intact or whether it seems possible that there has been a resection, and exactly what is the nature of any loop-reconstruction. This is an area where gastroduodenoscopy can be less accurate: the endoscopic appearances can be misleading, especially if the reconstruction was complicated and if the endoscopist happens not to be a surgeon.

Nevertheless, there is an important reason why endoscopy should not be excluded. This technique is by far the best way of diagnosing recurrence of peptic ulceration. Since the symptoms of dumping are postprandial and one of the possible symptoms is pain, it is not impossible that the pain of a recurrent ulcer starting after a meal could be confused with dumping.

PREOPERATIVE CARE AND INVESTIGATIONS

The patient, in the course of being selected for reconstruction of the pylorus, has undergone an upper gastrointestinal endoscopy, a barium meal series if there was doubt about the nature of the first operation, and some form of dumping provocation test. Most centres will not have routine access to facilities for measuring gastric emptying, but the reaction of the patient to a standard hypertonic glucose meal should always be observed and it is helpful to measure changes in haematocrit.

The patient enters the ward on the day before the operation, and preparation is routine, as for any other upper abdominal operation. Screening investigations such as blood count and chest x-ray are performed according to the usual protocol. A nasogastric tube is unnecessary at this stage, and while the patient's serum should be preserved for possible cross-matching of donor blood, it is unlikely that a transfusion will prove necessary and so routine cross-matching is not indicated. Physiotherapy for the chest, i.e. breathing exercises and, where necessary, postural percussion and drainage, are very important.

OPERATIVE DETAILS

Anaesthesia

General anaesthesia is the most comfortable for patient and surgeon. Good relaxation of the abdominal muscles is important because the freeing of adhesions may demand that the surgeon dissects high in the epigastrium, under overhanging ribs. Thus tracheal intubation, curarization and artificial ventilation are ideal.

46   GENERAL SURGERY

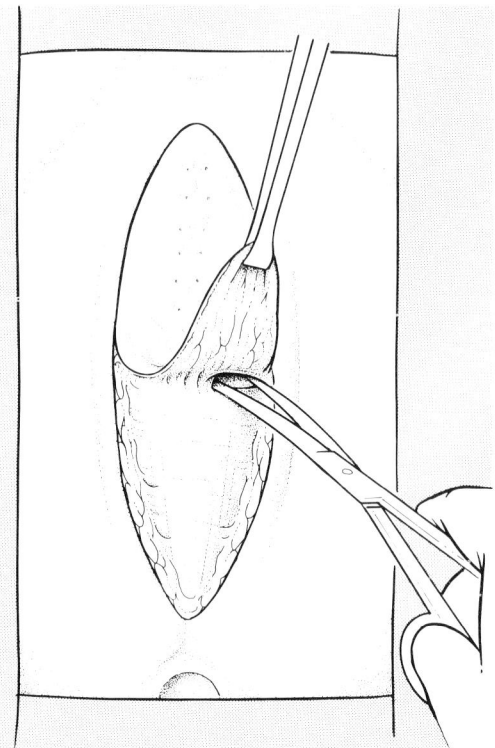

Figure 3.1 *The patient is lying supine and his head is towards the top of the page. The edges of the subcostal margins are indicated obliquely near the top of the frame. The old midline incision (note xiphisternum above and umbilicus below) is circumscribed by an oval incision through the skin. The lower end of the oval has been gripped in a pair of tissue-forceps and the skin island is being elevated by cutting the subcutaneous tissue with a pair of scissors.*

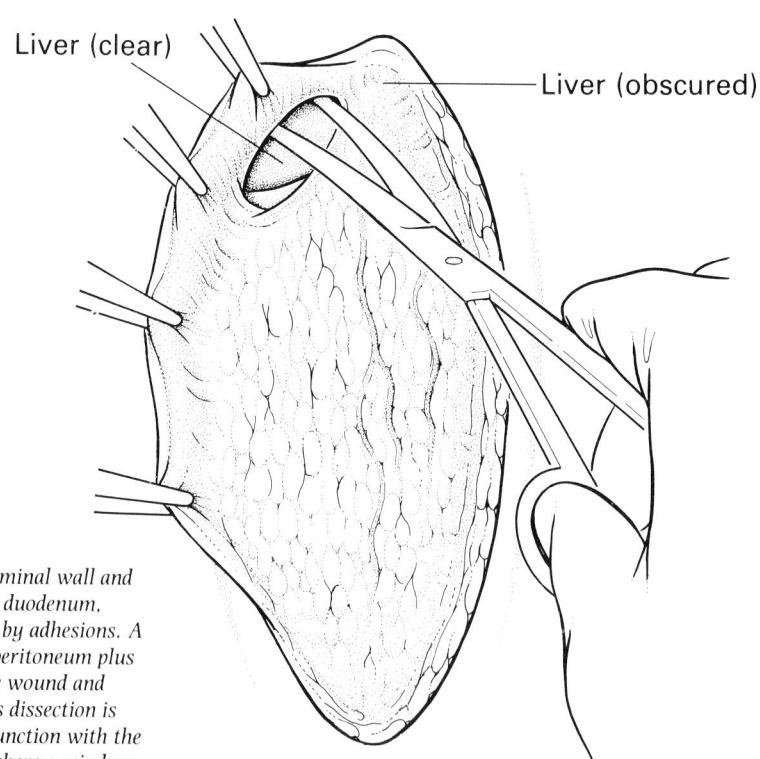

Figure 3.2 *Having cut through the abdominal wall and opened the peritoneum, the liver, stomach, duodenum, transverse colon, etc. are usually obscured by adhesions. A row of artery forceps have been placed on peritoneum plus rectus sheath along the right margin of the wound and traction has been put on that edge. Scissors dissection is then used to divide the adhesions at their junction with the peritoneum. The liver can be seen clearly where a window has been made in the adhesions, though less clearly to the left of the window.*

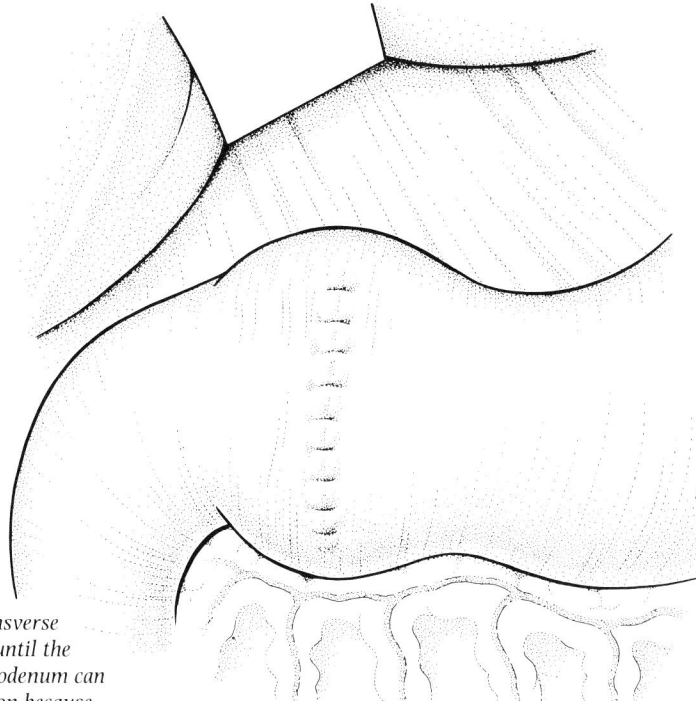

Figure 3.3 Adhesions are cleared and the transverse colon and mesocolon are mobilized downwards until the relevant anatomy of antrum and first part of duodenum can be seen. There is a bulbous distortion of the region because of the pyloroplasty, which is represented by a linear scar and a row of sutures.

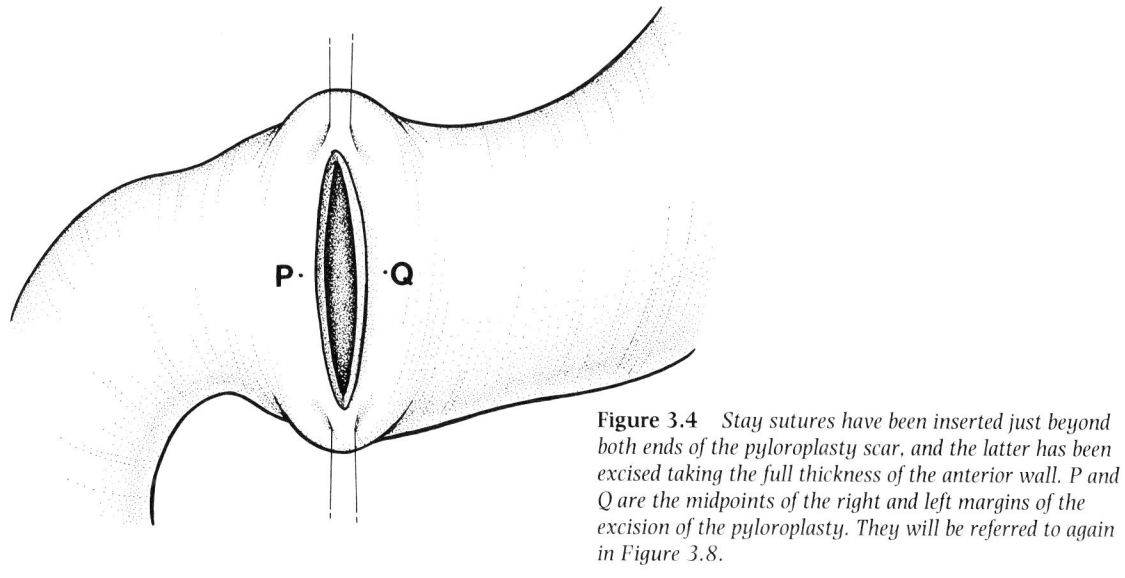

Figure 3.4 Stay sutures have been inserted just beyond both ends of the pyloroplasty scar, and the latter has been excised taking the full thickness of the anterior wall. P and Q are the midpoints of the right and left margins of the excision of the pyloroplasty. They will be referred to again in Figure 3.8.

Position

The patient lies supine, with a 5–10° tilt downwards from head to foot. The tilt encourages the transverse colon and small intestines to gravitate downwards away from the front of the stomach, and the transverse mesocolon tends to pull the stomach downwards from the rib cage.

If at any stage during the operation the surgeon experiences difficulty from distension of the stomach, he should ask the anaesthetist to pass a nasogastric tube so that the stomach contents can be aspirated.

Procedure

Incision (Figure 3.1)

The exact incision used naturally depends on the nature of the incision used at the first operation. Commonly the previous incision will have been upper midline or right paramedian. In either case, the scar in the skin is excised with an ellipse of surrounding skin. The incision is then deepened, through linea alba or rectus muscle, to and then through the peritoneum. The midline is virtually bloodless, but cutting through the rectus may produce some bleeding which will need to be controlled.

Division of adhesions (Figure 3.2)

On opening the peritoneum one usually meets a mass of intraperitoneal adhesions, binding the greater omentum to the anterior abdominal wall along the margins of the wound. These adhesions must be divided completely: a useful technique is illustrated. A row of artery forceps placed on the deepest layer of the margin of the incision is pulled on by an assistant, and the surgeon divides the fibrous adhesions as close as possible to the wound margin, a region in which they are usually bloodless.

When this process is complete, the surgeon can pass his hand deep to the abdominal wall at the top end of one side of the incision and sweep it all round the wound margins to the upper end of the other side of the wound.

The elevation of the abdominal wall reduces the risk of damaging the bowel or (in the upper part of the wound) the liver.

Completion of exposure (Figure 3.3)

Adhesions between the omentum and the underlying viscera have now to be divided so as to expose the stomach and duodenum. The transverse colon is gently pulled downwards off the front of the antroduodenal region, and the lower border of the liver retracted upwards so that the lesser curvature of the stomach can be exposed. The latter procedure is particularly difficult after a proximal gastric vagotomy; it is fortunate therefore that a drainage procedure is not often used in conjunction with that particular operation.

The dissection is continued until the whole of the relevant anatomy has been demonstrated. For the purposes of the present description it is assumed that the previous operation was the commonly performed Heineke–Mikulicz pyloroplasty. A description of how to proceed if the previous drainage was achieved with a Finney pyloroplasty is given subsequently (see page 53).

The relevant anatomy following Heineke–Mikulicz pyloroplasty is shown in Figure 3.3. The region of the antroduodenal junction is distorted by a bulbous deformity, at the centre of which lies a vertical scar. This scar represents the wound originally made in the front wall of the antroduodenal segment in an axial direction, and then sewn up at right angles to its original orientation.

The first key to the performance of an efficient reconstruction of the pylorus is to find this scar. If (as illustrated) a row of non-absorbable sutures can be seen the problem is simple. If not, it is necessary to identify by sight, touch, or both, what can be a hairline scar.

Excision of the pyloroplasty scar (Figure 3.4)

Stay sutures of a fine material, e.g. 000 chromic catgut or 2/0 silk, are inserted as shown through serosa and muscle at two points each 3 or 4 mm beyond the ends of the scar. An ellipse of the full thickness of the anterior wall of the pyloroduodenal segment, including the scar, has been excised.

The points marked P and Q are the midpoints of the right and left margins of the deficit resulting from the excision of the pyloroplasty. They will be referred to again in Figure 3.8 and subsequent figures.

Examination of the posterior wall (Figure 3.5)

The diagram shows in close-up a view of the posterior wall of the pyloroduodenal channel, as seen

Figure 3.5 *Close-up of the inside of the antroduodenal segment. At the junction of duodenum (fine corrugations) and antrum (coarser gastric rugae) is a band of muscle, the original pyloric ring.*

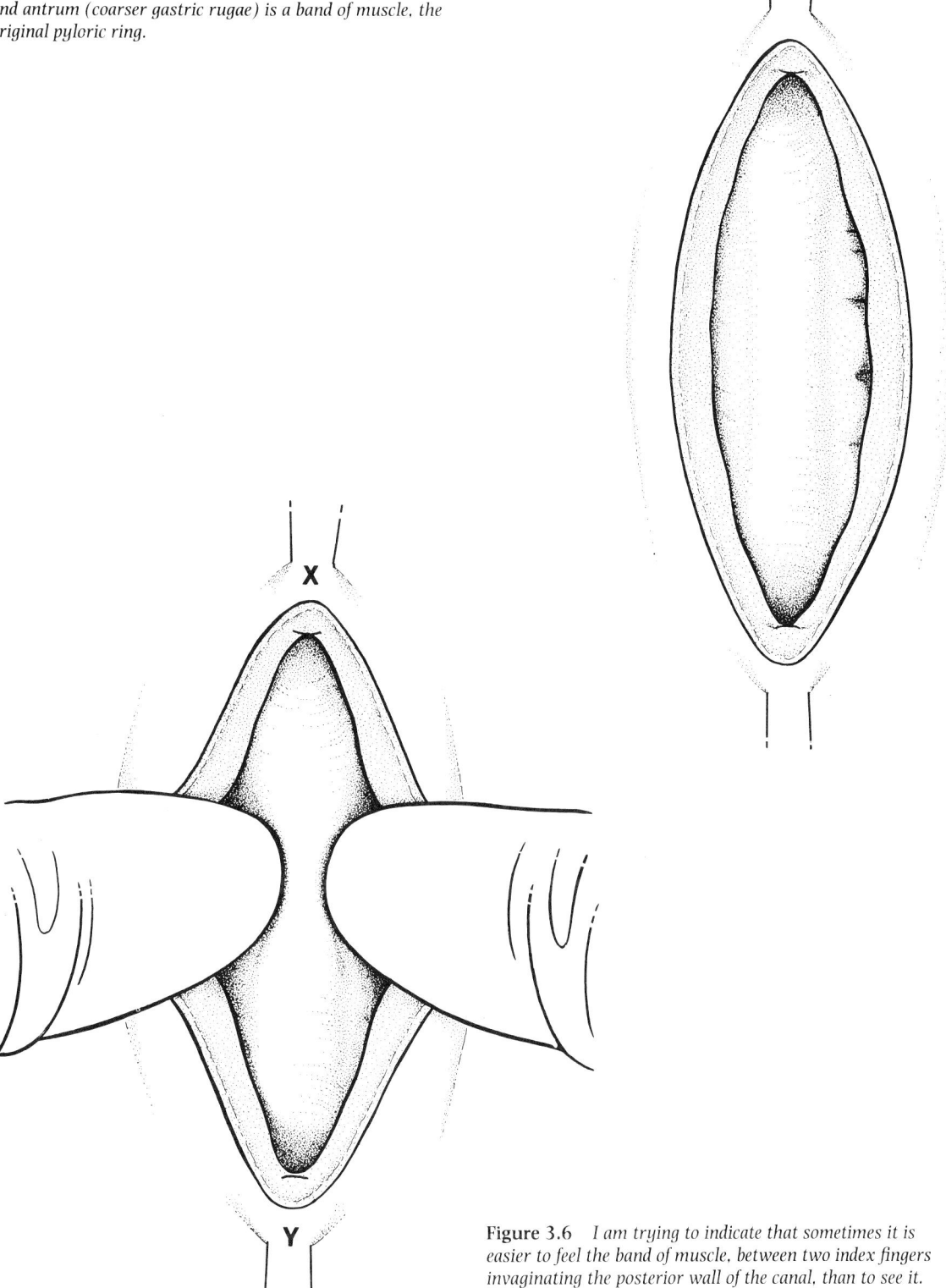

Figure 3.6 *I am trying to indicate that sometimes it is easier to feel the band of muscle, between two index fingers invaginating the posterior wall of the canal, than to see it. For explanation of points X and Y, see Figure 3.7.*

50 GENERAL SURGERY

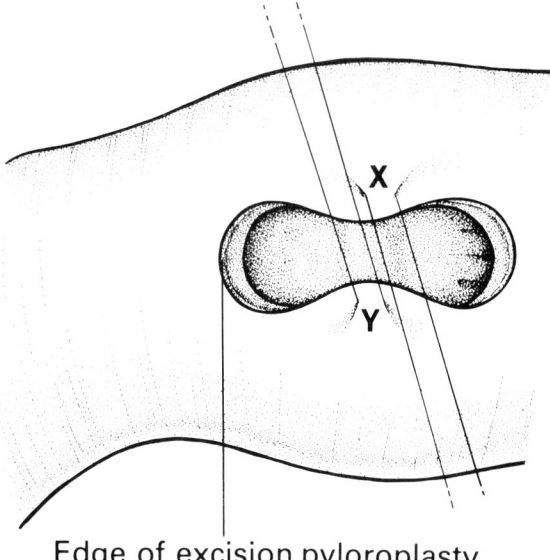

Edge of excision pyloroplasty

Figure 3.7 Points X and Y (shown on Figure 3.6) are now being approximated and will ultimately (Figure 3.8) meet in the front wall, i.e. they are returning to their original position of before the first operation.

Figure 3.8 Points X, Y have now been approximated with two sutures, one of which has already been tied. This has completed the repair of the pylorus. Stay sutures have been inserted at points P, Q, the midpoints of the right and left margins of the excision of the pyloroplasty (see Figure 3.9).

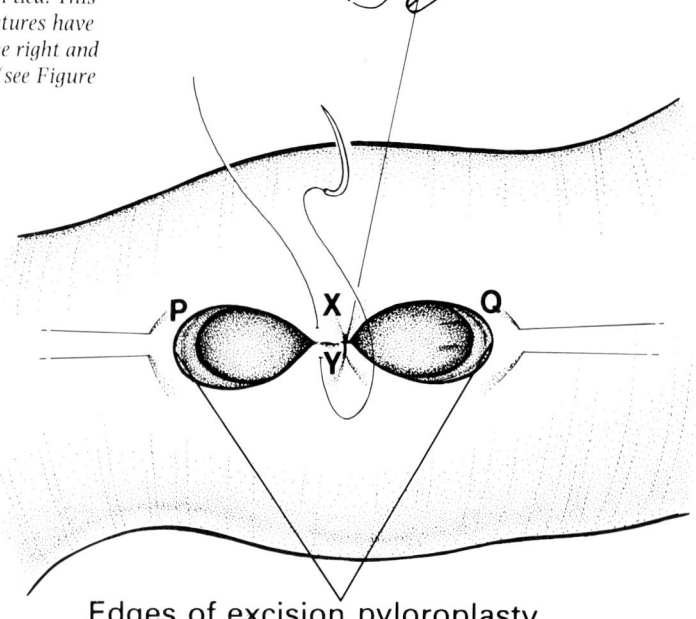

Edges of excision pyloroplasty

PYLORIC RECONSTRUCTION 51

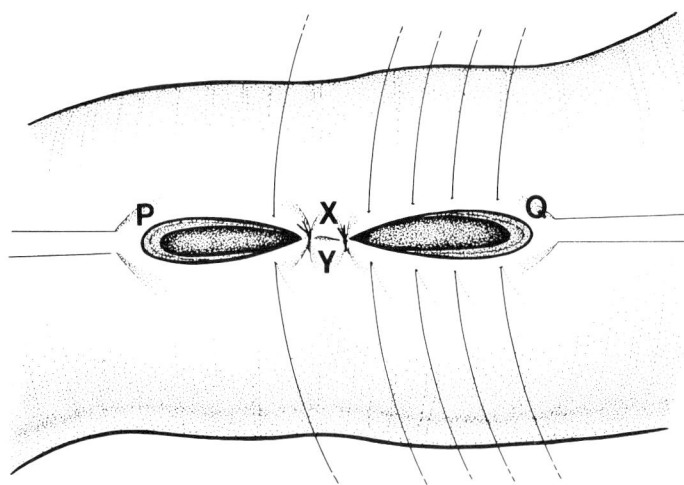

Figure 3.9 *Pulling points P and Q apart along the axis of the antroduodenal channel shows how the rest of the excision is to be repaired. A series of interrupted sutures has been inserted (but not tied) in the antral segment, and the first of a similar series has been inserted into the duodenal segment. Note the deformed outline of the antroduodenal channel has almost been restored to normal.*

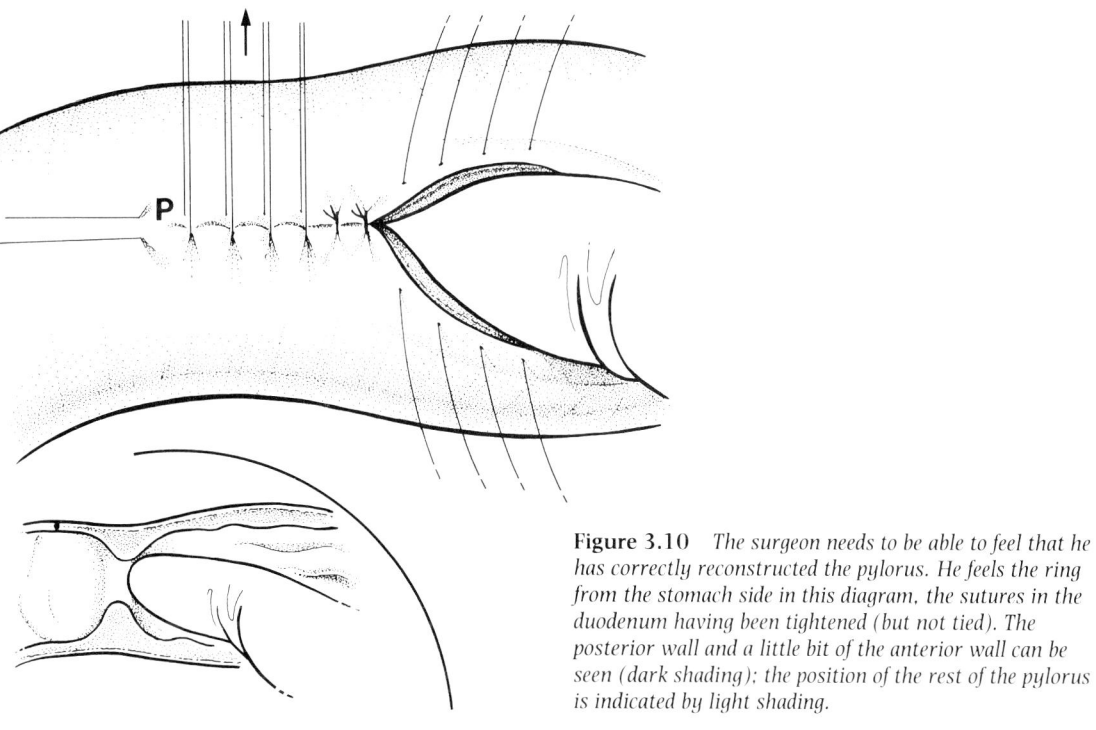

Figure 3.10 *The surgeon needs to be able to feel that he has correctly reconstructed the pylorus. He feels the ring from the stomach side in this diagram, the sutures in the duodenum having been tightened (but not tied). The posterior wall and a little bit of the anterior wall can be seen (dark shading); the position of the rest of the pylorus is indicated by light shading.*

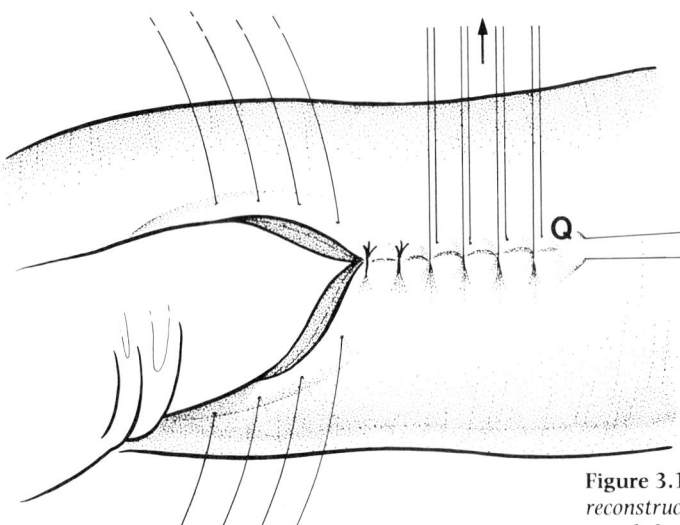

Figure 3.11 *The same as Figure 3.10 in reverse: feeling the reconstructed pylorus from the duodenal side. When the ring feels exactly right from both sides the sutures are tied.*

through the oval defect in the anterior wall. To the (patient's) right is the mucosa of the first part of the duodenum, showing numerous fine folds. To the left are the coarser rugae of the pyloric antrum. In the vertical midline, the mucosa of the transition area is heaped up over a vertical ridge of muscle, the pylorus itself.

The identification of the pyloric ring of muscle is the second key to the operation: once the pylorus has been identified, the rest of the operation is technically straightforward.

Identification of the pylorus (Figure 3.6)

Occasionally the pyloric ring is easy to see. When it is not immediately apparent, it may be easier to identify it by touch. In the first instance, the wall of the duodenum is thinner than that of the stomach, and this can be tested with a finger inside the gut and a thumb (or a finger of the other hand) behind the gut. The pylorus must lie at the transition between the two. However, the author finds that the method illustrated is usually the most efficient. The author uses the tip of the index finger of each hand gently to invaginate two areas of the posterior wall towards each other. The ring of thicker muscle of the pylorus then becomes apparent.

When the pylorus has been identified, the two stay sutures are checked to determine whether they have been placed accurately through the pyloric muscle ends. Any lack of correspondence must be due to the original surgeon having sewn up his axial pyloroplasty incision along a line that was not strictly at right angles to the line of the incision. If necessary, the position of the stay sutures are corrected. The accurately identified ends of the incision have been labelled X and Y in the diagram.

(For convenience of showing exactly where the stay sutures lie, they have been drawn as though they penetrated the full thickness of the gut wall: it is best, however, that they should be seromuscular only.)

A note of caution: while identifying the pyloric ring, it is unwise to pull apart the edges of the oval defect in the anterior wall of the gut because this act can distort the posterior wall and produce an artificial vertical ridge that feels like the pylorus.

Starting the reconstruction (Figure 3.7)

Having identified the pyloric ring, it must now be repaired by bringing the two cut edges of the ring together. In order to test how the tissues will lie, the two stay sutures are crossed over to draw the points X and Y towards each other. The pull on the stay sutures is adjusted until it appears that the correct position has been obtained, with the two edges of the pyloric ring in apposition.

PYLORIC RECONSTRUCTION 53

Repair of the pyloric ring (Figure 3.8)

The pyloric ring is now repaired with interrupted deep seromuscular sutures of a non-absorbable material (the author's preference is for fine silk). Usually only two such sutures are necessary: the pyloric ring is only 4–5 mm wide. The illustration shows the first such suture already placed and tied, and the second is being inserted. The stay sutures at X and Y have been removed, but one of the stitches of the repair is left long and held in an artery forceps to facilitate subsequent manipulations.

At this stage, a finger inserted along the channel from each side, gastric and duodenal, checks that the pyloric ring has indeed been reconstituted.

Only after this has been done, and the surgeon is confident that the ring has been well repaired, are stay sutures inserted near the points P and Q (see Figure 3.4), the midpoints of the oval defect that has been cut out of the anterior wall. Inaccurate identification of the points P and Q, and premature distraction along the P–Q axis can distort the pyloric ring and make it difficult to achieve an accurate repair.

Repair of the anterior wall

1. (Figure 3.9) The points P and Q are pulled apart along the axial line of the antroduodenal channel, using the stay sutures. This manoeuvre demonstrates the line along which the rest of the anterior wall has to be repaired. A series of interrupted full-thickness sutures of the same non-absorbable material have been inserted (but not tied) in the antral segment, and the first of a similar series has been inserted into the duodenal segment. The traction along the line P–Q has greatly reduced the deformity of outline of the antrum and first part of the duodenum.

2. (Figure 3.10) At all subsequent stages of the repair, it is crucial to check that any act performed to effect the repair does not distort the reconstructed pyloric ring. When all the sutures have been inserted (but not tied), the effect of tying the sutures in the duodenum is assessed by tightening them by traction on their ends. While the tension is maintained, the surgeon uses his right index finger from the gastric side to feel the pyloric ring.

3. (Figure 3.11) This diagram shows the complementary check of the ring from the duodenal end with the sutures in the antral wall held tight.

When the ring feels exactly right from both sides, the two sets of sutures are tightened and tied, thus completing the closure of the anterior wall.

4. (Figure 3.12) The upper illustration shows the anterior wall of the antrum and the first part of the duodenum after the repair has been completed. It shows the new positions of the points that were labelled P and Q, X and Y. The shaded area indicates the pyloric ring, lying in a plane perpendicular to the paper.

The lower diagram shows the same structures in longitudinal section: from left to right, the thick muscle of the stomach, the pyloric ring and the thin muscle of the duodenum.

The final check. (Figure 3.13) Finally, the surgeon uses the finger and thumb of his right hand to invaginate the front wall of the antrum and duodenum respectively, as a final check that the pyloric ring still feels normal and undistorted.

If the check is unsatisfactory, there is no alternative to taking down the whole repair of the anterior wall and starting again.

Procedure after the Finney pyloroplasty

1. (Figure 3.14) If the drainage procedure previously performed had been a Finney type of pyloroplasty, the appearance of the antroduodenal region would be as shown in the figure. At the previous operation the second and part of the third part of the duodenum would have been mobilized (by Kocher's manoeuvre) and the second part of the duodenum would lie in approximation to the antrum and the first part as shown.

The first step of the reconstruction is to take down the suture line in the anterior wall of the gut. This task is simple if a row of non-absorbable sutures is present as in the diagram. If it is not present, it helps if you ask your assistant to separate the free antrum and the free distal part of the third part of the duodenum from each other by gentle manual distraction with gauze swabs. This manoeuvre demonstrates the end of the suture line and shows the surgeon where to start his cut.

2. (Figure 3.15) In the diagram, the anterior wall suture line of Figure 3.14 has been opened, and the parting of the front wall of the antroduodenal segment and the front wall of the second part of the duodenum reveals the continuation of the anterior wall suture line onto the back wall of these two portions of gut. The anterior and posterior suture lines are of course continuous, and

Figure 3.12 (a) *The shaded area is the pyloric ring, viewed side-on.*

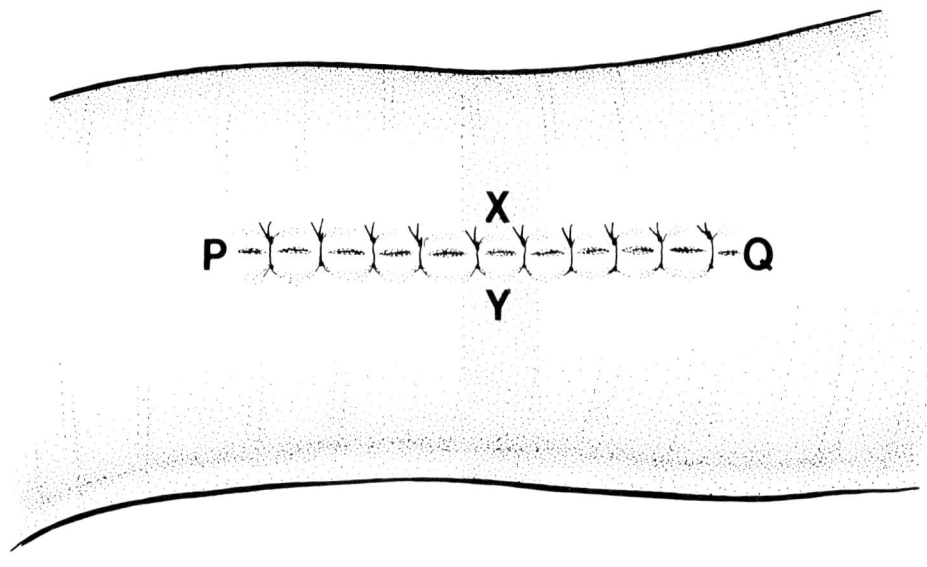

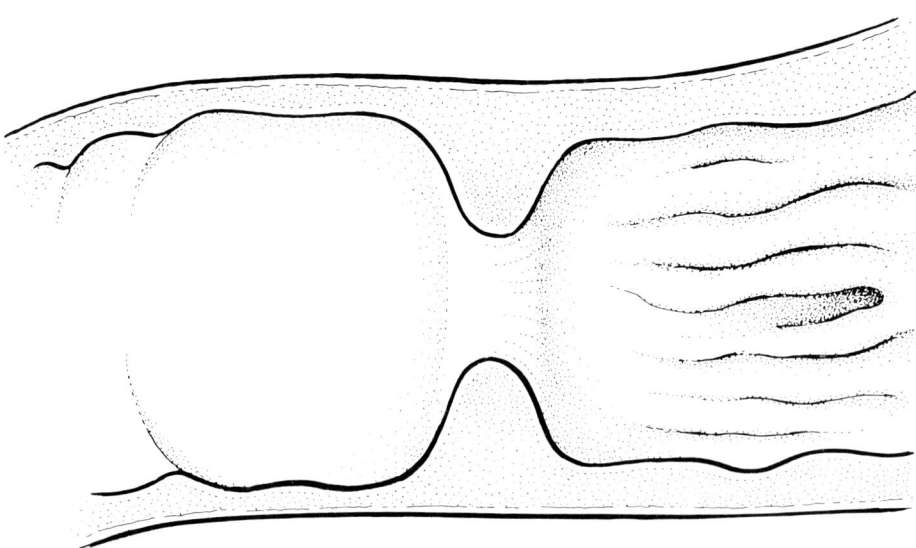

Figure 3.12 (b) *Longitudinal section. Note the muscle of the stomach is thicker than that of the duodenum.*

Figure 3.13 *Finally, invaginating the front wall of antrum and duodenum with thumb and index to make sure the ring is still of correct dimensions after tying the sutures.*

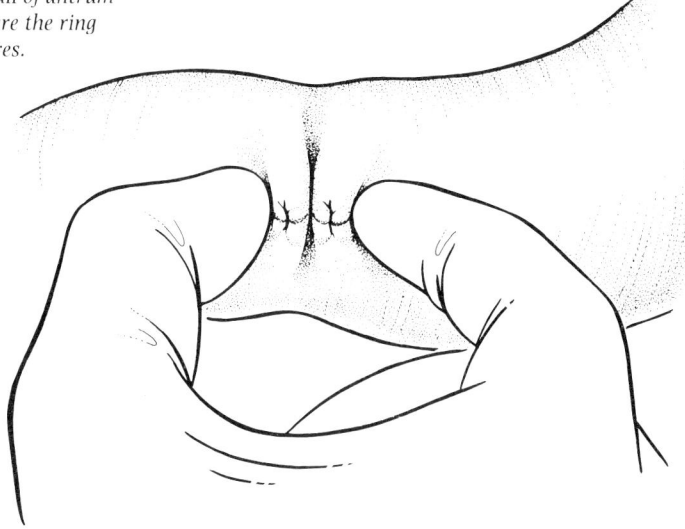

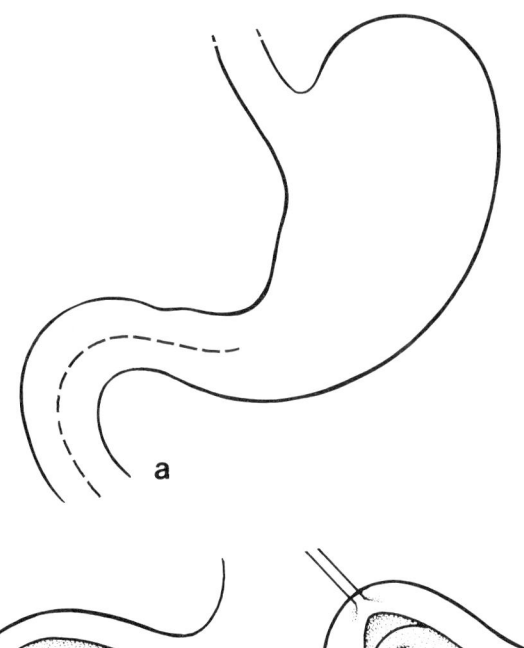

Figure 3.14 *The anterior suture line of a Finney pyloroplasty.*

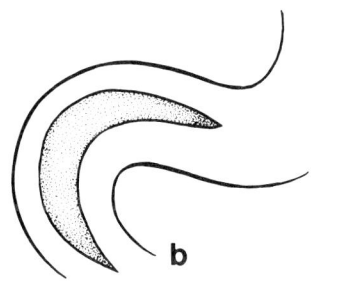

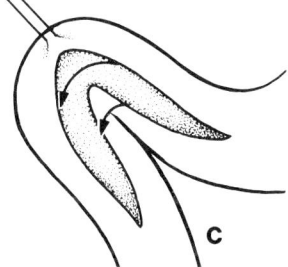

56 GENERAL SURGERY

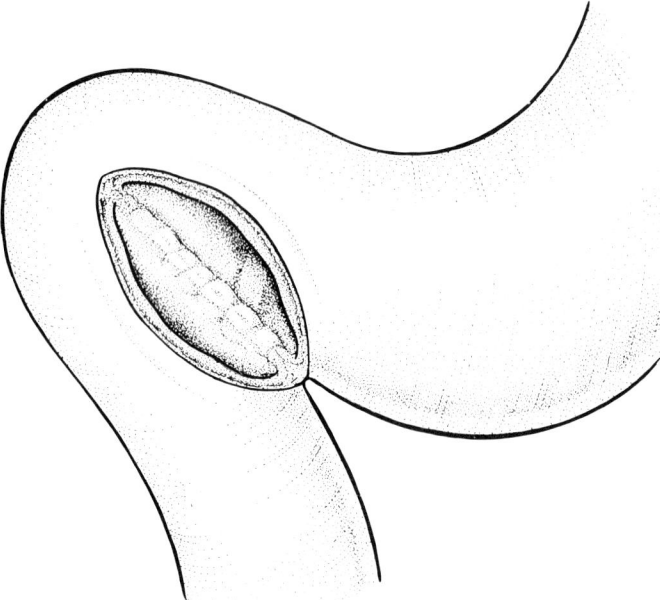

Figure 3.15 *The anterior suture line has been opened.*

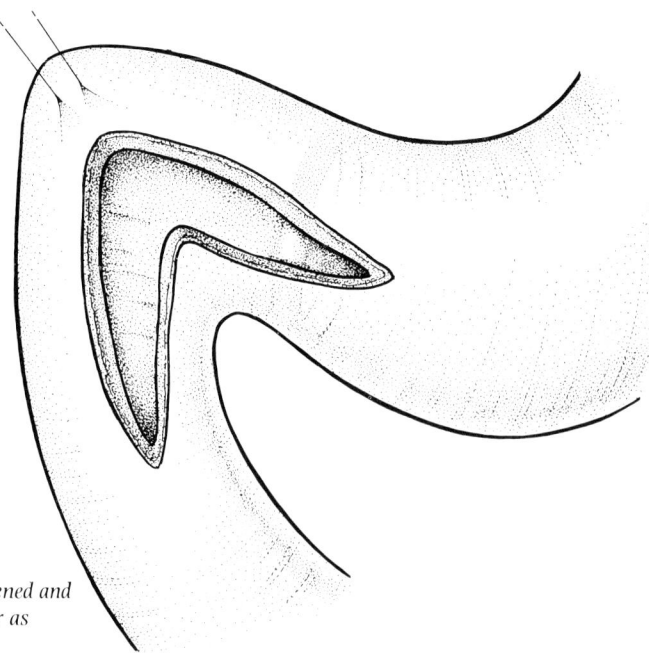

Figure 3.16 *The posterior suture line has been opened and the apex of the curve is being pulled towards the liver as shown.*

PYLORIC RECONSTRUCTION 57

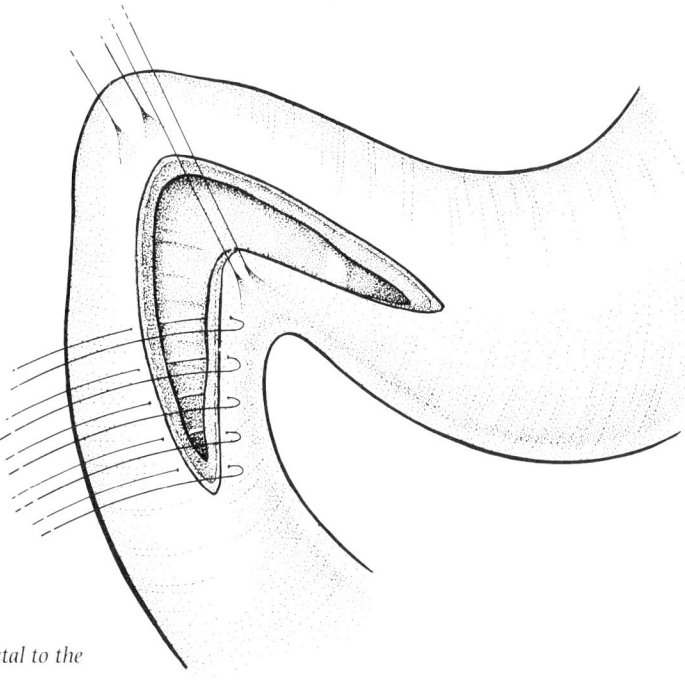

Figure 3.17 *The incision in the duodenum distal to the apical stay suture is being repaired.*

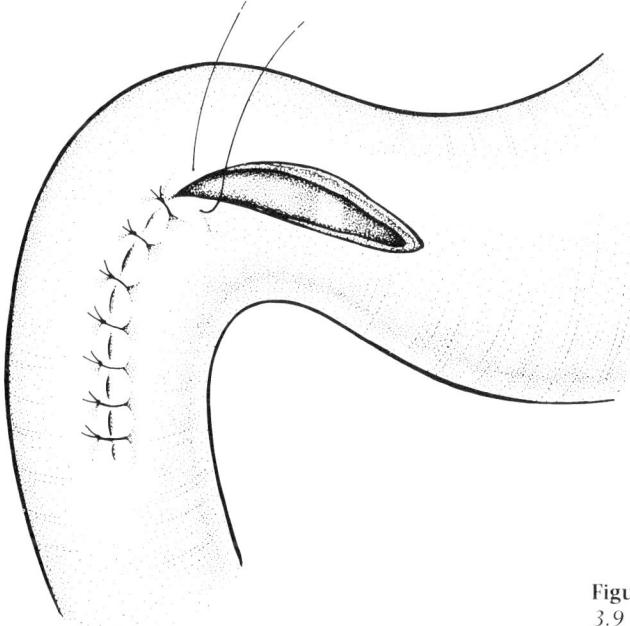

Figure 3.18 *The situation is now the same as in Figure 3.9 and repair proceeds as already indicated.*

represent the margins of the oval stoma that had previously been constructed between the antroduodenal segment on the one hand and the second part of the duodenum on the other. A part of the pyloric ring of muscle (shaded) may be seen in the posterior wall of the antroduodenal segment, but it may be very inconspicuous at this stage because the segment is still distorted by its posterior attachment to the second part of the duodenum.

3. (Figure 3.16) With the aid of further distraction of the stomach and third part of the duodenum away from each other, it becomes possible to complete the taking down of the previous side-to-side anastomosis by cutting along the posterior suture line. The position attained is that shown in the figure. The antrum and first part of the duodenum are no longer attached to the second part, and the whole of the U- or V-shaped incision that had been made in the anterior wall of the gut at the original operation becomes manifest.

A segment of the pyloric ring may now be visible on the posterior wall of the antroduodenal segment. It is heavily shaded in the diagram, and the position of the rest of the ring is indicated by light shading.

Note that a stay suture has been inserted near the apex of the incision in the gut. The position of this needs to be carefully chosen to prevent distortion of the tissues, and it may need subsequent modification (see next section).

4. (Figure 3.17) A careful decision is now made about the siting of a second stay suture at a point on the duodenum on the opposite side of the incision corresponding to the first stay suture. A series of full-thickness interrupted sutures is now inserted to approximate the distal limb of the incision. The figure shows the situation when about half of these sutures are inserted. They are tightened, but not tied until they are all in place and the surgeon is completely satisfied that the placing of the two stay sutures has been accurate and the repair of the second part of the duodenum is not deforming the antroduodenal segment.

5. (Figure 3.18) The diagram shows the previous row of sutures tied to complete the repair of the distal limb of the original incision. The situation is now exactly the same in principle as that shown in Figure 3.9 (although in this case the duodenal part of the incision, instead of being about the same length as the antral part, is usually much longer than the latter). The repair now proceeds as indicated in Figures 3.9–3.13.

Closure of the abdomen

After checking haemostasis and the swab count, the surgeon closes the abdomen by his preferred method, without drainage. Before doing so, and if it has not already been done to control gastric distension caused by gas, the anaesthetist is requested to pass a nasogastric tube into the stomach and the surgeon tests that its tip lies comfortably in the pyloric antrum. The anaesthetist secures the tube in position by taping it to the nostril.

POSTOPERATIVE CARE

In general, the care of the patient after the operation follows routine lines as for any upper abdominal procedure. Certain features however require emphasizing.

Gastric stasis

It will have been noted that a one-layer closure of the gut wall has been advocated. This is because the invaginating effect of a seromuscular second layer on the reconstructed pylorus cannot be checked once the deeper layer of sutures has been tied. The possibility of a leak at the suture line if the intragastric pressure is allowed to rise is therefore a real one.

For this reason it has been suggested that a nasogastric tube should be placed at the end of the operation. The author's regime is that at first this is aspirated once each hour. When the patient recovers consciousness completely, he is allowed sips of water by mouth if he wishes it. From the morning after the operation he is given 30 ml water each hour, immediately after the hourly aspiration. Each 12 hours the total volume aspirated from the stomach during the previous 12 hours is checked against the oral intake during that period. When the net balance is positive, i.e. when there is unequivocal evidence that the stomach is emptying itself because less has been aspirated than was given, the oral dose of water is increased to 60 ml hourly and the frequency of aspiration is reduced to every two hours. This schedule continues until the 12-hour net balance is again positive, whereon the schedule is altered to 90 ml hourly by mouth, with aspiration every three hours. When this schedule has been well tolerated for 12 hours, free fluids of any nature are offered, the nasogastric tube is removed and solid feeding is gradually introduced.

Until free fluids are commenced, water and electrolyte balance are maintained by the intravenous route.

The lungs

The patient who has originally needed an operation for his peptic ulcer is very likely to have been, or to still be, a smoker. This well-known association, together with the necessity to use a nasogastric tube in the early postoperative period, favour the development of postoperative pulmonary segmental collapse. The preoperative preparation of the chest has been mentioned: a postoperative regime of physiotherapy, adequate pain relief, bronchodilators when necessary, and the encouragement of expectoration by exhortation plus postural percussion and drainage (if the patient is producing sputum) should be enthusiastically pursued.

Antibiotics

The surgeon will naturally follow his usual policy. It is interesting that prophylactic antibiotics add little to the measures of the previous paragraph in preventing sputum retention and bronchopulmonary segmental collapse. With regard to wound infection, the subcutaneous tissues of patients with severe dumping symptoms are usually lean rather than fatty, so that even though the gastrointestinal tract has been widely opened during the operation, the incidence of wound infection is likely to be low. The author does not use prophylactic antibiotics in these patients.

Convalescence

Stitches are removed from the skin incision on the tenth day. Patients are usually ready to leave hospital by the seventh to tenth day. They are instructed to return to work between two and four weeks after discharge, depending on the nature of their occupations.

With regard to eating, they are advised to take a normal diet and not to try to eat large meals straight away. It seems a commonsense precaution to work gradually up to the size of meal they would ultimately like to be able to eat.

OUTCOME

Only one paper[12] about this operation has described the effect of the operation not only on the dumping symptoms, but also on the objective measurements of fall in plasma volume and rate of gastric emptying. The results reported in that paper are therefore of particular interest.

The pylorus was reconstructed in eight patients. Before reversal of the pyloroplasty, the dumping provocation test produced severe symptoms that matched their clinical complaints, and in every patient the maximal fall in plasma volume exceeded 10%. In every patient, the rate of gastric emptying was correspondingly rapid: half the test meal left the stomach in less than 20 minutes.

After the reconstruction, the dumping provocation test was repeated at three months and seven of the patients experienced no symptoms. The one who did have symptoms during the test (despite having no clinical complaint) had a fall in plasma volume of 18%, and the test meal had half left the stomach in only eight minutes. Clearly the operation had no physical effect on this patient, and the reduction in symptoms was probably due to the placebo effect of the operation combined with a voluntary reduction in food intake. By six months, the symptoms were as bad as ever.

Of the seven with no symptoms during the test at three months, six had a fall in plasma volume of less than 4% and the half-emptying time of the meal ranged between 45 and more than 60 minutes. The clinical improvement in these patients was maintained during the follow-up period of one to two years, and a repetition of the dumping provocation test at one year yielded the same results in all six as at three months, i.e. it was in the normal range. These six patients were the undoubted success of the operation.

The seventh patient without symptoms during the dumping provocation test at three months was particularly interesting in that although he too had no clinical symptoms at that time, his objective measurements were still partially in the dumping range—a fall in plasma volume of 11%, although the half-life of the meal in the stomach was 47 minutes. This patient redeveloped dumping symptoms about six months after the operation, and at 12 months the objective indices were unequivocally in the dumping range—10% for the maximal fall in plasma volume and 17 minutes for half the meal to empty.

It seems likely that the operation had no permanent effect on gastric emptying in this patient. The temporary reduction in emptying rate is unexplained, but it was suggested that oedema of the pyloric canal and non-specific reduction in gastric motility following laparotomy might have been responsible.

These detailed results suggest that reconstruction of the pylorus is feasible, and in the majority of patients it does work and it cures dumping symptoms. However, one patient did demonstrate the influence as a placebo of a major abdominal operation, and another demonstrated how temporary success can be achieved by an operation that has nevertheless produced no permanent change. Doubtless, factors such as these explain why so many operations have in the past been enthusiastically reported on in the short term, but never seem to be written about from the point of view of long-term results.

It is rather difficult to compare these results with those of other authors, not only because they did not use the dumping provocation test or any other objective index, but also because they usually express their results in terms of individual symptoms such as bile reflux, heartburn, diarrhoea or 'dumping' (by which it seems they mean the faintness, exhaustion, etc., here ascribed to the fall in plasma volume). Thus a patient may be reported as better with respect to one symptom but not with respect to others. Nevertheless, it seems that their results are on the whole similar to those reported by the author and his colleagues: about 75% of patients have a good to excellent response, and many of the remainder are complete failures.

Why should the operation give good results on some occasions yet completely fail on others? There is no proven answer to this question, but the author likes to think that his success rate from now onwards is likely to be greater than in the past. Several points of technique that have been stressed in this chapter had not been thought about at the time of the early operations in the series. It is not certain that the pyloric ring was accurately reconstructed in the earlier cases because the various techniques for demonstrating it had not been worked out. Again, the two stitches that actually reconstitute the ring were at first put in to include the full thickness of muscle until it was realized that they might be having a strangulating effect on the muscle ends, thus preventing union.

There is thus hope that, bearing all the technical details in mind, future success with this operation may more closely approach 100%. There is however no guarantee that this is true. In view of this uncertainty of success, it is apposite to finish this chapter by reminding the reader that, if a drainage procedure is considered by the surgeon to be essential to the type of vagotomy he has performed, such operations as antroduodenostomy and gastroenterostomy are much more readily and reliably reversible than pyloroplasty.

REFERENCES

1. Dragstedt LR & Owens FM Jr (1943) Supra-diaphragmatic section of vagus nerves in treatment of duodenal ulcer. *Proceedings of the Society for Experimental Biology and Medicine* **53**: 152–54.
2. Mix CL (1922) 'Dumping Stomach' following gastrojejunostomy. *Surgical Clinics of North America* **2**: 617–622.
3. Dragstedt LR, Harper PV Jr, Tovee EB & Woodward ER (1947) Section of vagus nerves to stomach in treatment of peptic ulcer; complications and results after four years. *Annals of Surgery* **126**: 687–699.
4. Herz AF (1913) The cause and treatment of certain unfavourable after-effects of gastroenterostomy. *Annals of Surgery* **58**: 466–472.
5. Goligher JC, de Dombal FJ, Duthie HL, Latchmore AJC, Smiddy FG, Pulvertaft CN, Conyers JH, Feather DB, Harrop Shoesmith J & Willson-Pepper J (1968) Five-to-eight year results of Leeds/York controlled trial of elective surgery for duodenal ulcer. *British Medical Journal* **ii**: 781–787.
6. Kay AW (1966) Review of the present position of vagotomy. In Thomson TJ & Gillespie IE (eds) *Postgraduate Gastroenterology* pp 213–222. London: Baillière, Tindall & Cassell.
7. Douglas M & Duthie HL (1972) Pyloroplasty alone in the management of patients with a negative exploration for duodenal ulcer. *British Journal of Surgery* **59**: 783–787.
8. Christiansen PM, Hart-Hansen O & Pedersen T (1974) Reconstruction of the pylorus for postvagotomy diarrhoea and dumping. *British Journal of Surgery* **61**: 519–520.
9. Frederiksen H-JB, Staehr-Johannsen T & Christiansen PM (1980) Postvagotomy diarrhoea and dumping treated with reconstruction of the pylorus. *Scandinavian Journal of Gastroenterology* **15**: 245–248.
10. Kelly KA, Baker JM & Van Heerden JA (1981) Reconstructive gastric surgery. *British Journal of Surgery* **68**: 687–691.
11. Martin CJ & Kennedy T (1982) Reconstruction of the pylorus. *World Journal of Surgery* **6**: 221–225.
12. Ebied FH, Ralphs DNL, Hobsley M & Le Quesne LP (1982) Dumping symptoms after vagotomy treated by reversal of pyloroplasty. *British Journal of Surgery* **69**: 527–528.
13. Faber RG, Russell RCG, Parkin JV, Whitfield P & Hobsley M (1974) Duodenal reflux during insulin-stimulated secretion. *Gut* **15**: 880–884.
14. Drumm J, Wolverson RL, Sorgi M, Donovan IA, Harding LD & Alexander-Williams J (1984) The

15. Hobsley M (1981) Dumping and diarrhoea. *British Journal of Surgery* **68**: 681–684.
16. Meurling S (1953) Post-cibal symptoms after partial gastrectomy for peptic ulcer. *Acta Societatis Medicorum Upsaliensis* (Supplement 3).
17. Roberts KE, Randall HT & Farr HW (1954) Cardiovascular and blood volume alterations resulting from intrajejunal administration of hypertonic solutions to gastrectomized patients. *Annals of Surgery* **140**: 631–640.
18. Hobsley M & Le Quesne LP (1960) The dumping syndrome. II Factors responsible for the symptoms. *British Medical Journal* **i**: 141–147.
19. Peskin, GW & Miller LD (1962) The role of serotonin in the 'dumping syndrome' *Archives of Surgery* **85**: 701–704.
20. Zeitlin IJ & Smith AN (1966) 5-Hydroxyindoles and kinins in the carcinoid and dumping syndromes. *Lancet* **ii**: 986–991.
21. Kaushik SP, Ralphs DNL & Hobsley M (1983) Gastric emptying and dumping after proximal gastric vagotomy. *American Journal of Gastroenterology* **77**: 363–367.
22. Ebied FH (1982) Clinical and objective evaluation of patients before and after surgical operations for duodenal ulcer. PhD Thesis, London University.
23. Ralphs DNL, Thomson JPS & Haynes S (1978) The relationship between the rate of gastric emptying and the dumping syndrome. *British Journal of Surgery* **65**: 637–641.
24. Lawson-Smith C, Thomson JPS & Hobsley M (1975) A dumping provocation test. *British Journal of Surgery* **62**: (Abstract) 153.
25. Howe CT, Candy J, Le Quesne LP, Hobsley M & Spence MP (1962) Effect of insulin on the dumping syndrome. *British Medical Journal* **ii**, 150–158.
26. Leeds AR, Ebied F, Ralphs DNL, Metz G & Dilawari JB (1981) Pectin in the dumping syndrome: reduction of symptoms and plasma volume changes. *Lancet* **ii**: 1075–1078.
27. Leeds AR, Ralphs DNL, Edge CJ & Ellis PR (1983) Guar bread in the dumping syndrome. *Abstracts of the 4th European Nutrition Meeting, 1983, Amsterdam.*

4
Reconstruction of the Gastric Reservoir

A. Cuschieri

The surgical reconstruction of the upper gastrointestinal tract after total or subtotal gastrectomy remains controversial. The most common procedure used is the Roux-en-Y jejunal[1,2] loop or modifications thereof such as the Tanner Roux 19[3] and the Hunt-Lawrence pouch.[4,5] The technique of loop jejunogastric/oesophageal anastomosis with an entero/enteric anastomosis performed further distally, is safer than the above in terms of its vascular supply and probably imparts the same functional results, although as usual in reconstructive surgical practice on the gastrointestinal tract there have not been any clinical trials comparing the efficacy and safety of the two approaches. Prevention of bile reflux into the stomach remnant and/or oesophagus entails fashioning the entero/enteric anastomosis of these reconstructions some 60 cm distal to the gastric/oesophageal anastomosis, wherein stems certain disadvantages of these procedures. The first is the creation of a long loop with its inevitable bacterial colonization in the long term. The second disadvantage results from the complete diversion of bile from the stomach remnant which enhances the risk of anastomotic ulceration. A further disadvantage that has been largely ignored concerns duodenal bypass which the procedures entail. The duodenum is a crucial area of initiation of digestive physiology essential to the adequate hormonal regulation of biliary and pancreatic secretions and furthermore, ensures adequate mixing of these secretions with food. Duodenal bypass therefore entails both an impairment of hormonal regulation in response to meals and an asynchrony or inadequate admixture of chyle with bilio-pancreatic juices.

Other more complex reconstructive procedures have involved the creation of reservoirs with loops of upper jejunum such as the Poth[6] and Hays pouches.[7] These were designed primarily to obviate early satiety and thereby increase the food intake. They have been abandoned largely because of stasis, dilatation of the reservoir and bacterial overgrowth. Furthermore, they are long and laborious procedures which add significantly to the operating time and are thus unrealistic as primary reconstructions at the time of a total or subtotal gastrectomy.

The use of a loop of interposed isoperistaltic jejunum between the stomach remnant and the duodenum was introduced by Henley in 1952,[8] but has been used since then almost exclusively as a remedial operation for some of the post-gastric surgery syndromes.[9,10] In recent years however the operation has been reintroduced as a primary reconstructive procedure at the time of total/subtotal gastrectomy with good results in terms of quality of life, maintenance of weight, absence of severe post-cibal symptoms and malabsorption from bacterial overgrowth.[11,12]

There is good evidence that an interposed isoperistaltic loop functions well. It is capable of sustaining segmental contractions resulting in a controlled intermittent emptying pattern.[11] However, its receptive capacity remains limited and accounts for the early satiety experienced by these patients which limits their food intake, necessitating frequent small meals. To some extent the capacity of the loop can be enhanced by interposing a longer jejunal loop but beyond 20 cm, problems are encountered with kinking which can lead to obstructive episodes.

These considerations have led the author to design a modification of the Henley's operation which involves the creation of a simple reservoir jejunal interposition with an isoperistaltic conduit.[13] The procedure has been evaluated over a period of 12 years and was initially used as a remedial operation in patients with severe symptoms after subtotal/total gastrectomy. Increasingly however the author has used it as a primary reconstruction at the time of gastrectomy in view of its superiority over the Roux-en-Y procedure in terms of nutrition and relative freedom from post-cibal symptoms.

PATIENT SELECTION AND PREOPERATIVE PREPARATION

Indications

1. Remedial operation. The operation is indicated in patients with severe and persistent postcibal symptoms after a high subtotal or total gastrectomy. It is the customary policy of the author not to offer reconstructive gastric surgery until $1\frac{1}{2}$–2 years have elapsed and when conservative management has failed to control symptoms. However, remedial surgery ought not to be delayed unduly and should be undertaken before the development of gross malnutrition and long-term metabolic consequences. In patients who have undergone resection for malignant disease, adequate investigations must be undertaken *to rule out local recurrence of the disease.*

2. Primary reconstruction. The procedure is indicated for all patients undergoing a subtotal/total gastrectomy as an alternative to Roux-en-Y reconstruction. It is unwarranted in patients undergoing partial gastrectomy or antrectomy.

Investigations

These concern those patients undergoing reservoir jejunal interposition for severe symptoms after subtotal gastrectomy. These patients are usually anaemic and malnourished largely from reduced dietary intake. In some, malabsorption will be confirmed on investigation. The malabsorption survey begins with a three-day faecal fat estimation. If steatorrhoea is confirmed in this way, primary small bowel disease, pancreatic exocrine insufficiency and bacterial overgrowth need to be excluded. By and large the most common cause of malabsorption in these patients is bacterial overgrowth. This is detected by performance of the ^{14}C-cholate breath test[14] or H_2 estimation of the

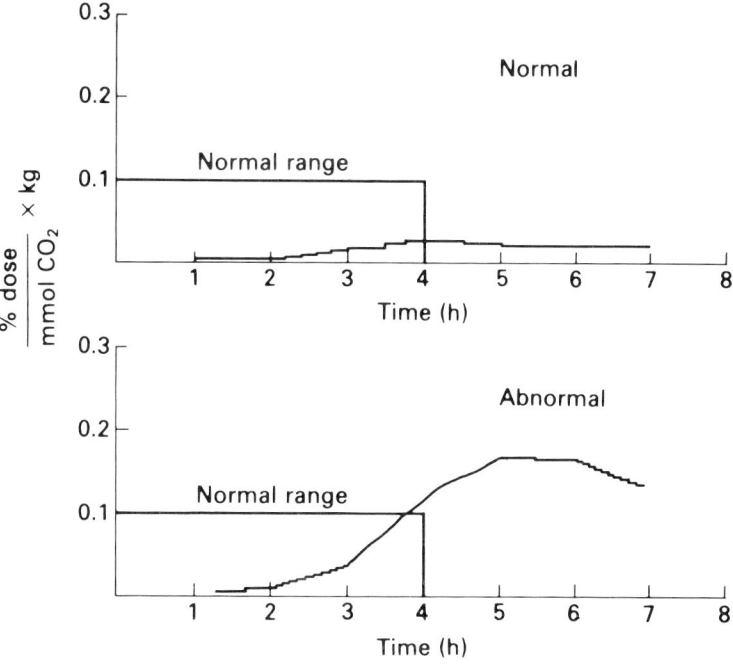

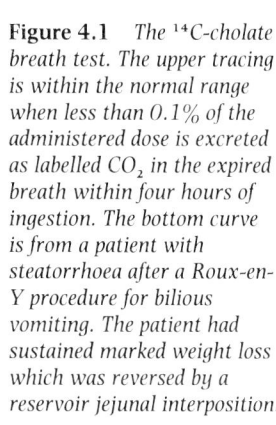

Figure 4.1 The ^{14}C-cholate breath test. The upper tracing is within the normal range when less than 0.1% of the administered dose is excreted as labelled CO_2 in the expired breath within four hours of ingestion. The bottom curve is from a patient with steatorrhoea after a Roux-en-Y procedure for bilious vomiting. The patient had sustained marked weight loss which was reversed by a reservoir jejunal interposition.

expired breath before and after the administration of lactulose.[15] An example of the ^{14}C-cholate breath test is shown in Figure 4.1. The principle of the test centres on the estimation of $^{14}CO_2$ in the expired air which depends on the extent of bacterial breakdown of the orally administered labelled cholate.

Aside from anthropomorphic measurements, the serum albumin, transferrin and total protein are necessary in all these patients. The anaemia is usually due to iron deficiency but mixed folate/B_{12} and iron deficiencies may be encountered. A full blood count is necessary together with estimation of serum iron, iron-binding capacity and if indicated, serum folate and B_{12} levels.

In the presence of a residual gastric stump, the gastric secretion of acid in response to maximal stimulation with pentagastrin is performed and if this exceeds 20 mmol/l, then a vagotomy is indicated as an integral part of the procedure. This consideration also applies to previously vagotomized patients since in the author's experience some 11% of patients undergoing remedial gastric surgery are found to have had an incomplete vagotomy.

Endoscopic assessment of the upper gastrointestinal tract completes the routine work up. Attention is paid to the presence of gastritis and reflux oesophagitis in particular.

Nutritional management

In the vast majority of patients with severe postcibal symptoms, malnutrition is severe and can reach life-threatening proportions (Figure 4.2). A period of nutritional management often extending to several weeks is essential to restore gross defects in lean body mass and serum proteins. If the serum albumin is very low (> 20 g/l) intravenous infusion of purified protein derivative, plasma or human albumin solution is necessary. Otherwise naso-intestinal feeding with elemental or pre-digested diets is usually possible and is preferable to intravenous hyperalimentation in these patients. Others are able to ingest food orally to a limited extent and in this group supplemental 'sip feeding' with pre-digested diets throughout the day can often result in an adequate daily caloric intake provided the patient is sufficiently motivated. Parenteral nutrition is reserved for those patients who cannot tolerate a naso-intestinal tube. A feeding jejunostomy is inadvisable in patients about to undergo reservoir jejunal interposition since it will compound the selection of the most appropriate jejunal loop for the construction of the reservoir and enhances the risk of sepsis.

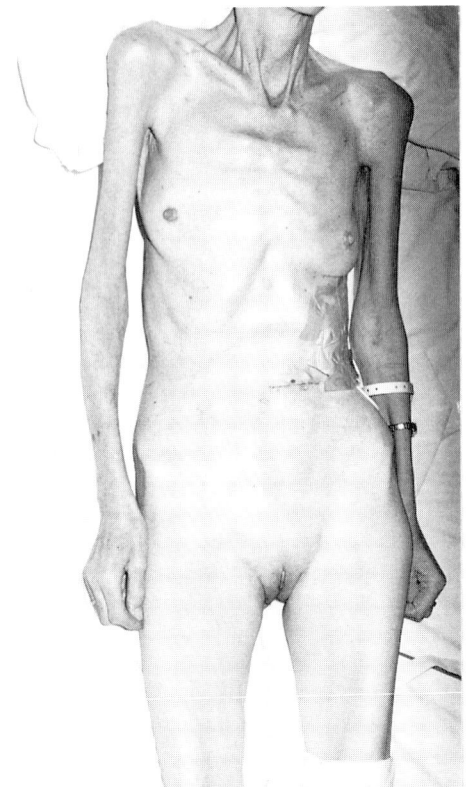

Figure 4.2 *Severe malnutrition after subtotal gastrectomy. The marked weight loss which can reach life-threatening proportions is largely due to a diminished dietary intake.*

OPERATIVE TECHNIQUE OF RESERVOIR JEJUNAL INTERPOSITION

Exposure

The operation can be conducted safely via the abdominal route and this is the approach used when the procedure is carried out to alleviate post-cibal symptoms in patients with a previous high to subtotal gastrectomy. The abdominal incision performed by the author depends on the nature of the subcostal angle (Figure 4.3). If this is narrow, a midline approach skirting to the right of the umbilicus gives the best exposure. An oblique incision extending across the epigastrium with a slight convexity upwards allows excellent surgical access in patients with a wide subcostal angle.

When the procedure is used as a primary reconstruction, the approach is dictated by the requirements for the gastric resection. Often this entails a left thoraco-abdominal approach since the

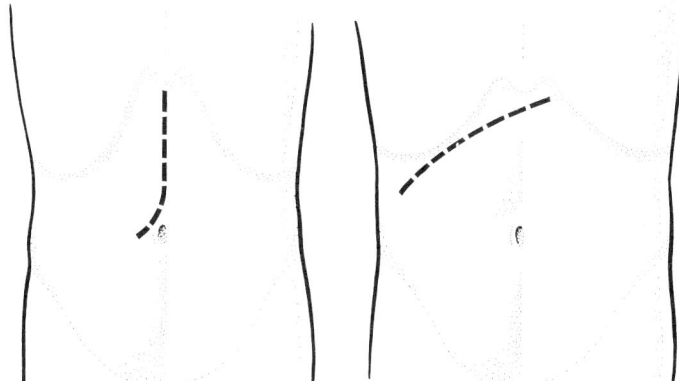

Figure 4.3 *The approach for gastric reconstructive surgery varies with the patient's build. In patients with a narrow subcostal a midline incision skirting to the right of the umbilicus inferiorly gives good access. By contrast in patients with a wide subcostal angle, the oblique epigastric incision is preferred.*

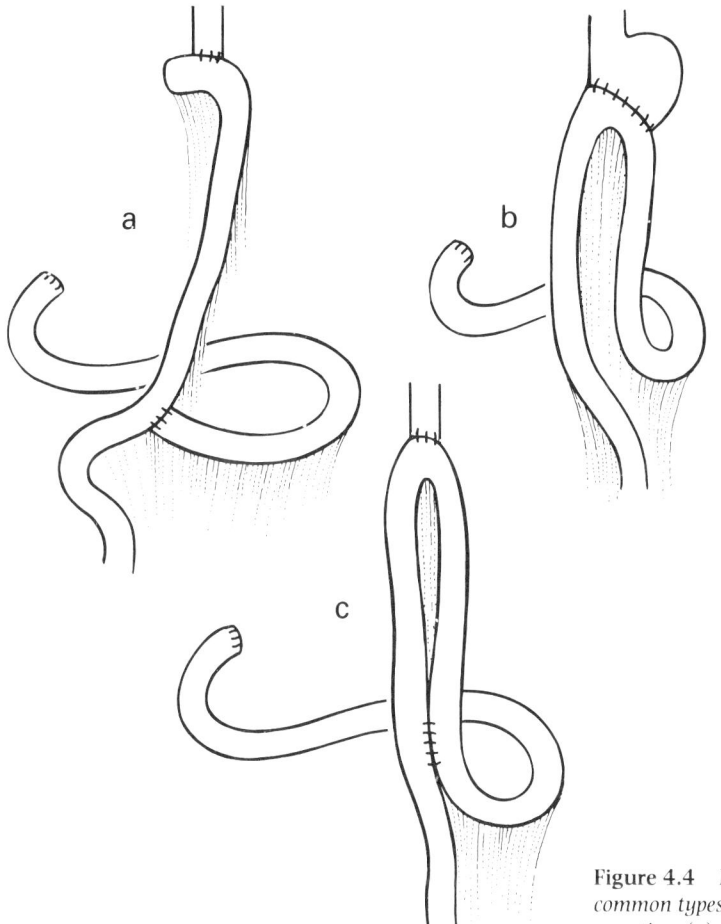

Figure 4.4 *Diagrammatic representation of the three common types of restoration of continuity after gastric resection.* **(a)** *Roux-en-Y;* **(b)** *Polya anastomosis;* **(c)** *Loop anastomosis with entero-enteric anastomosis.*

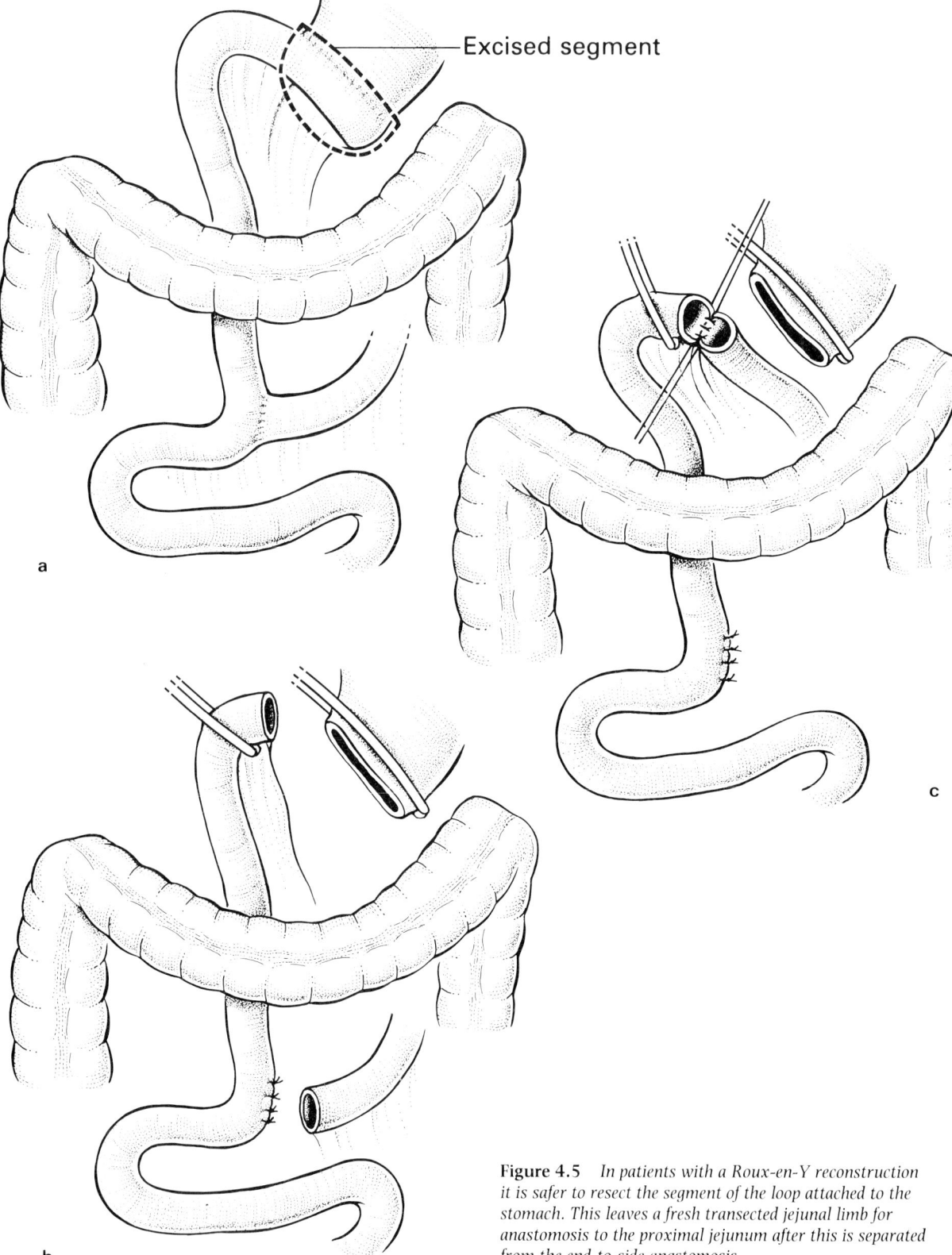

Figure 4.5 *In patients with a Roux-en-Y reconstruction it is safer to resect the segment of the loop attached to the stomach. This leaves a fresh transected jejunal limb for anastomosis to the proximal jejunum after this is separated from the end-to-side anastomosis.*

majority of gastric cancers occur in the upper third of the stomach and cardia.

Enterolysis and exploratory laparotomy

The anatomy is displayed by division of the adhesions which tend to be dense in the supracolic compartment. The stomach remnant and gastro-oesophageal junction are usually adherent to the undersurface of the left lobe of the liver and diaphragm. In addition, the gastrojejunal anastomosis should be displayed and the jejunal loop mobilized from the transverse mesocolon and colon. An adequate mobilization of the duodenum is essential for a safe anastomosis between it and the jejunal conduit. The mobilization is carried out by division of the lateral peritoneum followed by gauze dissection of the second part of the duodenum and head of pancreas from the inferior vena cava, and the third part from the transverse colon. It is a good policy to identify the common bile duct at this stage. A truncal vagotomy is performed after mobilization of the oesophagus and gastro-oesophageal junction.

Separation of gastrojejunal anastomosis

The three common types of gastrojejunal anastomoses performed after subtotal gastrectomy are shown in Figure 4.4.

The Polya anastomosis is easily taken down after the application of two curved non-crushing clamps on either side of the mobilized gastrojejunal anastomosis which is then disconnected by scalpel incision along the anastomotic scar. The detached jejunum is closed transversely with a single layer of 3/0 non-absorbable (black silk, polyamide) interrupted seromuscular sutures. In patients with a loop gastrojejunostomy and a distal entero–enteric anastomosis, the latter is also disconnected and the jejunal wound is closed with 3/0 non-absorbable sutures.

In patients with a Roux-en-Y reconstruction, it is safer to resect the portion of the jejunal loop attached to the stomach. This leaves a fresh transected jejunal limb for anastomosis to the proximal jejunum after this is separated from its end-to-side anastomosis (Figure 4.5). Again suturing is performed using a single layer technique with 3/0 non-absorbable interrupted deep seromuscular sutures.

Construction of the reservoir

1. **Selection of loop.** This is probably the most crucial part of the operation. Time should be spent in finding the best vascular pedicle available to sustain a 30 cm loop of isoperistaltic jejunum which is then transected at either end and its vascular pedicle separated from the rest of the mes-

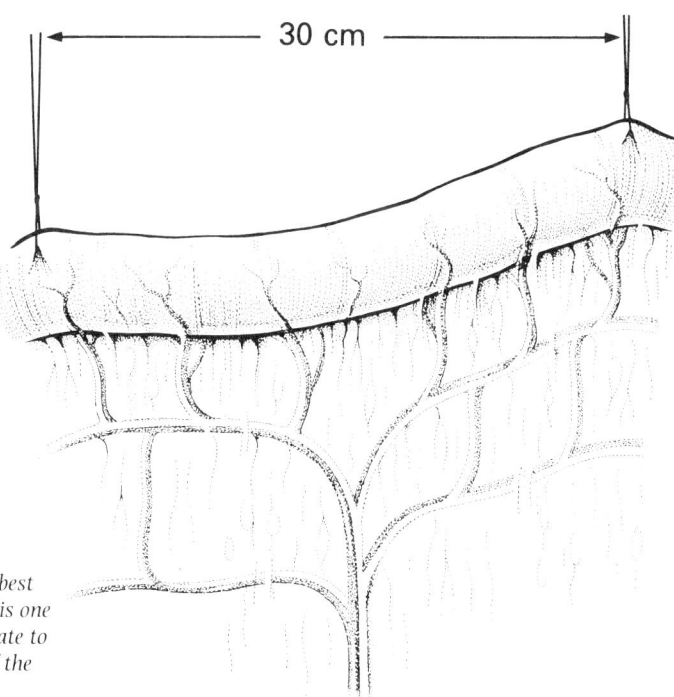

Figure 4.6 *A 30 cm loop is selected around the best available vascular pedicle. A good vascular pedicle is one containing a straight artery and vein which bifurcate to form an even arcade extending the whole length of the isolated segment.*

68 GENERAL SURGERY

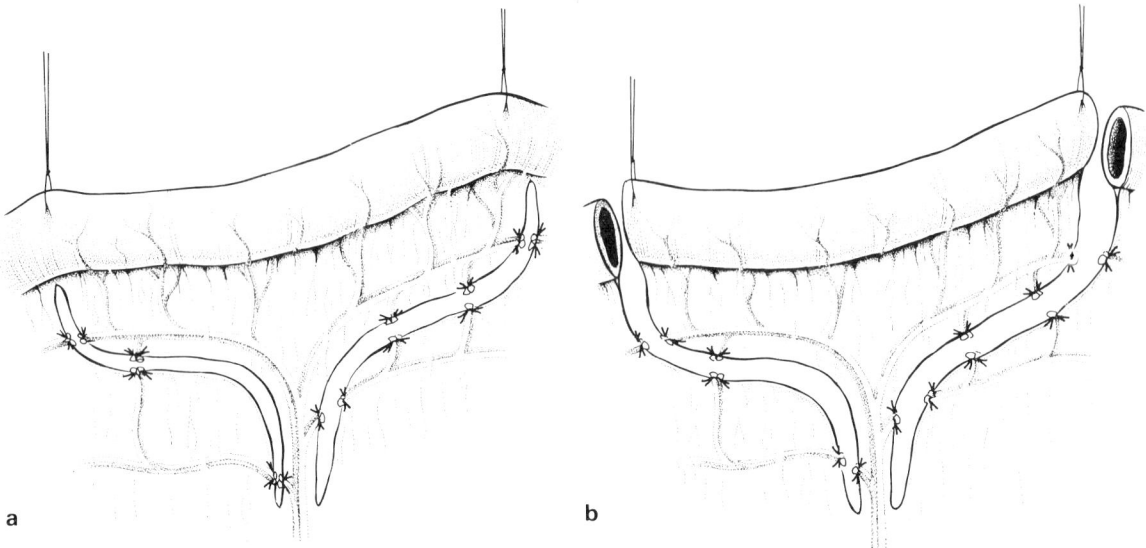

Figure 4.7 *Construction of vascular pedicle.* **(a)** *Division of anterior leaf of mesenteric peritoneum and ligature of branches from the vascular pedicle to adjacent arcades outwith the vascular territory of the selected loop.*
(b) *Complete separation of the vascular pedicle from the rest of the small bowel mesentery and transection of the isolated loop at either end.*

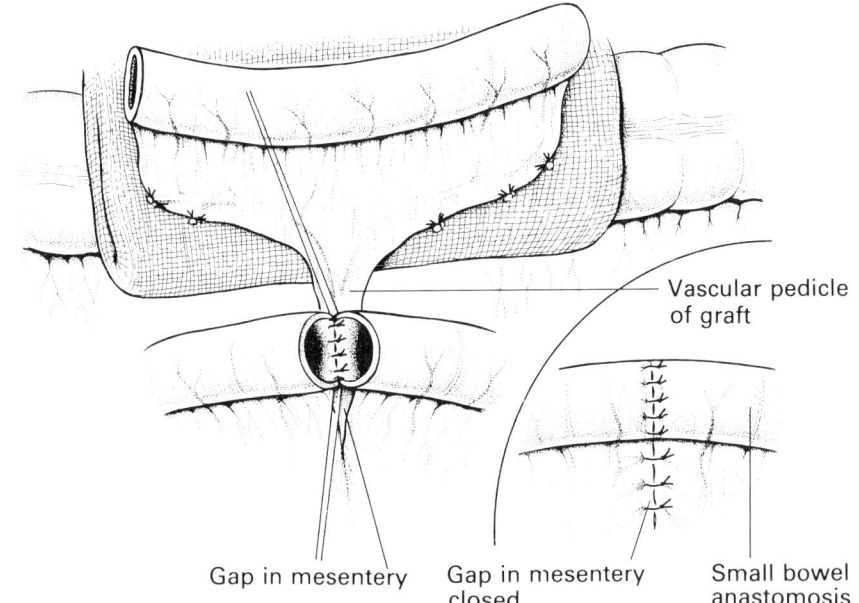

Figure 4.8 *Restoration of continuity of the small bowel by an entero-enteric anastomosis carried out below the vascular pedicle. The gap in the small bowel mesentery is closed with a few interrupted sutures.*

entery. A good vascular pedicle is defined as one containing a straight artery and an accompanying vein which bifurcate to form an even arcade extending along the whole length of the isolated segment. The selected loop is measured along its antimesenteric border and marked accordingly with stay sutures (Figure 4.6). The construction of the vascular pedicle is started by incising the first peritoneal layer on either side of the main feeder vessels. The incision of the peritoneum is then continued laterally on either side below and parallel to the primary vascular arcade until the proposed limits are reached. The incision of the peritoneum of the small bowel mesentery is then carried across the mesenteric arcades on either side until the bowel wall is reached (Figure 4.7). The vascular arcades are ligated with 3/0 black silk and then divided. Division of the second layer of peritoneum of the small bowel mesentery completes the separation of the vascular pedicle. After the loop is emptied by milking it in either direction, non-crushing clamps are placed on either side and the bowel is then transected at each end and is left covered by a moist swab. Restoration of continuity of the small intestine is effected by an end-to-end anastomosis using a single layer technique with 3/0 interrupted non-absorbable seromuscular sutures (Figure 4.8).

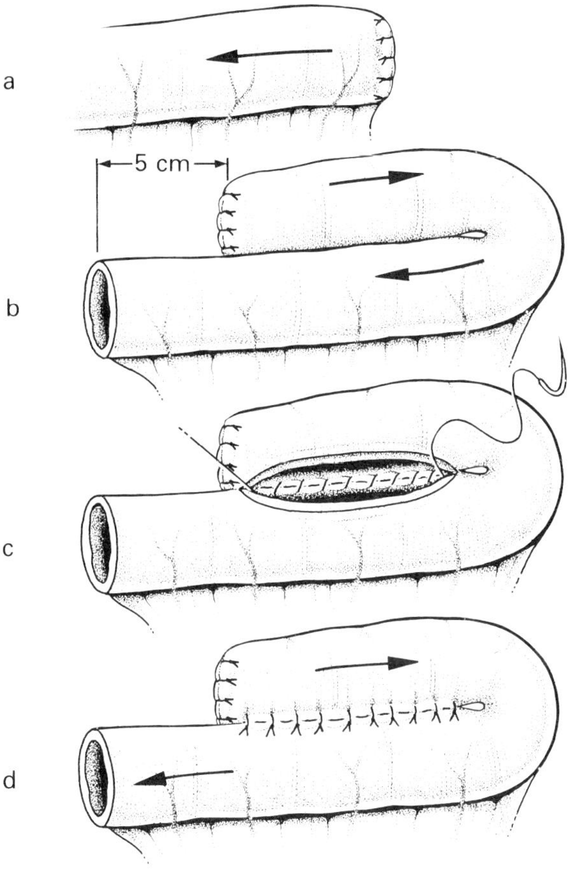

2. **Fashioning the reservoir.** The proximal end of the separated isoperistaltic loop is closed. The loop is then folded on itself such that the anterior limb is longer by 5 cm (Figure 4.9). A long entero-enteric anastomosis is next performed between the two limbs using a two-layer technique with interrupted 3/0 black silk or polyamide sutures and 2/0 chromic catgut (Figure 4.9).

3. **Anastomosis of reservoir to gastric remnant oesophagus.** The reservoir is brought up to the supracolic compartment through a gap in the transverse mesocolon. Care should be taken during this step to avoid twisting of the vascular pedicle (Figure 4.10). The gastric remnant is partially closed with interrupted 3/0 non-absorbable sutures, leaving a 2 cm orifice for anastomosis with the reservoir. A 2 cm incision is made in the apex of the reservoir which is then anastomosed to the gastric remnant using a single layer technique with 3/0 polyamide sutures. Two stay sutures are inserted one at either end, and the posterior part of the anastomosis is completed first. The posterior sutures are first inserted and then tied with the knots on the mucosal side (Figure 4.11). The suturing of the anterior wall of the anastomosis is similar except that the knots are tied externally (Figure 4.12). On completion of this anastomosis a Ryle tube is inserted and its tip left temporarily in the reservoir.

In the case of total gastrectomy, it is important that the oesophageal transection is conducted in such a way as to ensure optimal conditions for a safe anastomosis with the jejunal reservoir. The oesophageal musculature is incised all the way round to the mucosal tube which is then transected 1 cm further distally (Figure 4.13). This prevents retraction of the oesophageal mucosa inside the muscular layer and ensures mucosal approximation between the oesophagus and the jejunum.

Figure 4.9 *Construction of reservoir.* **(a)** *The proximal end of the isolated loop is closed in a single layer.* **(b)** *The loop is then folded on itself such that the distal end protrudes beyond the closed proximal end by 5 cm.* **(c)** *A long entero–enteric anastomosis is then performed between the adjacent 10 cm jejunal limbs. This anastomosis is carried out in two layers with continuous catgut and interrupted non-absorbable sutures.* **(d)** *The completed pouch with its 5 cm isoperistaltic conduit which will be anastomosed to the duodenal stump.*

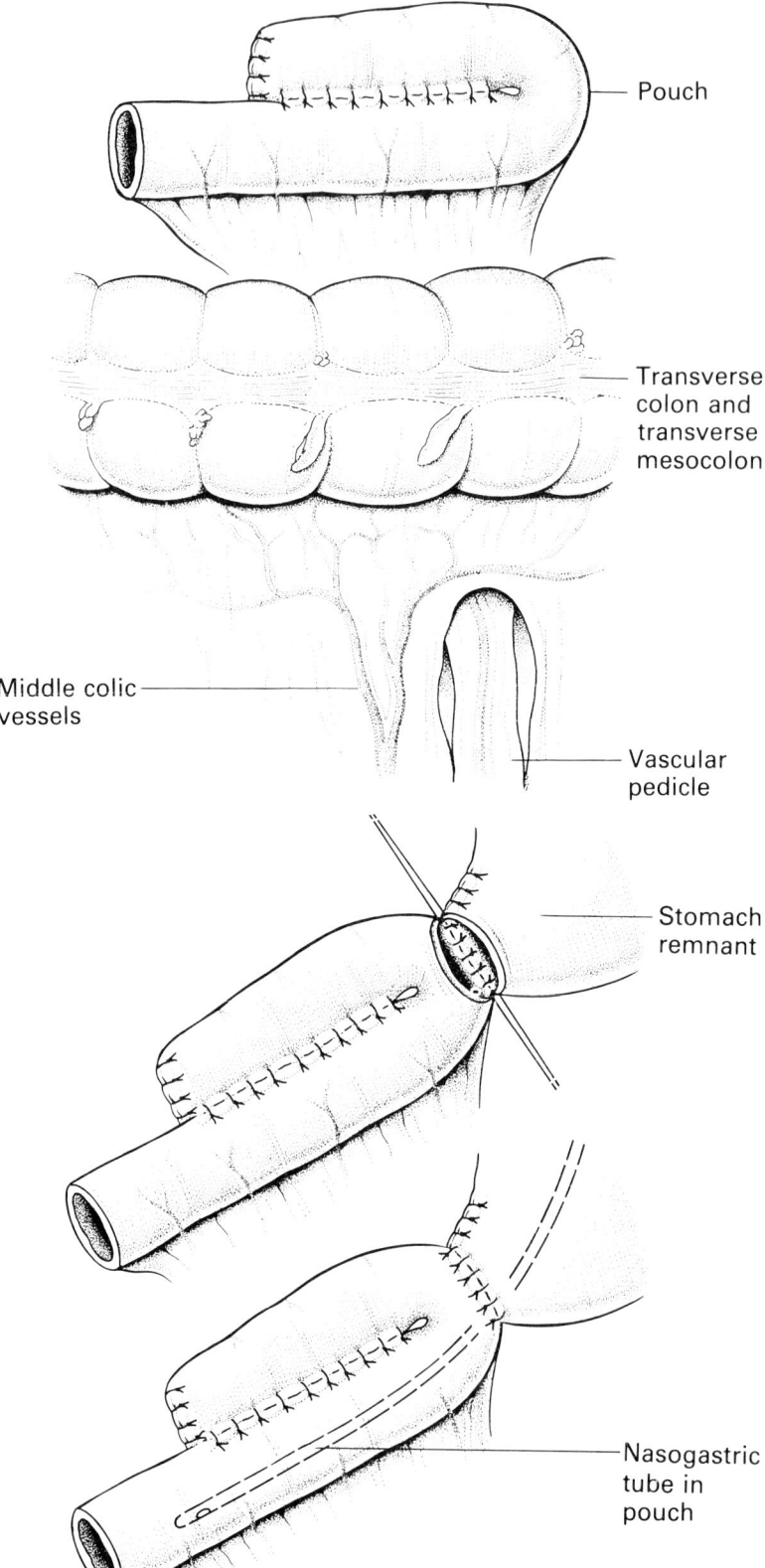

Figure 4.10 *The completed reservoir is transferred to the supracolic compartment through a gap in the transverse mesocolon to one side of the middle colic vessels. Care must be taken not to twist the folded pedicle during this manoeuvre.*

Figure 4.11 *Posterior part of the proximal anastomosis to the gastric remnant. The gastric remnant has been partially closed on the lesser curve side and a 2 cm incision performed on the apex of the reservoir. The anastomosis is performed in a single layer technique with interrupted sutures with the knots tied internally.*

Figure 4.12 *Completed anterior half of the proximal anastomosis to gastric stump. Again a single layer technique is used with interrupted non-absorbable sutures which are tied externally.*

RECONSTRUCTION OF THE GASTRIC RESERVOIR 71

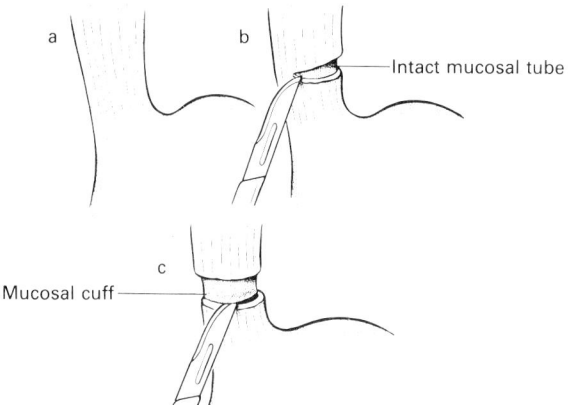

Figure 4.13 (a) *The mucosal layer is the crucial one for any oesophageal anastomosis. The technique illustrated ensures an adequate cuff of oesophageal mucosa at the transection site which does not retract inside the oesophageal musculature.* (b) *The muscular layers of the oesophagus are divided down to the mucosal tube.* (c) *The mucosa of the oesophagus is then divided 1 cm distal to the transected muscularis.*

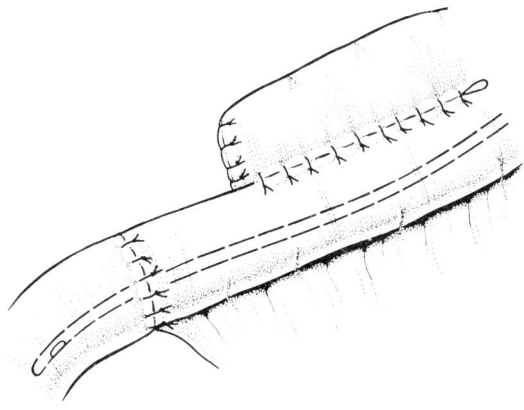

Figure 4.15 *Completed duodenojejunal anastomosis. The Ryle's tube has been threaded into the second part of the duodenum. If the duodenal stump is fibrotic, the anastomosis can be performed as an end-to-side one with the second part of the duodenum.*

Duodenojejunal anastomosis

By preference this anastomosis is carried out in an end-to-end fashion using a single layer technique with interrupted 3/0 non-absorbable deep seromuscular sutures. The posterior wall of the anastomosis is carried out initially with insertion of the sutures which are subsequently tied internally (Figure 4.14). At this stage the Ryle's tube is advanced beyond the anastomosis well into the duodenum. Thereafter the anastomosis is completed by suturing the anterior wall (Figure 4.15). If the duodenal stump is fibrosed or densely adherent to the head of the pancreas, the jejunal conduit from the reservoir is anastomosed to the second part of the duodenum in an end-to-side fashion. This procedure is feasible if adequate mobilization of the duodenum and head of pancreas is performed initially.

Closure and drainage

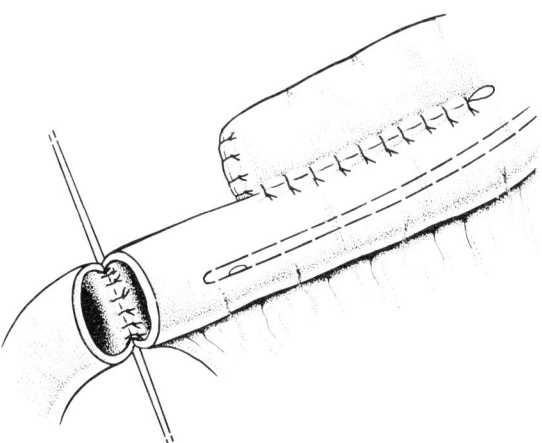

Figure 4.14 *Posterior wall of the anastomosis between conduit from the reservoir and duodenal stump. Wherever possible this should be performed in an end-to-end fashion. Again a single layer technique with interrupted non-absorbable sutures is used.*

The author uses a single silicone tube drain which has several side holes cut out and is attached to a drainage bag (closed system). The drain is brought out through a separate stab wound and made to lie alongside the reservoir and the two anastomoses. The abdominal wound is then closed in layers with 2/0 prolene.

POSTOPERATIVE CARE AND COMPLICATIONS

Postoperative management

The patients are kept on intravenous fluids with nil orally except for sips of water until a barium swallow confirms intact anastomotic suture lines on the 6th and 7th postoperative day. The Ryle's tube can be taken out earlier especially if it leads to excess discomfort. In those patients whose malnutrition necessitated pre-operative enteral or parenteral feeding, intravenous hyper-alimentation is continued until the patient has resumed an adequate oral intake.

Postoperative complications

Anastomotic leakage. With the technique used, the author has encountered only two minor (radiological) leaks, both at the proximal anastomosis, out of a series of 29 consecutive reservoir reconstructions. They were treated conservatively with nasogastric suction and progressed satisfactorily thereafter.

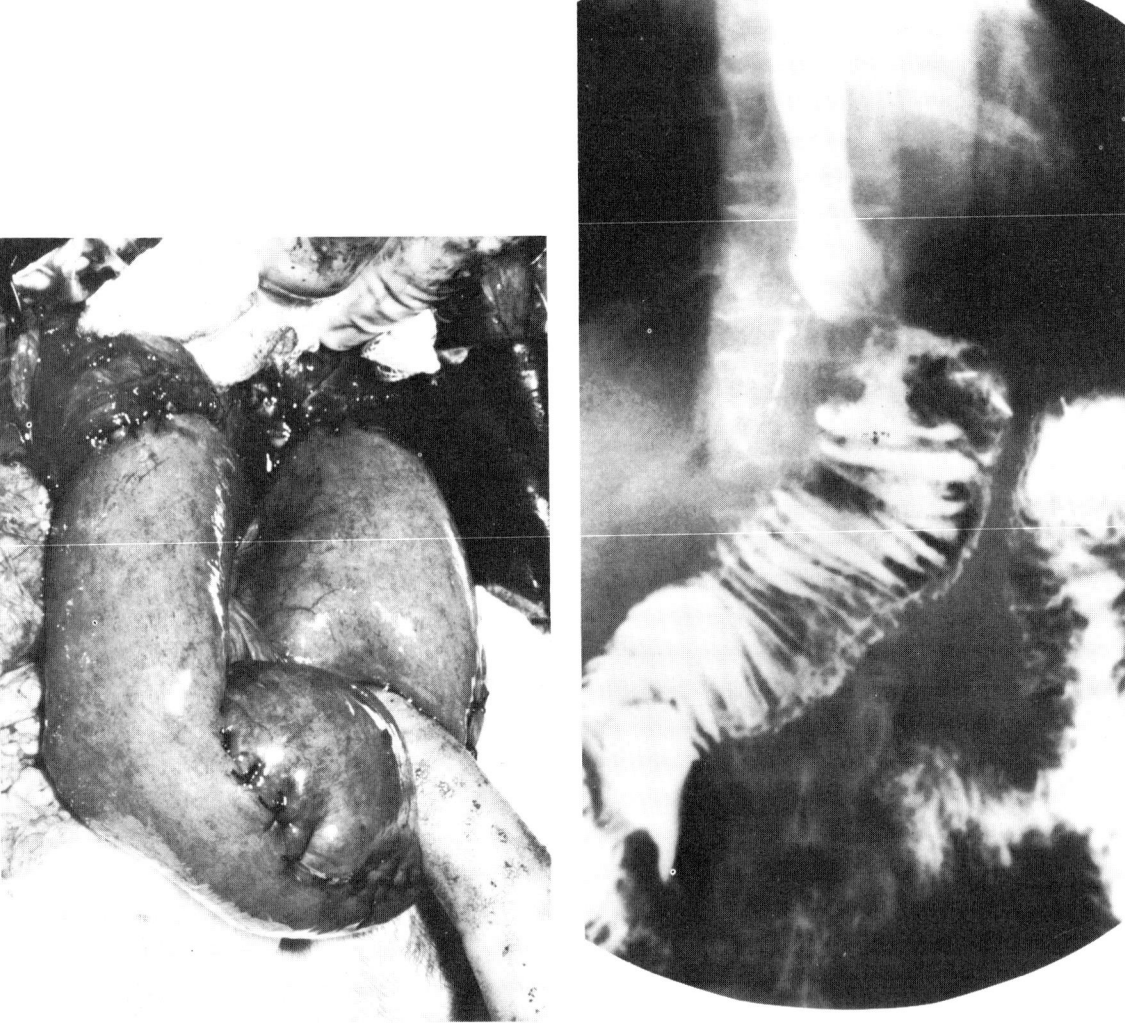

Figure 4.16 (a) *Operative photograph of the completed reconstruction.* (b) *Barium meal of the same patient two years after the operation.*

Stenosis. Stenosis of the proximal anastomosis with the onset of dysphagia was encountered in one patient six months after the operation. This required a local resection and re-anastomosis.

Necrosis of the reservoir. This is a theoretical complication which has not been encountered by the author. Provided care is taken during the construction of the pedicle and in ensuring against its twisting particularly during the transposition of the reservoir to the supracolic compartment, this complication should not occur since the vascular pedicle is merely folded on itself rather than rotated as happens in the fashioning of antiperistaltic interposed segments.

LONG-TERM OUTCOME

Nutritional state. All patients have gained weight (range 24–59%) and have been able to maintain a haemoglobin above 12 g/dl and an albumin at above 35 g/dl.[13] The maximum nutritional benefit has been encountered in patients with severe post-cibal symptoms after previous subtotal gastrectomy. When used as a primary method of reconstruction, the patients have been able to reach their preoperative within three to four months of the operation. There has been no evidence of bacterial overgrowth during a follow-up period extending to 12 years.

Changes in the reservoir. Long-term dilatation of the reservoir has not been encountered (Figure 4.16). The emptying of a liquid isotope meal is expressed by a single experimental pattern with a $T_{\frac{1}{2}}$ or 31 min $\pm$ 4.9. Intermittent vomiting is encountered in 10% and results from inspissated vegetable food residue. All the patients are now advised to take fizzy drinks after each meal. No dietary restriction has been found necessary.

Histology. Examination by light microscopy of repeated endoscopic biopsies has demonstrated maintenance of a normal villous architecture. There is however hyperplasia of the Paneth cells and an infiltrate of eosinophils and plasma cells. These changes have also been reported in patients with isoperistaltic jejunal interposition.[11] The accumulation of eosinophils and plasma cells is thought to result from exposure of the mucosa to a variety of antigens.

REFERENCES

1. Roux C (1879) De la gastro-enterostomie. *Revue de Gynecologie Chirurgie Abdominale* i: 67–122.
2. Earlam R (1983) Bile reflux and the Roux-en-Y anastomosis. *British Journal of Surgery* 70: 393–397.
3. Tanner NC (1954) Surgery of peptic ulceration and its complications. *Postgraduate Medical Journal* 30: 448–465.
4. Hunt CJ (1952) Construction of a food pouch from segment of jejunum as a substitute for stomach in total gastrectomy. *Archives of Surgery* 64: 601–608.
5. Lawrence WJ Jr (1962) Reservoir construction after total gastrectomy—an intensive case. *American Surgery* 155: 191–198.
6. Poth EJ (1957) The dumping syndrome and its surgical management. *Annals of Surgery* 23: 1097–2013.
7. Hay RP (1953) Anatomic and physiologic reconstruction following total gastrectomy by the use of a jejunal food pouch. *Forum* 4: 291–296.
8. Henley FA (1952) Gastrectomy with replacement. *British Journal of Surgery* 40: 118–213.
9. Sawyers JL & Herrington JL Jr (1973) Superiority of antiperistaltic jejunal segments in management of severe dumping syndrome. *Annals of Surgery* 178: 311–321.
10. Cuschieri A (1977) Isoperistaltic and antiperistaltic jejunal interposition for the dumping syndrome. A comparative study. *Journal of the Royal College of Surgeons, Edinburgh* 22: 319–324.
11. Landi E, Fianchini A, Landa L, Maniscalco L & Cutini G (1981) The interposed isolated loop following total gastrectomy: functional results. *Italian Journal of Surgical Science* 11: 227–234.
12. Zannini G, Renda A, Zotti GC, Fimmano A & Santini M (1981) Jejunal interposition with EEA stapler after total gastrectomy. *Italian Journal of Surgical Science* 11: 104–106.
13. Cuschieri A (1982) Long term evaluation of a reservoir jejunal interposition with an isoperistaltic conduit in the management of patients with the small stomach syndrome. *British Journal of Surgery* 69: 386–388.
14. Gilat T, Ben Hur H, Gelman-Malachi E et al (1978) Alterations of the colonic flora and their effect on the hydrogen breath test. *Gut* 19: 602–605.
15. King CE & Toskes PP (1979) Small intestinal bacterial overgrowth. *Gastroenterology* 76: 1035–1055.

5

Conservative Surgery of the Spleen

Leon Morgenstern

The spleen, until recently considered an organ of little significance and insurmountable surgical difficulty, is no longer thought easily expendable nor surgically inviolable. It is the largest single aggregate of reticuloendothelial and lymphoid tissue in the human body. The importance of its immunological function is only now being increasingly demonstrated and recognized.[1] Its role in the prevention of overwhelming sepsis by such organisms as pneumococcus, meningococcus and *Haemophilus influenzae* has been well defined.[2] Not until the development of new haemostatic materials and special surgical techniques, however, has it been possible to consider splenic repair or partial splenectomy technically feasible or safe. It is the purpose of this chapter to define the indications for the conservative approach to splenic surgery, describe the operative technique involved and indicate the results achieved by such surgical procedures.

INDICATIONS AND PATIENT SELECTION

Trauma

The most frequent indication for splenic repair or partial resection is trauma.

1. Trauma may be minor, consisting of one or more capsular avulsions. The most frequent of such injuries occurs during operations in the left upper quadrant when the surgeon or his assistant unwittingly exerts undue traction on the peritoneal folds attached to the spleen. One of the most constant of these and the one that most frequently results in capsular avulsion injuries is the lienoomental fold (Figure 5.1), coursing from the lower pole of the spleen to the nearby omentum (the 'criminal fold'). In the past, most such iatrogenic injuries were treated by splenectomy. More recent experience, however, has shown that splenectomy is rarely necessary. Minor capsular avulsion injuries may cease bleeding spontaneously or with pressure alone; most others will respond to the application of some topical haemostatic agent such as microcrystalline collagen,[3] oxidized cellulose or analogous topical agents.

2. Major trauma may be blunt or penetrating. Both are amenable to repair or partial resection (Figure 5.2). Only complete avulsion of the spleen from the hilar vessels or severe fragmentation make repair or partial resection impossible. Most major centres now report one-third to one-half of all splenic injuries amenable to repair or partial resection.

The younger the patient, the more pressing the need for splenic preservation. Infants and children are most susceptible to overwhelming post-splenectomy sepsis,[4] although splenectomized individuals of all ages may be affected.[5] Splenic repair is more easily accomplished in infants and in children because of the firmer consistency of the splenic parenchyma, greater contractility of the vasculature and, in the opinion of the author, more efficient natural coagulation mechanisms. Conversely, older patients are more difficult subjects for conservative surgery. Nevertheless, they should be given the benefit of splenic salvage if it does not prolong operating time unduly nor increase

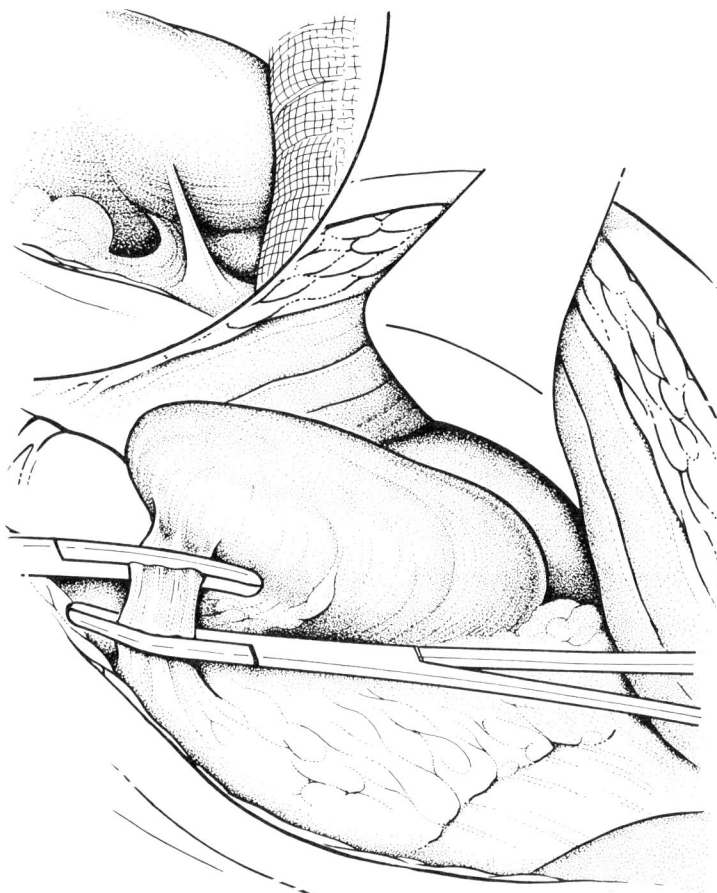

Figure 5.1 *The lieno-omental fold extends from the lower pole of the spleen to the greater omentum in the left upper quadrant. Both the spleen and greater omentum are derivatives of the embryonic dorsal mesogastrium hence this almost constant association between the two structures. Traction on this lower pole fold is the most common cause of iatrogenic injury during surgical procedures in the left upper quadrant. Since the fold usually contains sizeable vessels it should be clipped or ligated before division.*

operative risk. This is a matter of judgement for the individual surgeon. It makes little sense to persist in saving the spleen of an octogenarian if this is not accomplished in the simplest manner. In aged patients, the risk of untoward immunological sequelae from splenectomy is negligible considering natural life expectancy.

The presence of associated intra-abdominal injuries also should influence the choice of patients for splenic salvage. In the presence of associated visceral perforation with peritoneal contamination, extensive hepatic, pancreatic or renal injury, or severe vascular injury, splenic preservation is indicated only if the simplest manoeuvres will accomplish it. The only exception to this rule is the infant or young child.

The most important principle in splenic preservation following trauma is that the risk of attempted salvage should never exceed the risks attendant on total splenectomy. Although the immunological sequelae of splenectomy are indisputable, the incidence of such sequelae, with our present state of knowledge, is still quite low.

Splenic cysts

The non-parasitic splenic cyst which is symptomatic can be removed without sacrificing the entire spleen.[6] The precise aetiology of such cysts is not known, although previous trauma has been implicated more than any other factor. Lymphogenous, haemangiomatous and epidermoid cysts are also amenable to removal by either enucleation or partial splenic resection. Partial resection or unroofing of the cyst without sacrifice of the spleen has also been performed as an alternative technique.[7]

Miscellaneous non-malignant hypersplenic states

Splenic enlargement from any cause can result in significant hypersplenism which can pose a risk to the life or well-being of the patient. Excluding malignant hypersplenism (leukaemias and lymphomas) where partial resection is not indicated, there have been a number of conditions for which partial splenectomy has been either suggested or

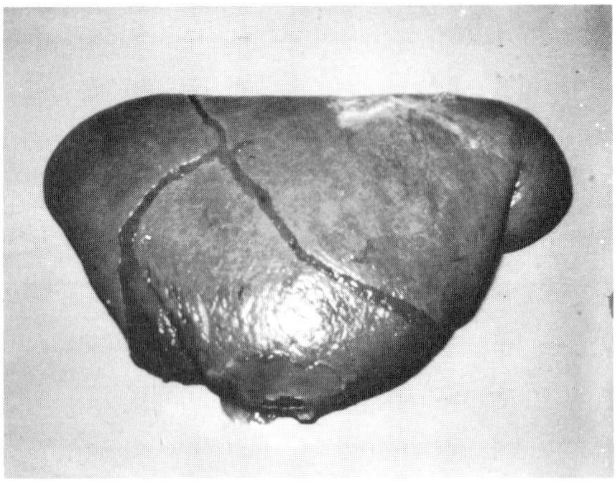

Figure 5.2 *A spleen resected for a typical stellate laceration which would have been amenable to repair or partial resection. Note the adherent blood clot at the left. Such a clot should not be removed until the spleen is fully mobilized in case massive bleeding occurs before control of the splenic circulation has been achieved.*

performed. These include myeloid metaplasia,[8] Gaucher's disease,[9] thalassaemia major[10] and schistosomiasis.[11] However, the numbers and results of such operations are not yet sufficient to firmly establish the rationale of conservative surgery in these conditions.

Partial resection is contraindicated in idiopathic thrombocytopenic purpura and autoimmune haemolytic anaemias. It has no place in the management of primary or metastatic malignancies.

PREOPERATIVE CARE AND INVESTIGATIONS

Trauma

History

The nature of the trauma is an important determinant of management. In general, trauma localized to the left upper quadrant favours attempts at splenic salvage. Left upper quadrant pain and shoulder tip pain (Kehr's sign) suggest the diagnosis of splenic injury.

Laboratory and imaging studies

The initial haemoglobin and haematocrit determinations are laboratory guides to the rate of intra-abdominal bleeding. Patients in whom these remain stable may be candidates for non-operative management, as will be described in the next section. Hypotension unresponsive to volume replacement, progression of abdominal symptoms or findings of an acute surgical abdomen are an indication for immediate surgical intervention.

Confirmation of the diagnosis of splenic injury is highly desirable unless operation is so urgent that further investigation is precluded. In patients who are obtunded we have used emergency laparoscopy under local anaesthesia with a miniature laparoscope.[12] Blood in the left gutter or a bulging haematoma in the left upper quadrant are generally indicative of splenic rupture; at times the splenic injury itself may be seen when located on the lower pole.

The technetium-99 scintiscan is a very reliable means of assessing splenic trauma; we have used this imaging technique in preference to others for diagnosing the degree and location of the splenic injury. CT scan does not always show parenchymal disruptions, but visualizes perisplenic extravasation and haematoma more accurately than the scintiscan. Ultrasound is of no value. Arteriography is reserved for those patients in whom the study is being done for associated intra-abdominal injury, kidney, liver or major vessels.

Splenic cysts

History

Splenic cysts may be discovered incidentally during x-ray studies performed for some other reason since the wall of the splenic cyst is not infrequently totally or partially calcified. In most cases of larger splenic cysts, the patient complains of nagging left upper quadrant discomfort. Pressure on or adherence to the left hemidiaphragm may evoke left shoulder tip pain.

It is important to obtain a history of exposure to the cyst-forming parasite echinococcus, if such exposure exists. A history of trauma is of little significance since it may or may not be aetiologically related; in 10 splenic cysts resected by the author or his staff, a definite history of trauma was obtained in half the cases.

Any or all of the imaging techniques are useful in the study of splenic cysts. Technetium-99 scintiscan confirms the splenic aetiology, defines the anatomical location and the amount of residual functional splenic tissue. CT scan delineates the cyst precisely, and can also identify any solid intracystic components if they exist. Ultrasound confirms the liquid nature of the cyst contents, but is not absolutely necessary in the presence of the preceding two studies. Arteriography does not materially aid diagnosis or management, but by showing the anatomical distribution of the splenic vessels may make the dissection of the splenic vessels easier in the performance of a subtotal splenectomy.

Miscellaneous haematological conditions

Previous history and laboratory examinations have usually established the diagnosis of the underlying disease and the degree of hypersplenism. Sequestration studies are of little value in planning partial resection, but arteriography may be useful in demonstrating the vascular anatomy so the most feasible site of transection may be chosen. In some centres, arteriographic embolization is used as a means of non-operative partial splenic ablation for hypersplenism.[10] Further study is required to establish this as an acceptable method of treatment.

When the contemplated operative procedure is elective, it is advisable to use preoperative immunization measures in the event splenic salvage is impossible and total splenectomy becomes necessary. Polyvalent pneumococcal vaccine effective against 23 serotypes is now available and should be given. Meningococcal vaccine is also available, although effectiveness has not yet been thoroughly demonstrated. A vaccine against *Haemophilus influenzae* is now being developed. There is evidence to show that preoperative immunization mounts a better antibody response than when done postoperatively.

NON-OPERATIVE MANAGEMENT

Selective patients with splenic injury may be managed non-operatively, providing special criteria are adopted.[13] The non-operative approach has been widely accepted as a mode of management in children,[14,15] but similar management in adults is a more recent development.

In adults, those patients selected should be patients whose trauma is limited to the left upper quadrant and in whom the diagnosis of isolated splenic injury is reasonably certain. Patients with severe abdominal trauma in whom associated visceral injuries may warrant exploration are excluded.

The diagnosis is made by scintiscan or CT scan. Defects which appear substantially large, involving an entire pole for example, are not indications for surgical intervention. If the patient's abdominal signs remain unchanged or improve on close observation, and if the haemoglobin and haematocrit remain stable on serial determinations, the patient may be observed without resorting to operation. We have set an arbitrary limit of two transfusions for correction of the red blood cell and volume deficit due to the splenic injury; beyond this limit, if the haemoglobin and haematocrit continue to fall, operation is indicated.

Patients are kept at bed rest initially, and are observed in an intensive care unit for the first 48 hours. After 48 hours they are observed on routine ward care, with ambulatory privileges. After one week a repeat scan is performed and if unchanged or improved, the patient may be discharged. Strenuous physical activity such as contact sports, jogging, bicycling or any jarring abdominal exercises are forbidden. Periodic scintigrams (e.g. at three, six and 12 months) are helpful to assess splenic healing and provide a guide to the resumption of normal activity.

In summary, isolated splenic injuries which have ceased bleeding as shown by clinical observation and laboratory studies may be observed rather than treated by operation, since such injuries have been shown to heal uneventfully. Younger patients are more amenable to this approach since their coagulation and repair mechanisms appear more suited to this type of management. Should the serial scintiscan show evidence of an expanding extracapsular haematoma, even in the absence of symptoms, the indication is for elective operation.

To date, no late complications of splenosis or splenic cyst formation have been reported. If the criteria of high patient selectivity and close observation are followed this should remain an acceptable form of treatment for adults as well as children.

OPERATIVE TECHNIQUES

Minor trauma

Capsular avulsion injuries, whether incurred by operative injury or by blunt trauma, may be treated by application of topical haemostatic

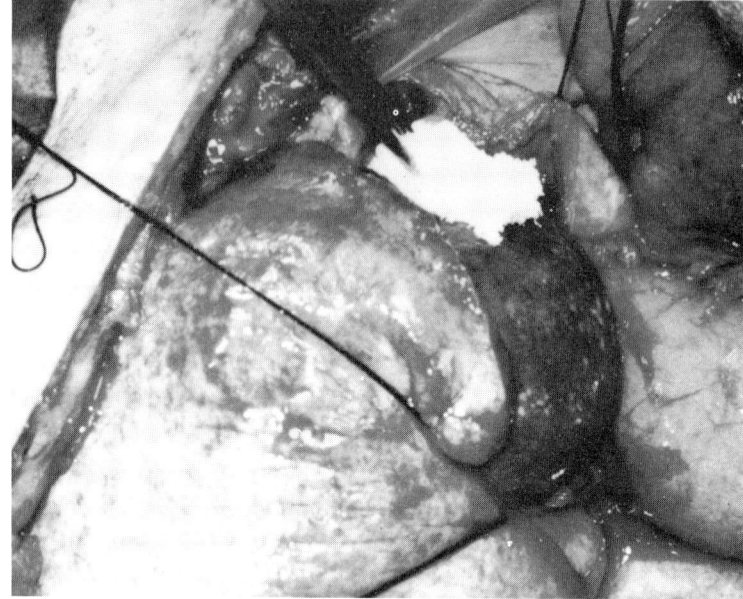

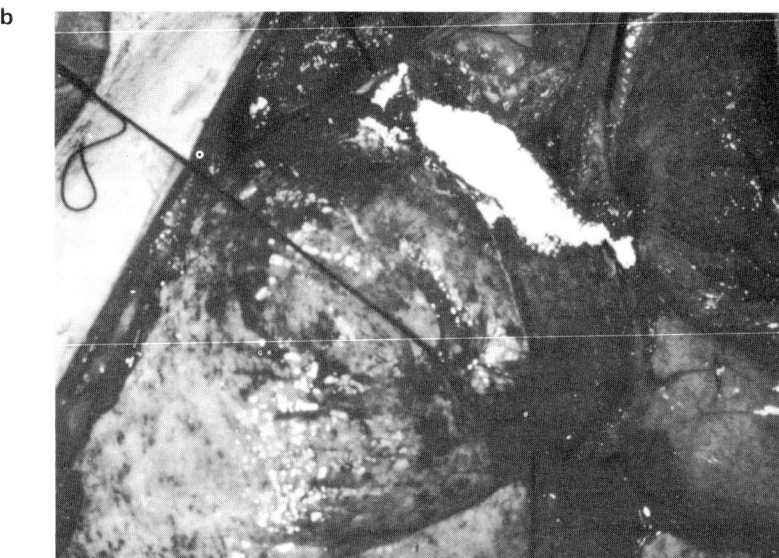

Figure 5.3 *Microcrystalline collagen is being applied to a capsular avulsion injury of the spleen incurred during an oesophagogastrectomy. The correct mode of application is shown and in (b) the appearance of the compressed microcrystalline collagen is illustrated.*

agents if the capsular avulsion is not too extensive. If the capsule has been stripped extensively to involve a large expanse of bare parenchyma, topical haemostasis is rarely successful. We have discouraged the use of electrocoagulation in the management of avulsion injuries since the thermal eschar has a tendency toward late separation and increases the risk of delayed bleeding.

The two most important factors in topical haemostasis are time and patience. The most effective agent, in our opinion, is the powdered form of microcrystalline collagen. This is applied with a dry forceps to the bleeding site in a quantity sufficient to form a 2 or 3 mm layer of collagen after compression with a dry sponge (Figure 5.3). Pressure should be applied evenly for three minutes, after which the sponge or laparotomy pad is slowly and carefully removed to avoid dislodgement of the coagulum. Breakthrough bleeding is managed by application of another thin layer of microcrystalline collagen. Should the coagulum become loosened, partially dislodged, or prematurely wet, it should be totally removed and the application process repeated. The collagen should adhere firmly and conform to all contours of the injured surface. Excess collagen beyond the borders of the injury should be removed.

Splenorrhaphy and partial splenic resection

The incision

Excellent exposure and access to the spleen is the *sine qua non* for conservative surgery of the spleen. If the abdominal injury is suspected of involving other intra-abdominal organs or structures, the standard incision for major trauma is the vertical midline incision. Splenic mobilization through this incision is more difficult than with the left subcostal incision, particularly in obese patients or those with narrow costal angles.

If the injury is thought or known to be limited to the spleen, the best incision for access and exposure is the left subcostal incision, extending from the midline to the anterior axillary line. Division of the falciform ligament affords more room and makes mobilization easier.

If the left subcostal incision appears inadequate, because of a very high lying spleen or unusual adhesions, the best means of extending the incision is by adding a vertical midline component upward towards the xiphoid (the Kehr incision) (Figure 5.4). This opens the left upper quadrant widely, and is well suited for all operative manoeuvres on the spleen.

Control of splenic artery

Unless bleeding from the spleen is massive, in which case rapid mobilization is required, the preliminary control of splenic arterial inflow is of great assistance in conservative splenic surgery.

The splenic artery, fortunately, is easily accessible for such preliminary occlusive control. The gastrocolic omentum is entered preferably to the left of the midportion of the greater curvature. Whether the individual branches of gastroepiploic vessels are taken close to the stomach, or the omentum is divided serially below the gastroepiploic vessels, care is taken not to injure or ligate the main gastroepiploic arteries and veins. The window in the omentum should be large enough to visualize the splenic artery clearly as it courses above the pancreas. The splenic artery is tortuous in all but the youngest of infants and children, becoming more tortuous and brittle with advancing age. The apex of one of the tortuous loops is chosen for the site of occlusion, the overlying peritoneum is incised and the artery encircled by a double loop of Silastic (vessel loop) (Figure 5.5). Pulling this encircling loop taut occludes splenic arterial inflow, lessening bleeding from the splenic surface and allowing for controlled dissection. The temporary 'ligation' can be periodically loosened to allow for some splenic circulation or to assess adequacy of haemostasis. At the conclusion of the splenic procedure, it is removed.

Ligation of the splenic artery as an adjunct to splenorrhaphy or partial resection is not recommended.

Mobilization

Adequate and atraumatic mobilization of the spleen so that it lies comfortably on the operative field is mandatory for successful splenorrhaphy or resection. Only topical haemostatic measures are feasible on the unmobilized spleen in the left upper quadrant. Suture repair of the spleen in this position is neither feasible nor safe.

Mobilization of the injured spleen is no different from that of the uninjured spleen except that it should be done more expeditiously. Blood clot in the left upper quadrant should be removed, but

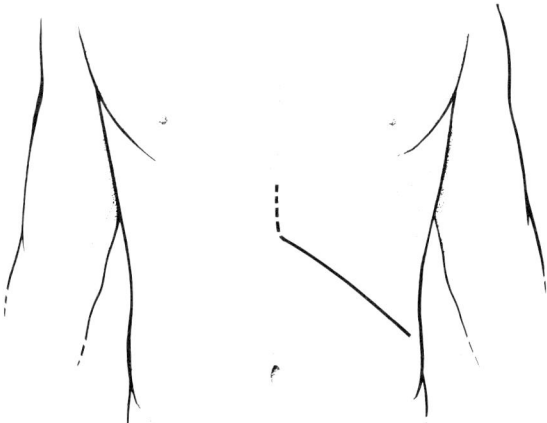

Figure 5.4 *The left upper quadrant subcostal incision is the most suitable for conservative splenic operations since it affords the greatest access and the best means of atraumatic mobilization. Shown also is the upward vertical extension which adds greatly to exposure of the left upper quadrant structures (Kehr incision).*

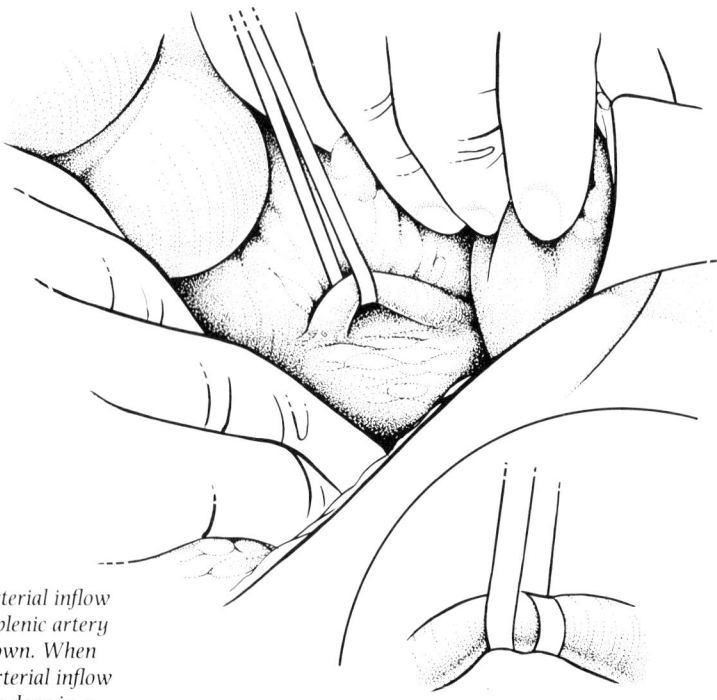

Figure 5.5 *To secure control of the splenic arterial inflow during splenorrhaphy or partial resection the splenic artery is encircled by a Silastic loop in the manner shown. When this is made taut by upward traction, splenic arterial inflow is occluded and procedures on the spleen may be done in a relatively bloodless manner. The splenic artery should not be occluded with any type of clamp since it is brittle and may be easily injured.*

blood clot adherent to the spleen should be left undisturbed since its removal can initiate massive bleeding. Control of the splenic arterial inflow is very useful should this occur.

The objectives in mobilization are two-fold. First, to move the spleen forward and anteriorly so that all surfaces can be inspected and dealt with as necessary, and to make all vessels accessible for selective ligation. Secondly, to mobilize the spleen in such a manner that its capsule remains intact. A capsule which is extensively stripped during mobilization makes repair or partial resection virtually impossible.

To avoid capsular avulsions and stripping, the spleen should be handled with 'egg shell' delicacy. The anterior peritoneal attachments (lieno-omental, lieno-colic, lieno-gastric) should be divided and ligated first. It helps considerably if the division of the lower portion of the lieno-gastric vessels is done before any mobilization commences. Once the anterior attachments are freed the spleen is cupped in the left hand and the retroperitoneum behind the spleen incised parallel to the spleen from below the level of the lower pole to the level of the diaphragm. The spleen is then gently mobilized anteriorly together with the distal portion of the pancreas; gentleness does not preclude rapidity. A point of particular danger for capsular avulsion is the extreme upper pole. Here the lieno-gastric vessels are short and taut; care must be taken that the vessels are divided and ligated (or clipped) before they are torn or before the capsule of the upper pole is stripped.

With the spleen completely mobilized so that it now occupies 'central stage' (Figure 5.6), splenorrhaphy or partial resection may be done.

Selective devascularization

The spleen has a segmental circulation dividing it into from two to five or more segments (Figure 5.7). The superior polar branch seems to be the most constant branch supplying the major portion of the upper pole. This branch usually has its origin outside the hilus of the spleen whereas the others are often intrahilar.

In cases of trauma, the injury itself may have avulsed the segmental vessel and the devitalized

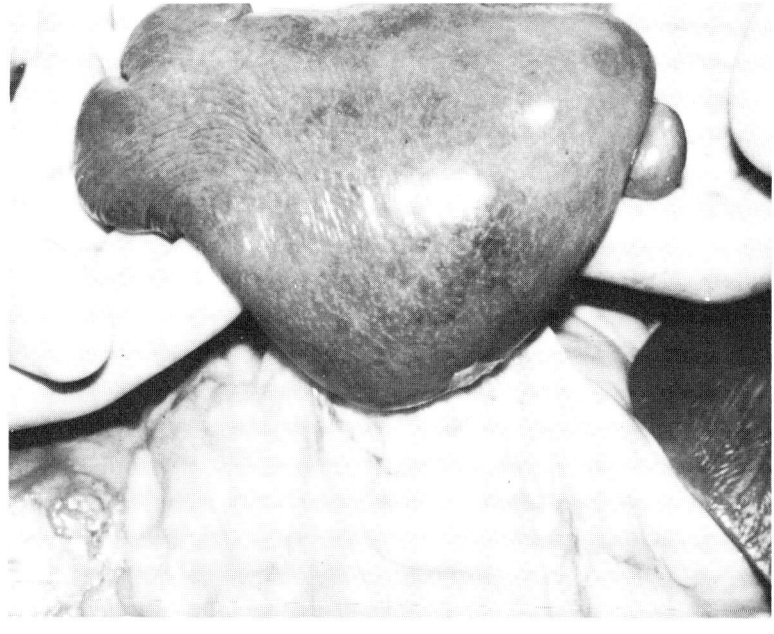

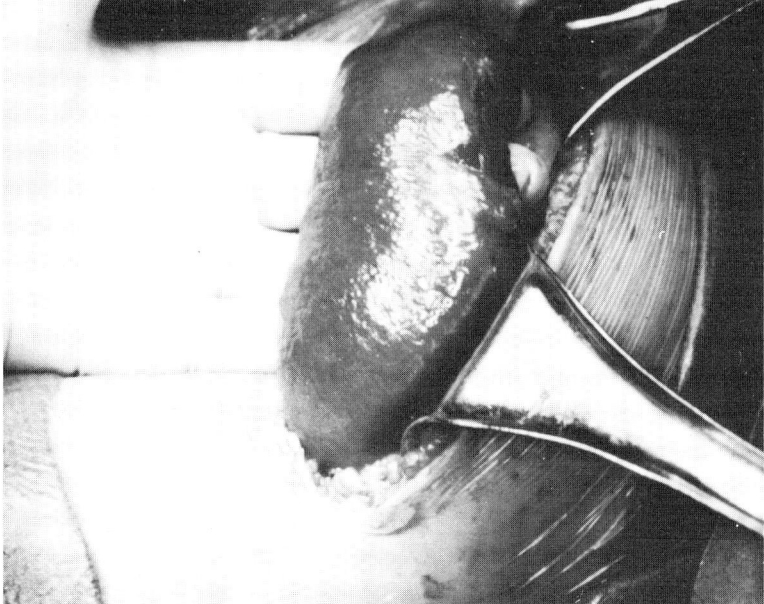

Figure 5.6 *The mobilized spleen occupies 'centre stage' and is fully exposed for any surgical manoeuvres including splenorrhaphy, partial resection or topical haemostasis.*

fragment or fragments can be clearly recognized by their dark bluish discoloration. The disrupted vessels are individually secured and ligated as encountered.

In cases where the site of resection is to be chosen electively, such as localized trauma, splenic cysts and haematological conditions, the vessels supplying the segment to be resected are dissected out and selectively ligated. In some instances this cannot be done and the segmental vessels must be sought intraparenchymally, ligating them as encountered.

When the segmental vessels are ligated (Figure 5.8), the devascularized splenic segment assumes a sharply defined dark bluish hue with a clear line of demarcation (Figure 5.9). It is through this line of demarcation that the resection is done, if that is the procedure elected.

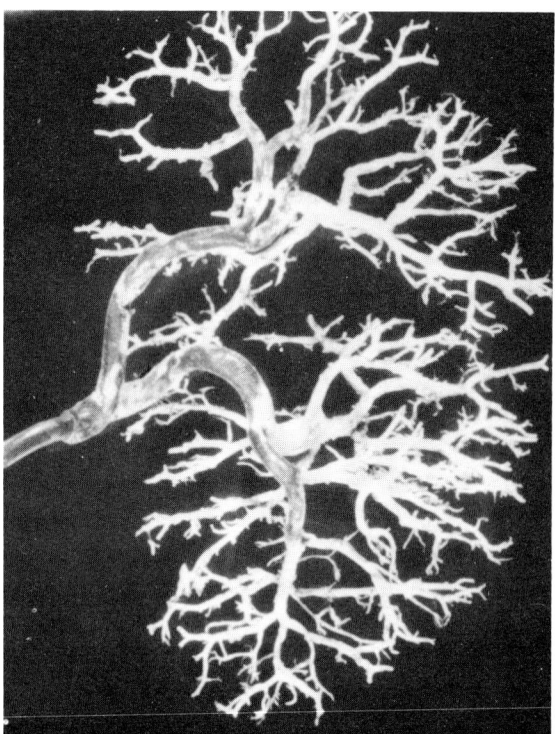

Figure 5.7 *Latex cast prepared from arterial circulation of a human spleen. The large superior polar artery is seen arising from the main splenic artery near the hilum. This particular spleen has two major segments and several minor segments along which a dissection plane could have been developed.*

Splenorrhaphy

If lacerations are relatively superficial and there is no devascularization or separation of splenic fragments, suture repair or splenorrhaphy is the procedure of choice.

The splenic parenchyma is an unforgiving tissue; unless handled with extreme gentleness, it responds with maceration and irreparability. In general, young spleens can be sutured with greater ease than old spleens. Spleens in which the nature of the pathological process is infiltrative or incites fibrosis are also more easily amenable to suture (e.g. myelofibrosis, Gaucher's or schistosomiasis).

The most preferable suture material in my experience has been 2/0 chromic catgut on an atraumatic needle, wetting and slightly stretching the suture before use. Polypropylene monofilament sutures are too stiff; other synthetic sutures are too rough and tear the splenic parenchyma.

The suture can be applied in one of several fashions. I prefer the simple running suture (Figure 5.10). Alternatives are the running locked suture (Figure 5.11) or closely placed interrupted sutures. In all methods the secret of successful suturing is the maintenance of the proper degree of tension. Too little tension does not hold the divided splenic parenchyma well and continued oozing results; too much tension tears the splenic parenchyma and bleeding from the suture holes themselves can be very troublesome.

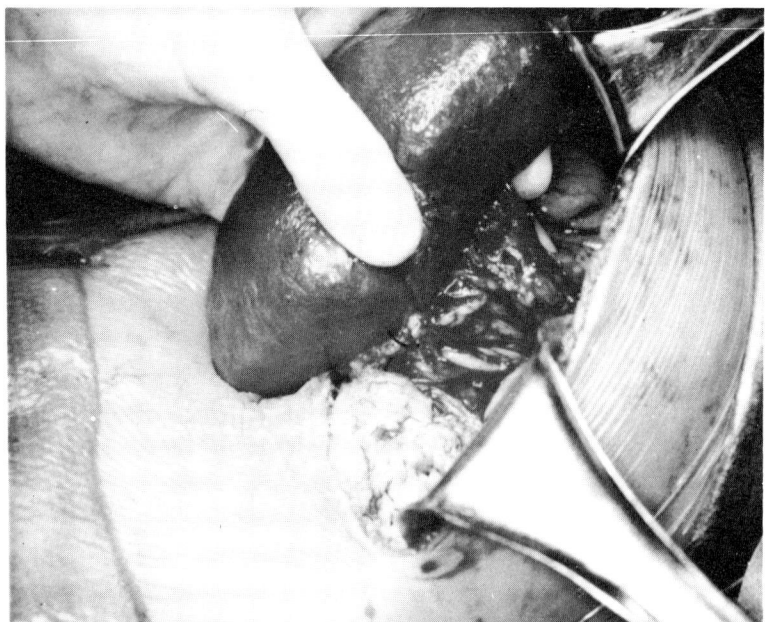

Figure 5.8 *With the spleen fully mobilized the segmental vessels can be identified and selectively ligated.*

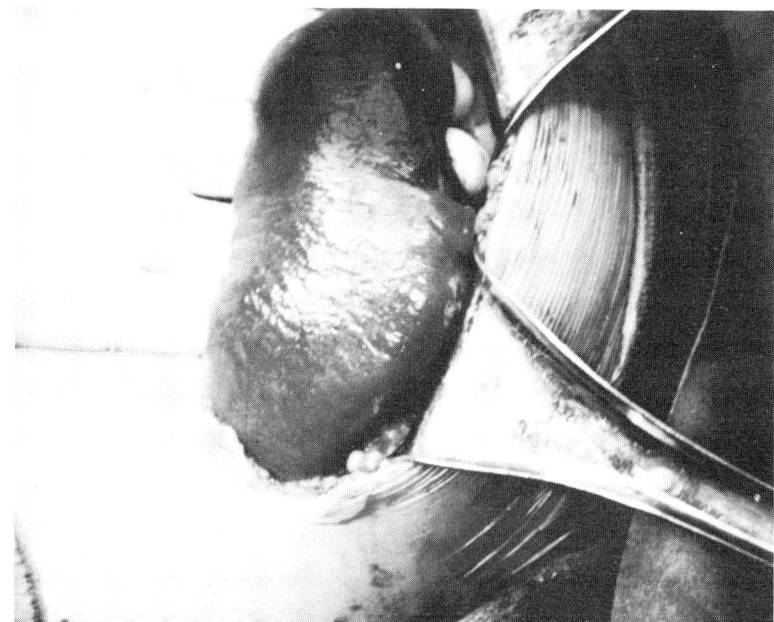

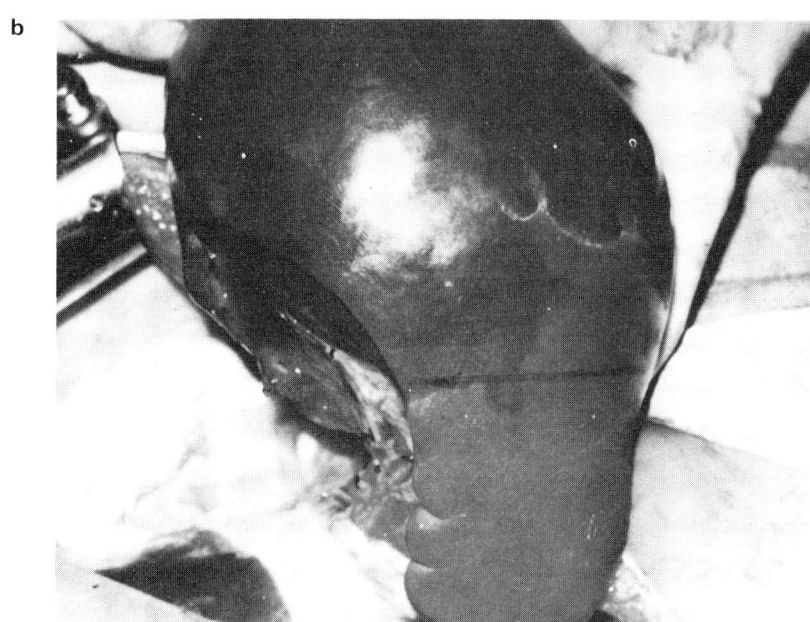

Figure 5.9 *Examples of selective ligation of superior polar vessels:* **(a)** *the line of demarcation appeared at the level of the operator's second digit, although it is not clearly evident in black and white, while in* **(b)** *the clear line of demarcation between the vascularized and devascularised segments is well illustrated. Resection is done through the line of demarcation.*

Frequently, there is some bluish discoloration in the vicinity of the suture repair. This is of no significance and does not denote devascularization. We have seen no problems after repair, although we have frequently seen this discoloration.

Bleeding from suture lines, if not controlled by simple pressure, may be controlled by application of a topical haemostatic agent, such as microfibrillar collagen.

All surfaces of the spleen should be inspected for lacerations, which should then be appropriately sutured. Lacerations which extend into the hilum do not preclude successful suture. A combination of suture and topical haemostatic agent in this location can be successful in splenic salvage.

84 GENERAL SURGERY

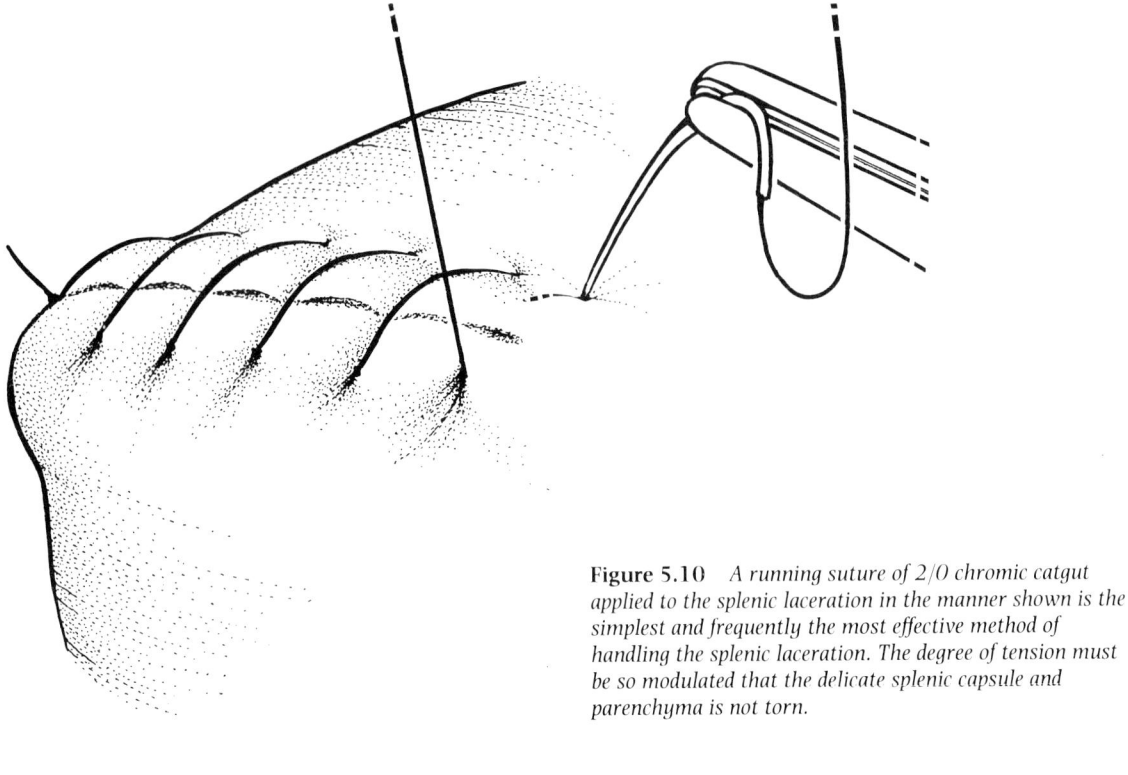

Figure 5.10 *A running suture of 2/0 chromic catgut applied to the splenic laceration in the manner shown is the simplest and frequently the most effective method of handling the splenic laceration. The degree of tension must be so modulated that the delicate splenic capsule and parenchyma is not torn.*

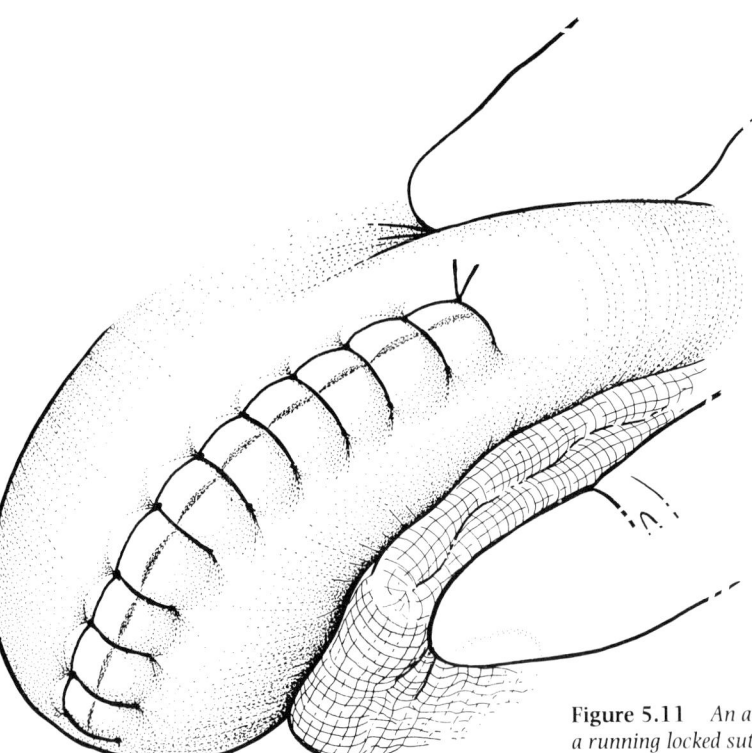

Figure 5.11 *An alternative to the simple running suture is a running locked suture which is a little more difficult to place without tearing the parenchyma. However, it can be very effective in obtaining excellent haemostasis and is the suture of choice with some surgeons.*

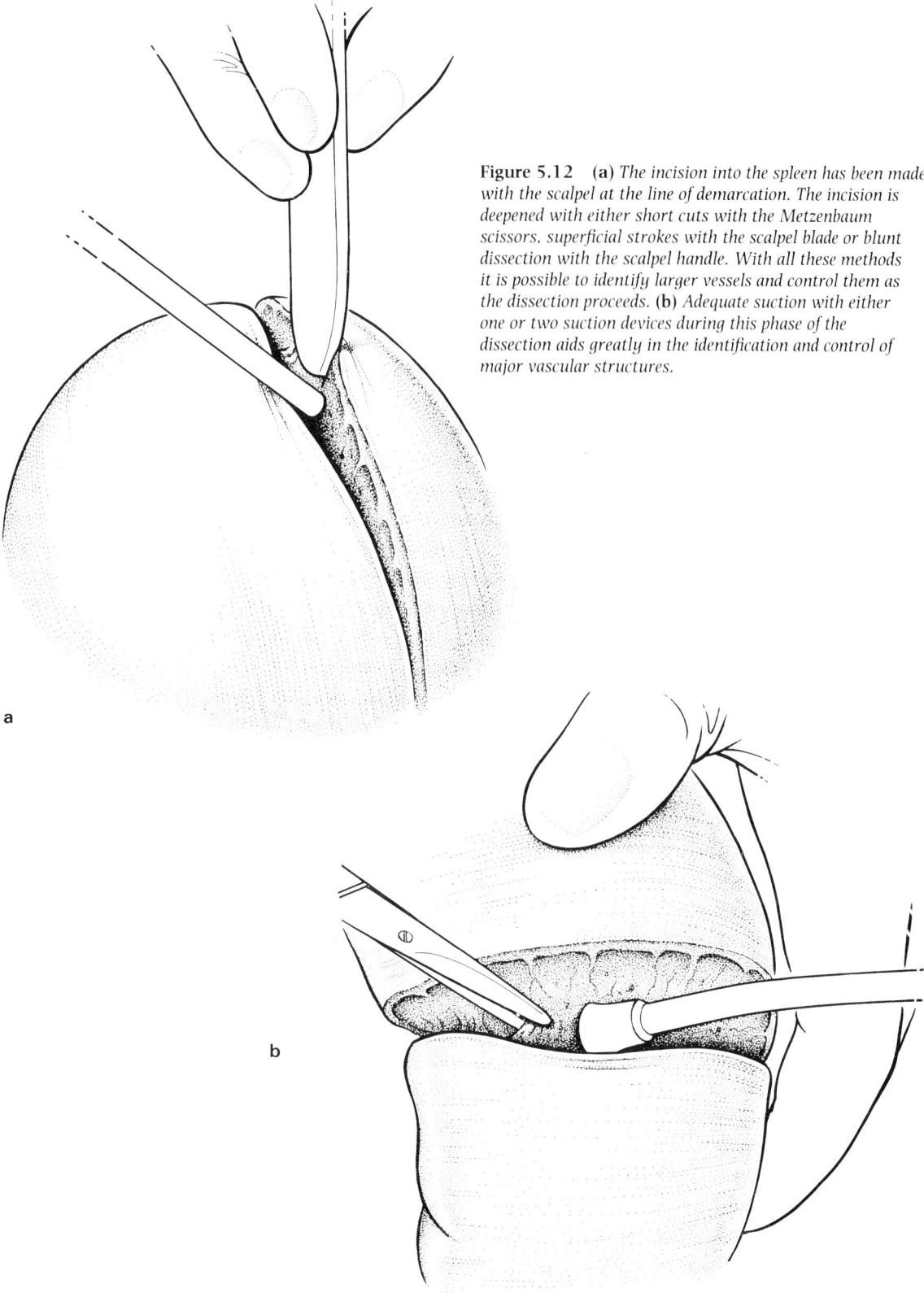

Figure 5.12 (a) *The incision into the spleen has been made with the scalpel at the line of demarcation. The incision is deepened with either short cuts with the Metzenbaum scissors, superficial strokes with the scalpel blade or blunt dissection with the scalpel handle. With all these methods it is possible to identify larger vessels and control them as the dissection proceeds.* (b) *Adequate suction with either one or two suction devices during this phase of the dissection aids greatly in the identification and control of major vascular structures.*

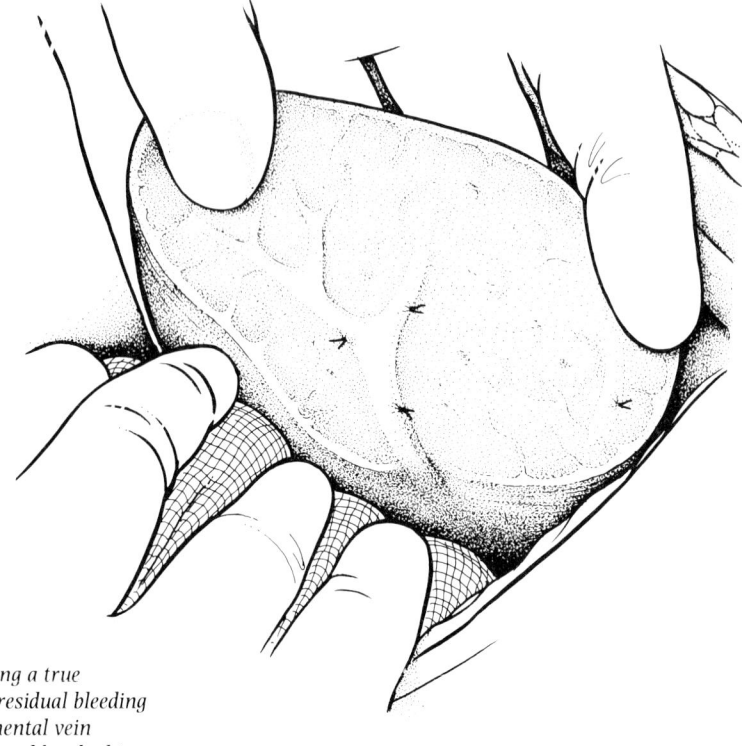

Figure 5.13 *If the dissection has been along a true segmental plane, there should be very little residual bleeding at the conclusion of the dissection. The segmental vein traverses the surface of the splenic remnant and has had its branches tied. Arterial branches have been controlled by small or medium haemoclips.*

Figure 5.14 *Bleeding arterial vessels are easily identified and grasped with the neurosurgical Adson forceps and clipped as shown in Figure 5.13.*

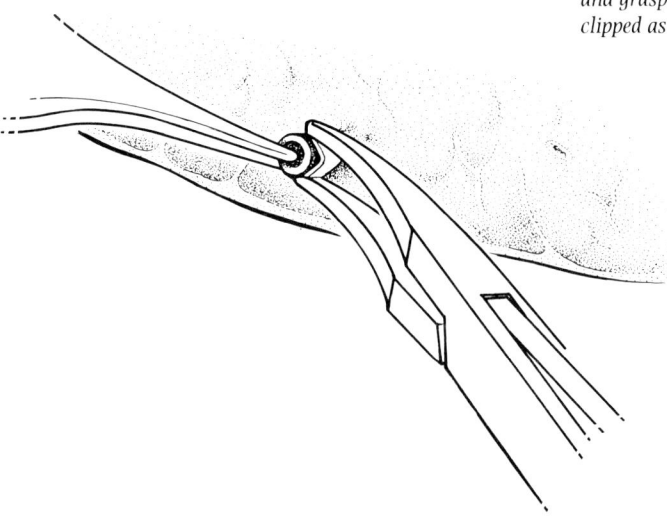

Partial splenectomy

For partial splenectomy, careful mobilization is performed as has been described above. If not torn or avulsed by injury in traumatized spleens, the segmental vessels are doubly ligated and divided. Within minutes this results in the sharp demarcation between vascularized and devascularized parenchyma.

The incision into the spleen is made at the line of demarcation, using a scalpel to divide the splenic capsule. Instruments necessary for this dissection include two (Frazier) neurosurgical suction tips, small and medium haemoclips on short clip holders and fine vascular 4/0 or 5/0 silk sutures.

The incision is deepened as shown in Figure 5.12 and the dissection proceeds using blunt dissection with the knife handle or short superficial strokes with the blade. As vascular structures are encountered or felt they are clipped and divided. Continued and accurate suction is a great help at this stage. As the dissection is carried deeper, larger vessels may be encountered and dealt with appropriately. This dissection should be slow and meticulous with the objective of securing as many vessels as possible in a controlled fashion as the parenchyma is divided.

When the parenchymal division is accomplished through a proper plane it should appear as in Figure 5.13. The segmental vein is clearly visible and preserved. All major bleeders should have been divided and ligated as the plane of incision was deepened.

Residual surface oozing may be capillary (sinusoidal) in origin or from small arterioles and venules. Arteries usually project from the divided parenchyma, allowing them to be elevated by a neurosurgical (Adson) forceps and clipped (Figure 5.14). Venules are flat and thin-walled, appearing frequently in a V-shaped configuration (Figure 5.15). Bleeding from venules is best controlled by a figure-of-eight or running suture of 4/0 arterial silk. Finally, if the sinusoidal ooze from the raw splenic parenchyma does not cease, we apply a thin layer of microcrystalline collagen.

Some authors have advocated section of the spleen in a V-shaped fashion at the line of resection to allow coagulation of the two 'halves' of the V with sutures. We have not found this necessary, and do not believe it adds any substantial advantage over leaving a raw splenic surface which quickly becomes covered with omentum or adjacent viscera. Likewise, we have found it unnecessary to employ pledgets of foreign material to prevent sutures from cutting into the spleen. With proper tension, pledgets and bolsters are not required.

There are alternative ways of dealing with the divided splenic parenchyma, depending on the thickness of the parenchyma at the line of division, the consistency of the spleen and ability to identify the segmental vessels accurately. We have sutured the divided parenchyma in some instances with interrupted mattress sutures of 2/0 chromic catgut (Figure 5.16) or even a running suture of 2/0 chromic catgut (Figure 5.17) if the parenchyma is not too thick and its consistency will accept a running suture. Residual ooze is handled in similar fashion in all instances, namely by the application of a topical haemostatic agent in as minimal quantities as possible to prevent excessive foreign body reaction.

The splenic remnant is then carefully reposited in the left upper quadrant (Figure 5.18). Upper pole remnants lie more naturally in the old splenic fossa, but lower pole remnants also seem to find their place without difficulty. We have had no instances of torsion of a remnant and see no need to fix the remnant to adjacent structures or to parietal peritoneum.

The exact amount of intact splenic parenchyma necessary to preserve full immunological competence is not known with certainty since experimental results vary and clinical evidence is still sparse. Viable remnants of any size with intact circulation should be preserved. If more than one remnant is vascularized, is obviously viable and is not bleeding, it should be preserved. Separated remnants will adhere naturally if juxtaposed. They may also be held together in an omental pocket. A synthetic mesh for holding multiple fragments coapted has been described.[16] The surgical objective is to preserve as much viable spleen as possible. Twenty-five per cent seems to be the minimal amount necessary for preservation of function; an amount approaching 50% is undoubtedly better.

New adjuncts to splenic preservation recently described include 'gluing' with highly concentrated human fibrinogen,[17] coaptation with fibrin tissue adhesive and collagen fleece[18] and a seemingly endless number of absorbable topical haemostatic agents. It is as yet too early to evaluate the 'fibrin glue' method, and the new haemostatic agents seem to offer no improvement over those already in use.

Drains

There is no indication for the use of drains following conservative surgery on the spleen unless there

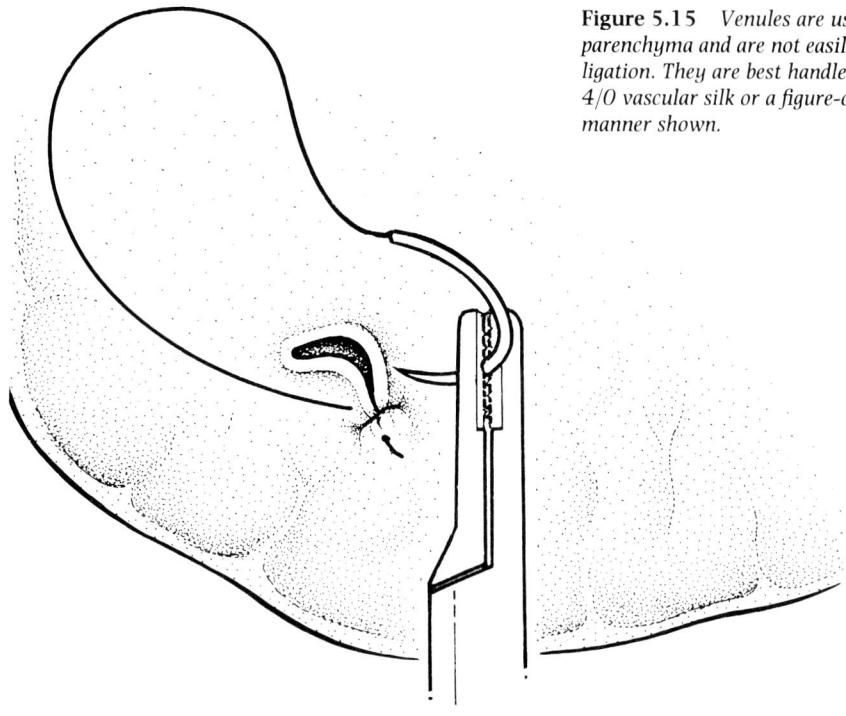

Figure 5.15 *Venules are usually flattened in the splenic parenchyma and are not easily grasped for clipping or ligation. They are best handled with a running suture of 4/0 vascular silk or a figure-of-eight suture applied in the manner shown.*

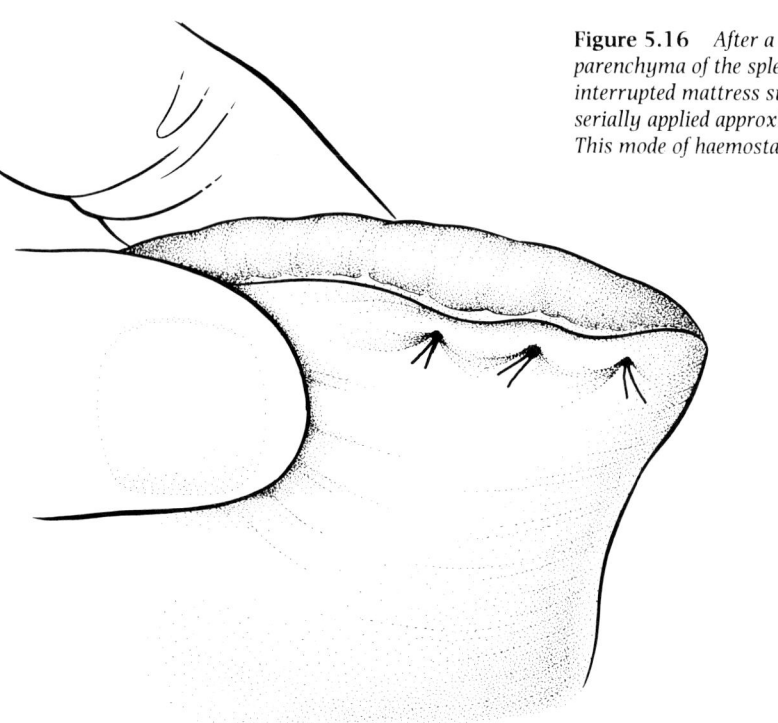

Figure 5.16 *After a segmental resection, if the divided parenchyma of the splenic remnant is thin enough, interrupted mattress sutures of 2/0 chromic catgut may be serially applied approximately 1 cm from the raw surface. This mode of haemostasis is depicted above.*

CONSERVATIVE SURGERY OF THE SPLEEN 89

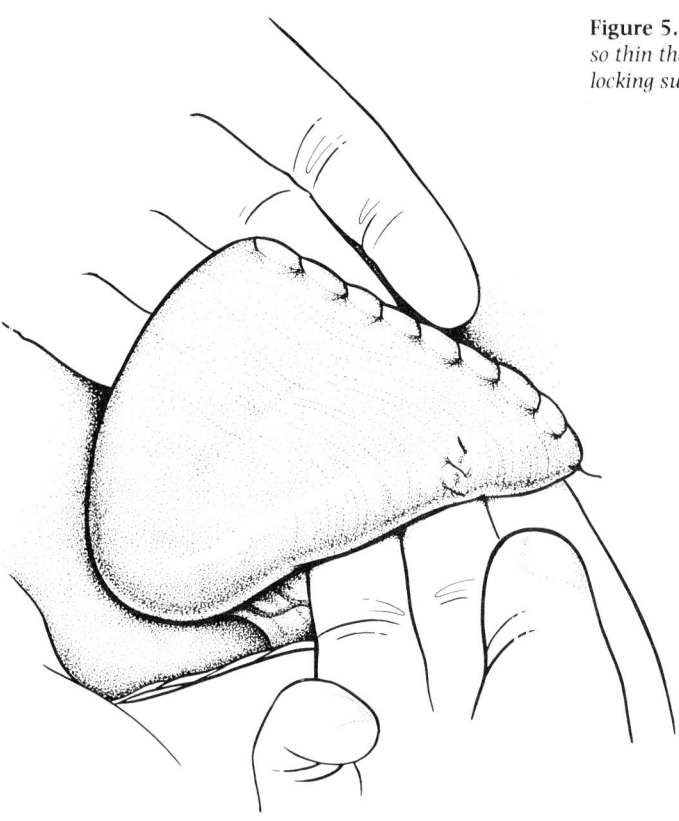

Figure 5.17 *In selected cases the transected parenchyma is so thin that it lends itself to a running suture or a running locking suture applied along the divided splenic surface.*

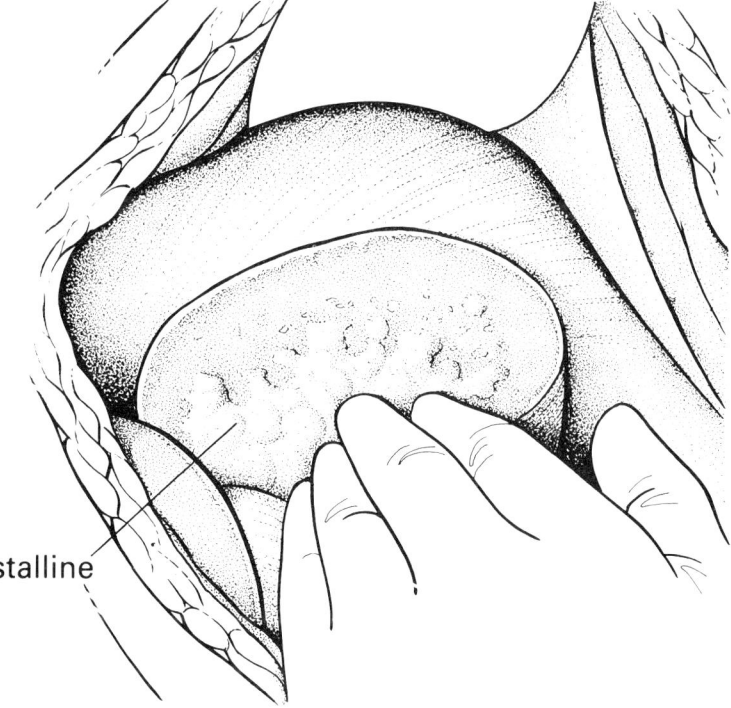

Figure 5.18 *With all major bleeding vessels controlled by ligation or clipping, any residual surface ooze is controlled by the application of a topical haemostatic agent such as microcrystalline collagen and the spleen is carefully reposited in the left upper quadrant of the abdomen. It is best to observe the reposited spleen for five, or 10 minutes in its final position to make sure that no ooze occurs after replacement.*

Microcrystalline collagen

is associated pancreatic injury. If the pancreas is not injured and the pancreatic tail is well protected during the procedure, drainage is unnecessary. The drain is not a good indicator of haemorrhage; in fact it may be deceptive since major bleeding may occur without any manifest sanguineous drainage via the drain site.

When drainage is employed for suspected associated injury, either a soft rubber drain (Penrose) or a silicone drain (Jackson–Pratt) may be used. Drainage should be collected in sterile drainage bags rather than allowed to drain onto bulky dressings. Since they allow for ingress of bacteria as well as external drainage, they should be removed as soon as possible.

SPLENIC IMPLANTS

In the event that splenic repair or partial salvage is impossible, an alternative is the planned implantation of fragments of spleen into an omental pocket or bursa, constituting a 'controlled splenosis'. There has been considerable controversy regarding the immunological competence of such implants,[19,20] with no apparent decisive resolution of the problem to date. There is no question that implants can eventually be demonstrated to be viable splenic tissue by scintiscan; whether or not they are truly functional is still disputable. Overwhelming postsplenectomy sepsis has been known to occur in patients with known splenosis.[21] There is some evidence that suggests that an intact splenic circulation is necessary for effective immunological function.

Since the matter is in doubt, I see little disadvantage in employing a safe technique of splenic implantation when splenic salvage is impossible.

The technique is simple. The excised spleen or splenic fragments are used to fashion implants which measure $20 \times 20 \times 1.0$ mm in size. The implants are made thin since they parasitize the omentum for a new blood supply. Their immediate fate is almost total degeneration and then a slow regeneration from neovascularized focal remnants. The regenerated implant does not have normal architecture but does exhibit some semblance of the red pulp sinusoidal pattern. Regeneration of the white pulp is less prominent.

The splenic implants are individually sutured to a predetermined segment of omentum which is then fashioned into an omental pouch. A simple suture or clip will suffice to keep the fragments suitably separated. To achieve an aggregate splenic mass equivalent to 25 g of spleen or more it is necessary to use about 25 implants. The implants are placed on the omentum as shown in Figure 5.19; when the requisite number of fragments has been placed, the omentum is folded over the implants, sandwiching the implants between the two layers of omentum.

Other methods have been employed such as fragmenting the spleen with an ordinary vegetable grater,[22] or using a pocket of peritoneum for the

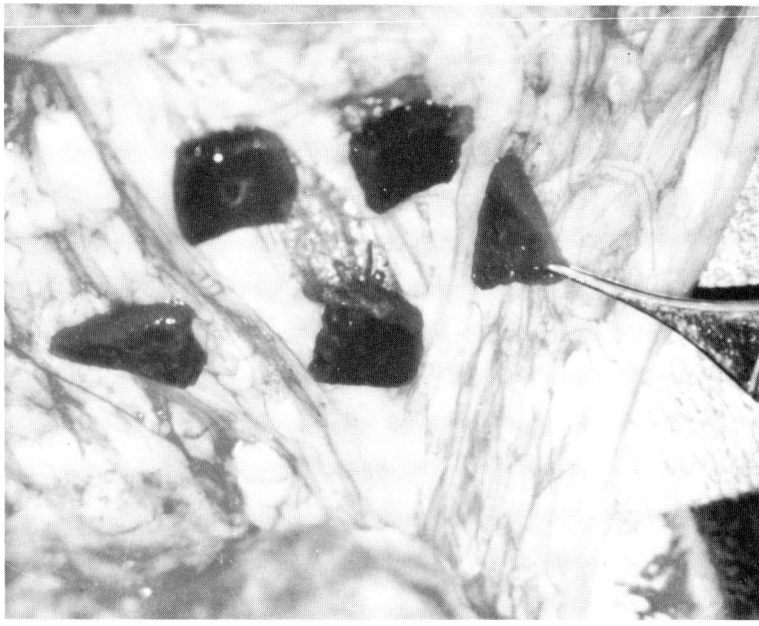

Figure 5.19 *Fragments of splenic tissue fashioned from the intact spleen and measuring approximately $20 \times 20 \times 1$ mm are placed in the omentum as shown. Each splenic fragment should be held in position with a single clip or atraumatic suture of 4/0 silk. After all the fragments have been placed in position the omentum is folded on itself over the fragments to form an omental pouch.*

implant. These methods have no advantage over the omental-implant technique.

Splenic implants cannot be completely relied on as yet to offer protection against overwhelming sepsis to encapsulated pathogens. Hence, patients who have had splenic implantation should, nevertheless, be immunized with the polyvalent pneumococcal vaccine and with the other vaccines against meningococcus and *Haemophilus influenzae* as they become available. Antibiotic prophylaxis should also be continued in these individuals.

POSTOPERATIVE CARE

Care and observation in the intensive care unit for 24 or 48 hours is advisable for patients who have had splenorrhaphy, or partial resection. Abdominal examination for distension or ileus and serial haemoglobin and haematocrit determinations are the best guides to untoward postoperative sequelae such as bleeding. I prefer to retain the nasogastric tube (placed before operation) for suction drainage for a period of 24 hours to preclude any complications from postoperative gastric dilatation or emesis. Some surgeons feel this is unnecessary.

Antibiotics are not administered unless there is a reason other than the splenic operation itself, such as contamination, pneumonitis or some other extrasplenic cause.

Deep breathing is encouraged but vigorous respiratory therapy (especially physiotherapy) is not. Nearly all patients will develop a transitory minor left pleural effusion which clears in a matter of days or weeks.

Leukocytosis following splenic surgery may be marked and in itself is no cause for alarm. We have also observed that some patients develop a marked thrombocytosis (over one million) following splenorrhaphy or partial resection. This is transitory and does not require drug therapy.

OUTCOME

Conservative procedures on the spleen have become standard practice in most major surgical centres. In children's hospitals, either non-operative management or attempted salvage, for all splenic injuries, has met with remarkable success. Only 10–20% of splenic injuries result in total splenectomy. In adult trauma centres as well, the practice of non-operative management is gaining increasing popularity in carefully selected cases, and the success rate for attempted splenic salvage is between 30% and 50%. More operations are also being done for such benign conditions as splenic cysts, and the benign hypersplenic conditions described above in the text.

Considering the large numbers of such procedures now being done worldwide, there have been remarkably few published reports of treatment failures. No doubt, there have been instances of bleeding following conservative splenic surgery, but there is doubt in the mind of the author that the instances of bleeding following total splenectomy exceed those following lesser procedures on the spleen. With careful attention to operative technique, and special handling of the delicate splenic parenchyma, it is possible to do the procedures described above with maximal safety and minimal operative risk. In the author's experience with over 100 cases of splenic salvage, there has not been one instance where reoperation has been necessary for rebleeding or any other complication related to the spleen or splenic remnant.

The theoretical risks of non-operative management are the late development of traumatic splenic cysts and disseminated splenosis. Neither of these complications has as yet been reported in the literature as significant factors in morbidity or mortality. Two verbal reports have reached the author about the necessity for reoperation on splenic remnants which have become devitalized and cystified because of inadequate blood supply. Such complications are exceedingly rare and should be non-existent with increased experience in the handling of the splenic remnant.

The true value of splenic implantation, whatever method is used in preserving the fragments, remains in doubt. The experimental work, based mainly on pneumococcal challenge in splenectomized and non-splenectomized experimental animals, is as yet inconclusive. Nevertheless, this method is a non-harmful alternative to total splenic extirpation; and only increasing experience and careful patient follow up will answer the unresolved issues.

A major problem in supporting the rationale for conservative splenic surgery has been the difficulty in documenting the true incidence of the immunological sequelae which occur in the asplenic individual. Most reports which now exist in the literature on the subject are retrospective reports[2,4,23] which are fraught with statistical pitfalls. There have been some attempts at prospective case-gathering studies, but as yet, the numbers are too small to be significant. Nevertheless, the combined anecdotal evidence for the existence and prevalence of overwhelming post splenectomy sepsis is undeniable.

Enthusiasm in any surgical procedure must be tempered with good surgical judgement. The incidence of overwhelming post-splenectomy sepsis is low, particularly when the splenectomy is performed for trauma. Hence, no undue risk should be taken if the risk of salvage exceeds the risk of future complications. In this author's opinion, such occasions are exceedingly rare.

Iatrogenic injuries occurring during left upper quadrant surgery used to account for approximately 20% of all splenectomies performed in most large hospitals. With the newer knowledge of splenic anatomy, the vulnerability of the spleen to minor trauma, and the successful methods of treatment of minor iatrogenic trauma, the incidence of 'accidental splenectomy' should be reduced to near zero.

In summary, the spleen is an organ which has suffered a long winter of surgical neglect. Only recently have techniques and materials grown equal to the demanding technical skills necessary for splenic salvage. The growing literature on the increasing immunological importance of the spleen demands that the modern surgeon should be qualified and capable of saving all or part of this organ in those patients where its salvage can be performed safely, and without undue risk.

Acknowledgement

The author expresses his grateful appreciation to Ms Deena Bailey, Ms Judi Lippe and Mr James Rosenberg for their invaluable assistance in the preparation of this chapter.

REFERENCES

1. Witte MH, Witte CL, Van Wyck DB & Farrell KJ (1983) Preservation of the spleen. *Lymphology* 16: 128–137.
2. Francke EL & Neu HC (1981) Postsplenectomy infection. *Surgical Clinics of North America* 61: 135–155.
3. Morgenstern L (1977) The avoidable complications of splenectomy. *Surgery, Gynecology & Obstetrics* 145, 525–528.
4. Singer DB (1973) Postsplenectomy sepsis. *Perspectives in Pediatric Pathology* 1: 285–311.
5. O'Neal BJ & McDonald JC (1981) The risk of sepsis in the asplenic adult. *Annals of Surgery* 194: 775–778.
6. Morgenstern L & Shapiro SJ (1980) Partial splenectomy for nonparasitic splenic cysts. *American Journal of Surgery* 139: 278–281.
7. Millar JS (1982) Partial excision and drainage of post-traumatic splenic cysts. *British Journal of Surgery* 69: 477–478.
8. Christo MC (1984) Personal communication. Brazil, April 20, 1984.
9. Govrin-Yehudain J & Bar-Maor JA (1980) Partial splenectomy of Gaucher's disease. *Israel Journal of Medical Sciences* 16: 665–668.
10. Pringle KC, Spigos DG, Tan WS, Politis C, Pang EJ, Reyez HM & Georgiopoulou P (1982) Partial splenic embolization in the management of thalassemia major. *Journal of Pediatric Surgery* 17: 884–891.
11. Kamel R & Dunn MA (1982) Segmental splenectomy in schistosomiasis. *British Journal of Surgery* 69: 311–313.
12. Berci, G, Dunkelman D, Michel SL, Sanders G, Wahlstrom E & Morgenstern L (1983) Emergency mini-laparoscopy in abdominal trauma: an update. *American Journal of Surgery* 146: 261–265.
13. Morgenstern L & Uyeda RY (1983) Nonoperative management of injuries of the spleen in adults. *Surgery, Gynecology & Obstetrics* 157: 513–518.
14. Wesson DE, Filler RM, Ein SH, Shandling B, Simpson JS & Stephens CA (1981) Ruptured spleen—when to operate? *Journal of Pediatric Surgery* 16: 324–326.
15. King DR, Lobe TE, Haase GM & Boles ET (1981) Selective management of injured spleen. *Surgery* 90: 677–682.
16. Delany HM, Porreca F, Mitsudo S, Solanki B & Rudavsky A (1982) Splenic capping: an experimental study of a new technique for splenorrhaphy using woven polyglycolic acid mesh. *Annals of Surgery* 196: 187–193.
17. Brands W, Mennicken C & Beck M (1982) Preservation of the ruptured spleen by gluing with highly concentrated human fibrinogen: experimental and clinical results. *World Journal of Surgery* 6: 366–368.
18. Scheele J, Gentsch HH & Matteson E (1984) Splenic repair by fibrin tissue adhesive and collagen fleece. *Surgery* 95: 6–13.
19. Oakes DD & Sherck J (1982) Splenic trauma, splenosis, and death from sepsis (letter). *JAMA* 247: 1404–1405.
20. Patel J, Williams JS, Shmigel B & Hinshaw JR (1981) Preservation of splenic function by autotransplantation of traumatized spleen in man. *Surgery* 90: 683–688.
21. Scully RE, Galdabini JJ & McNeely BU (1975) Case records of the Massachusetts General Hospital. Weekly clinicopathological exercises. Case 36–1975. *New England Journal of Medicine* 293: 547–553.
22. Seufert RM, Böttcher W, Munz D & Heusermann U (1981) Erste klinische Erfahrungen mit der heterotopen Autotransplantation der Milz. *Chirurg* 52: 525–530.
23. Oakes DD (1981) Splenic trauma. *Current Problems in Surgery* 18: 341–401.

6

Segmentectomy 4

Henri Bismuth
Denis Castaing

According to the functional anatomy,[1] the liver is divided into two livers (or hemilivers) by the main portal scissura, also called Cantlie's line. These right and left livers are themselves divided into two parts by two other portal scissurae which, according to Couinaud's nomenclature,[2] are called sectors. These four sectors are themselves divided into seven segments. In total, with the spigelian lobe which represents an additional segment, the liver is divided into eight segments. Figure 6.1 shows these eight segments.

Therefore, according to Couinaud, a segment is the smallest anatomical unit of the liver. The segment described by Couinaud corresponds approxi-

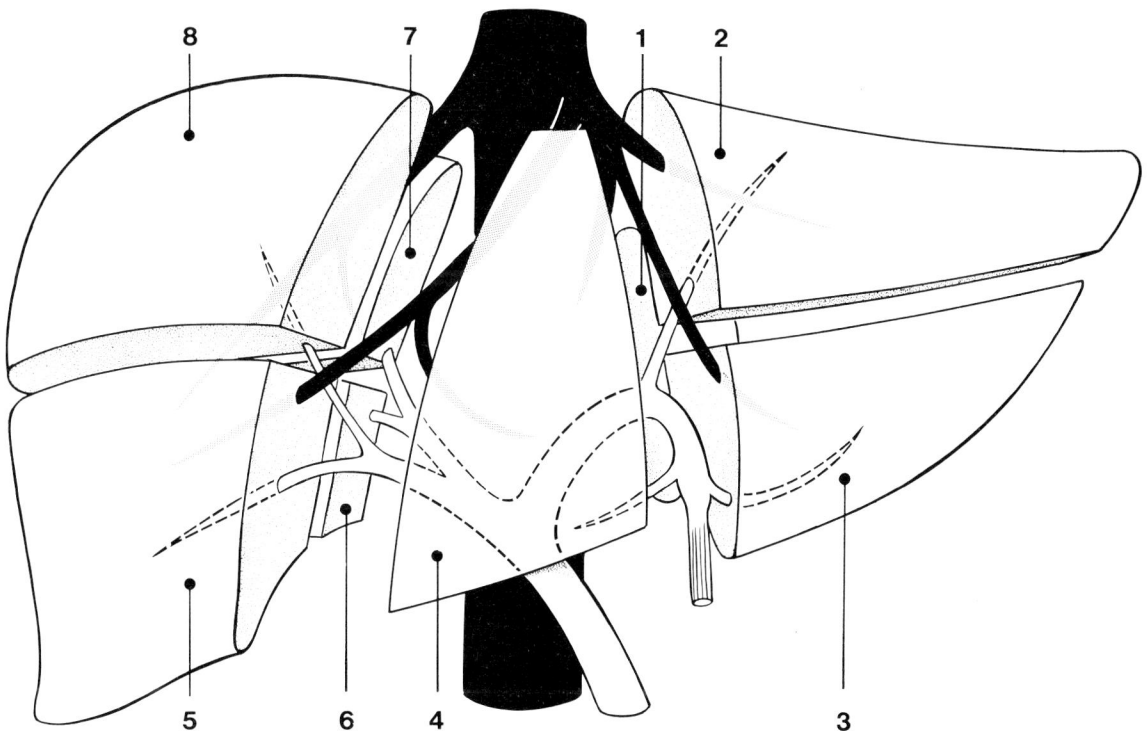

Figure 6.1 *Anatomy of the liver: the eight segments, according to Couinaud.*[2]

mately to the subsegment described by Goldsmith and Woodburne.[3] It is different from the area described by Healey and Schroy,[4] which is based on the biliary distribution rather than on the portal distribution.

The resection of one of the eight segments of the liver is called a segmentectomy: unisegmentectomy when one segment is removed, plurisegmentectomy when two or more segments are removed. Liver segmentectomies are intermediate procedures between the four common hepatectomies and the small atypical wedge resections. Segmentectomies are 'réglées' because they follow exclusively the anatomical liver scissurae that separate the different segments of the gland. Respect of these scissurae during segmental excisions prevents impairment of the vascularization of the remaining parenchyma and excessive bleeding. A thorough knowledge of the anatomical structure of the liver is a prerequisite to carrying out liver segmentectomies.[5]

Segment 4 is the right part of the medial sector of the left hemiliver (medial sector = segments 4 and 3). It lies between the middle hepatic vein, which lies in the main hepatic scissura, and the round ligament scissura. As the middle hepatic scissura represents the separation between the two hemilivers (functional division of the liver) and the round ligament scissura represents the separation between the two lobes (morphological division of the liver), the segment 4 represents the difference between the right hemihepatectomy and the right lobectomy. Its inferior surface has two parts: one is free and appears limited by the gallbladder fossa, the hilus and the round ligament fissura, and the other, situated behind the hilus, is in front of the segment 1; there is not an apparent line of division between segment 4 and segment 1.

Segmentectomy 4 permits the anatomical resection of hepatic lesions without the unnecessary removal of a large amount of normal parenchyma. It is particularly useful (a) in some benign tumours; (b) for some carcinomas of the gallbladder; (c) for removal of small central hepatocarcinomas and hilar cholangiocarcinoma; (d) for liver resections in cirrhotic patients; and (e) more rarely for biliary surgery above the hilus.

SEGMENTECTOMY 4 (Figure 6.2)

Anterior segmentectomy 4

Usually, only the anterior and mobile part of segment 4 is removed. This anterior portion is located anteriorly to the liver hilus and corresponds to the

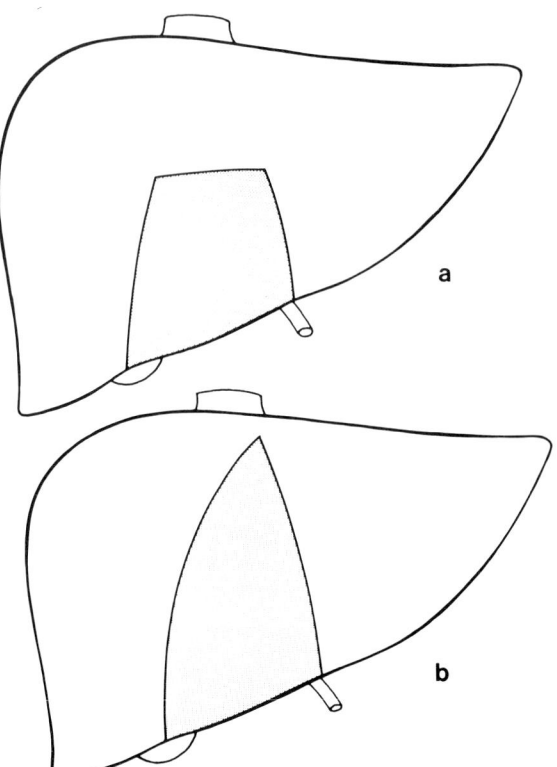

Figure 6.2 (a) *Anterior segmentectomy 4: resection of quadrate lobe;* (b) *total segmentectomy 4.*

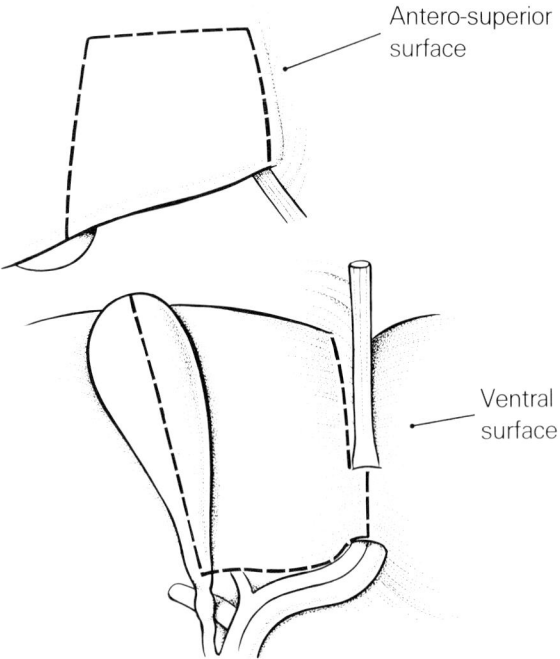

Figure 6.3 *The limits of anterior resection of segment 4.*

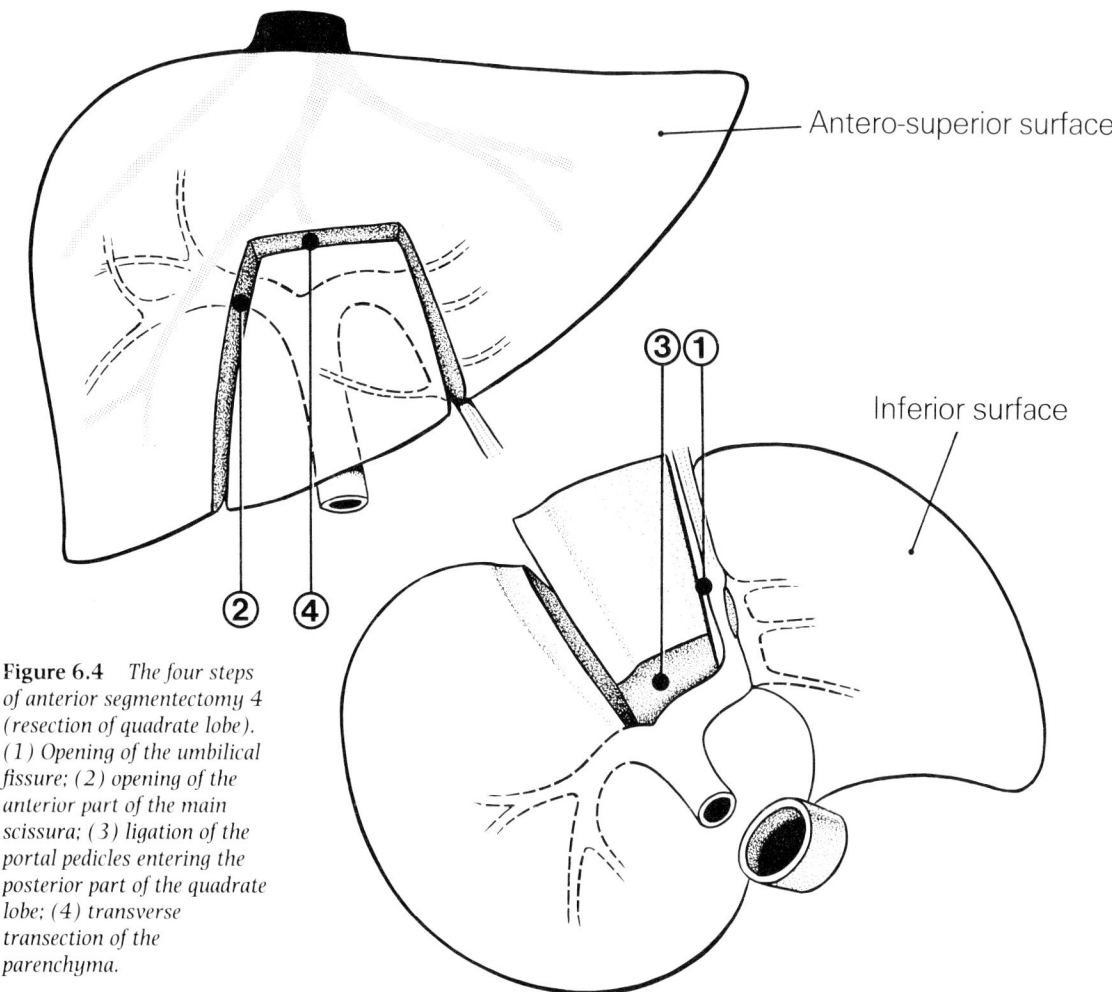

Figure 6.4 *The four steps of anterior segmentectomy 4 (resection of quadrate lobe). (1) Opening of the umbilical fissure; (2) opening of the anterior part of the main scissura; (3) ligation of the portal pedicles entering the posterior part of the quadrate lobe; (4) transverse transection of the parenchyma.*

quadrate lobe. This lobe is limited to the left by the umbilical fissure and to the right by the main scissura (Figure 6.3).

Anterior segmentectomy 4: resection of quadrate lobe

Performed for the first time by Caprio,[6] this technique was fully described by Champeau and Pineau[7] who extended its use to biliary surgery by proposing either the mobilization or the resection of the quadrate lobe for gaining access to the superior part of the biliary confluence. The four steps of the operations are summarized in Figure 6.4.

Through a midline or right subcostal incision, the round ligament and the anterior part of the falciform ligament are divided (Figure 6.5). The first step of the resection consists of dividing the bridge of parenchyma which frequently joins segments 3 and 4 below the round ligament (Figure 6.5). The round ligament is pulled upward, exposing the inferior surface of the quadrate and the left lobes. The bridge of parenchyma is transected by crushing it down with a Kelly clamp and by electrocoagulation or ligation of the small vessels. Then, the peritoneum is divided at the inferior part of the round ligament and the underlying vascular elements are dissected to the right. The vessels going to the left must be respected because they vascularize the left lobe. Two or three arterial and portal pedicles are usually dissected. The portal pedicles are behind the arterial pedicles which are superficial. In depth, there is a fibrous tissue, which constitutes the superior limit of the umbilical portion of the round ligament and in which two biliary ducts are usually present.

Figure 6.5 *First step: opening of the inferior surface of the round ligament, after section of the bridge of parenchyma which lies over the ligament. Ligation of the vessels towards the quadrate lobe is carried out.*

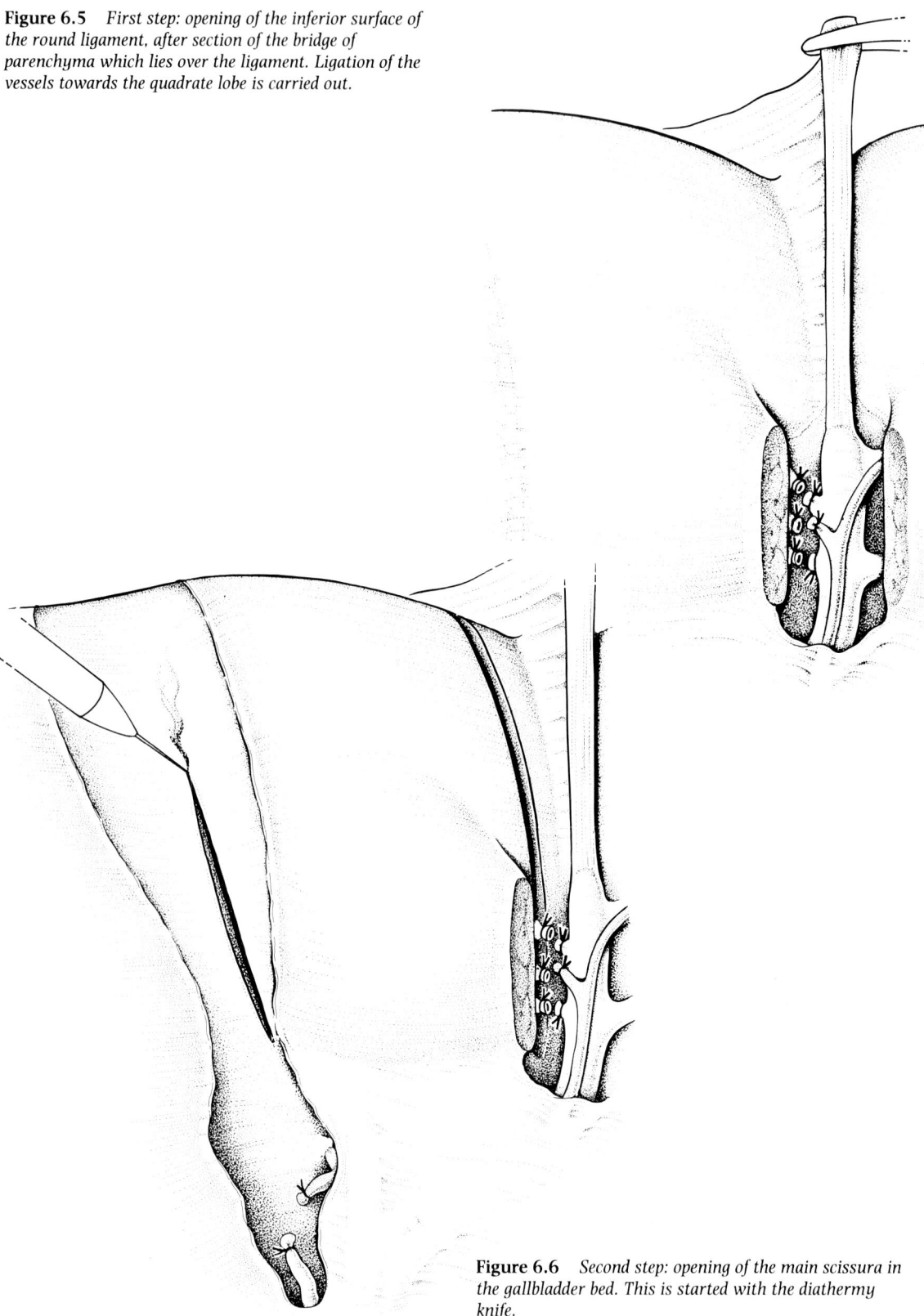

Figure 6.6 *Second step: opening of the main scissura in the gallbladder bed. This is started with the diathermy knife.*

The liver parenchyma is then opened on the right of the falciform ligament without trespassing the level of the left border of the hilus.

The next step is the opening of the main scissura (Figure 6.6). The gallbladder is removed or if cholecystectomy is not necessary the gallbladder bed is exposed on its left side until the middle of the fossa has been exposed.

From the anterior border of the liver and along the main scissura, the liver is transected up to the vertex of the hilus. There are no portal branches in this scissura and the only major vascular elements requiring ligation are the left branches of the middle hepatic vein. It is preferable to transect the liver a little to the left of the main scissura to avoid the middle hepatic vein.

The third step is the ligation of the vessels coming from the hilus to the posterior border of the quadrate lobe (Figure 6.7). At the inferior part of the liver, the capsule of Glisson is incised in front of the peritoneum of the hilus and some small arterial and portal branches of the quadrate lobe are ligated and divided.

Subsequently, a transverse incision of the capsule of Glisson is made at the anterior surface of the liver, which joins the posterior ends of the right and left liver transections. This posterior liver transection is performed progressively by crushing down the parenchyma (Figure 6.8 and 6.9). During this transection, three to five branches of the middle hepatic vein are divided. Cautious haemostasis of the opened parenchyma must be obtained

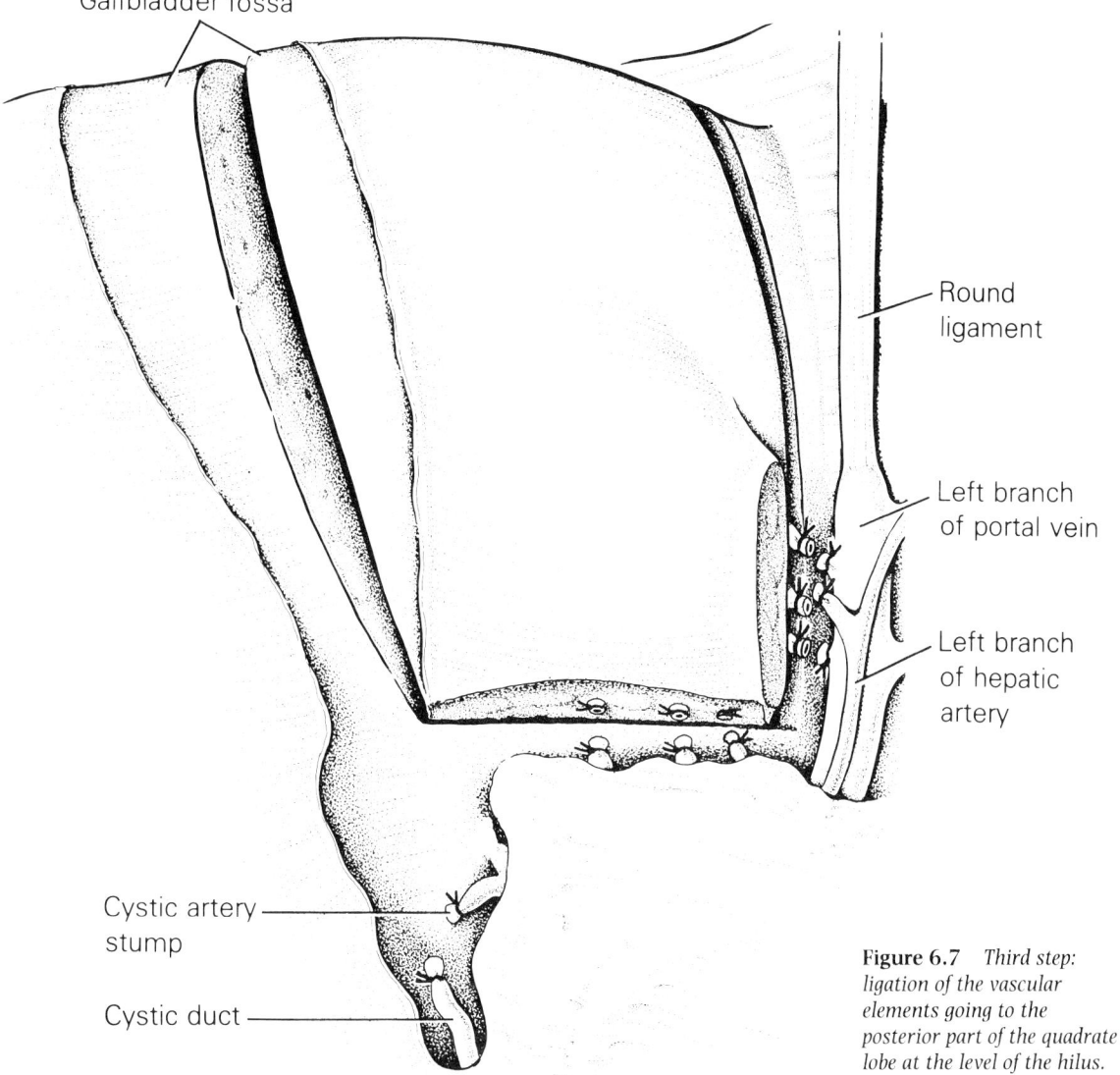

Figure 6.7 *Third step: ligation of the vascular elements going to the posterior part of the quadrate lobe at the level of the hilus.*

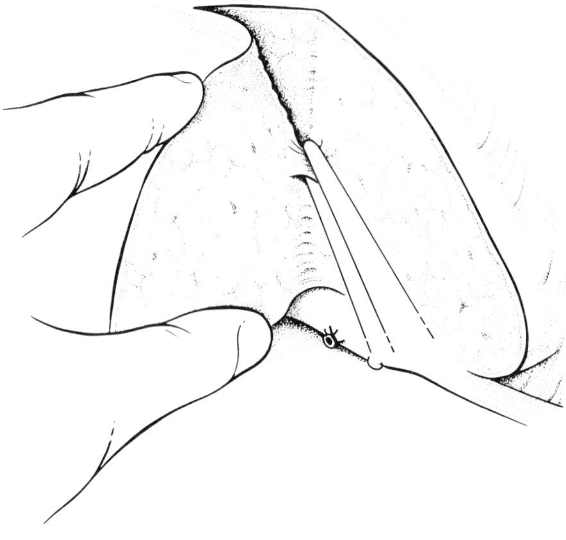

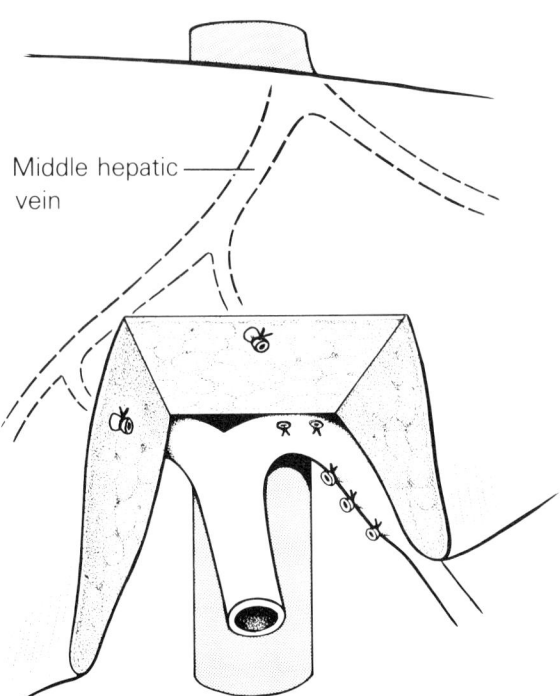

Figure 6.8 *Fourth step: transverse incision of the liver joining the left and the right incisions.*

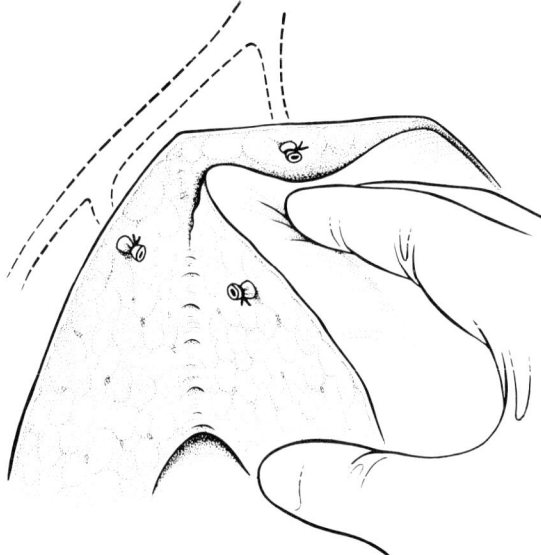

Figure 6.9 *Fourth step: ligation of the branches of the middle hepatic vein.*

and has to be controlled after removal of the quadrate lobe (Figure 6.10).

Anterior segmentectomy 4 for intrahepatic biliary anastomosis (Figure 6.11)

For palliative treatment of carcinoma of the hilus, if biliary drainage of the two lobes is indicated, we have been able to achieve a double intrahepatic cholangioanastomosis by resection of the quadrate lobe.[8]

Figure 6.10 *Completion of the anterior segmentectomy 4.*

By opening the hepatic parenchyma to the right of the round ligament, one or two portal pedicles are found: only the portal and arterial branches are ligated and the bile ducts are open. Completion of the anterior segmentectomy is performed as in the usual technique described above. Since this opening of the parenchyma on the right follows the main scissura, there is no biliary duct in this hepatic section: to expose the duct of segment 5, an additional wedge-shaped incision has to be made perpendicular to the wedge sissura to the right. The duct of segment 5 is incised longitudinally. On the left, the larger duct is kept intact whereas the other is ligated. Therefore, two intrahepatic ducts are used for the double anastomosis: one on the right, the duct of segment 5, in communication with the right lobe, and one on the left, the duct of the excised segment 4, which is in communication with the left liver. The two anastomoses are performed on the same jejunal loop which lies in the space created by excision of the quadrate lobe (Figure 6.11).

With the help of intra-operative ultrasound, a more elegant technique can be used. After ultrasound detection of the dilated duct of segment 5, the parenchyma is opened according to the hepatic scissura (and not the portal scissura), leading directly to the duct of segment 5 (Figure 6.11b).

SEGMENTECTOMY 4   99

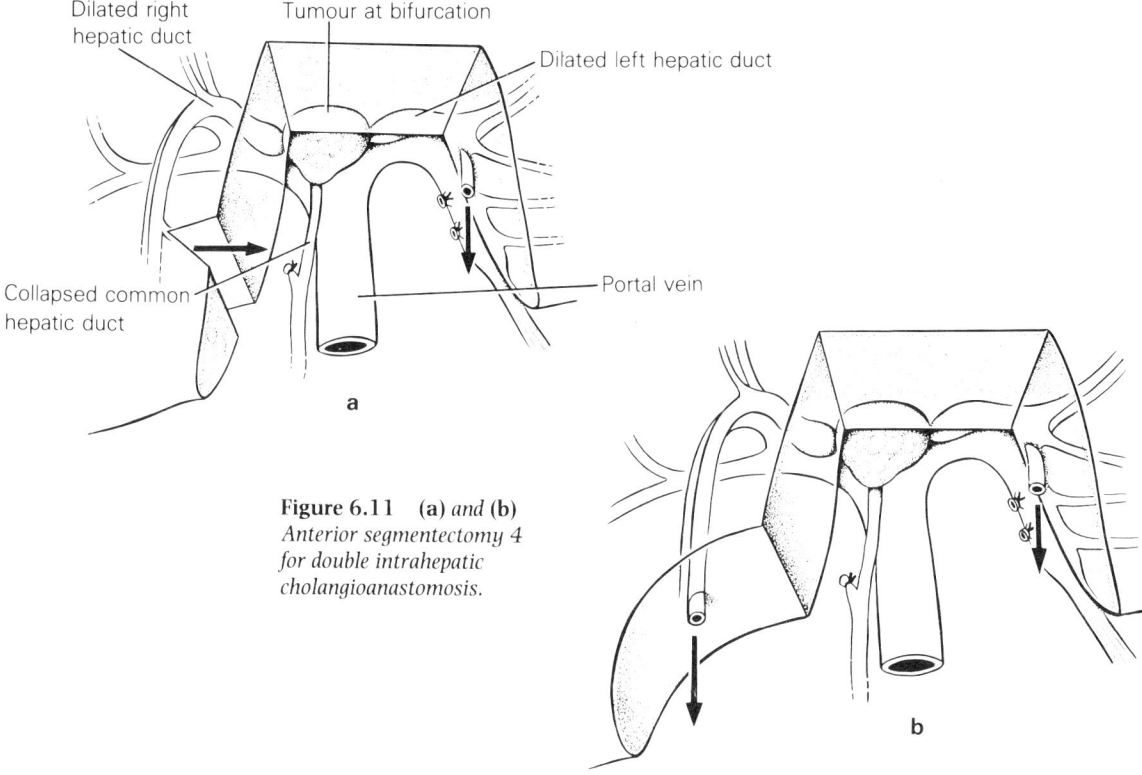

Figure 6.11 (a) *and* (b) *Anterior segmentectomy 4 for double intrahepatic cholangioanastomosis.*

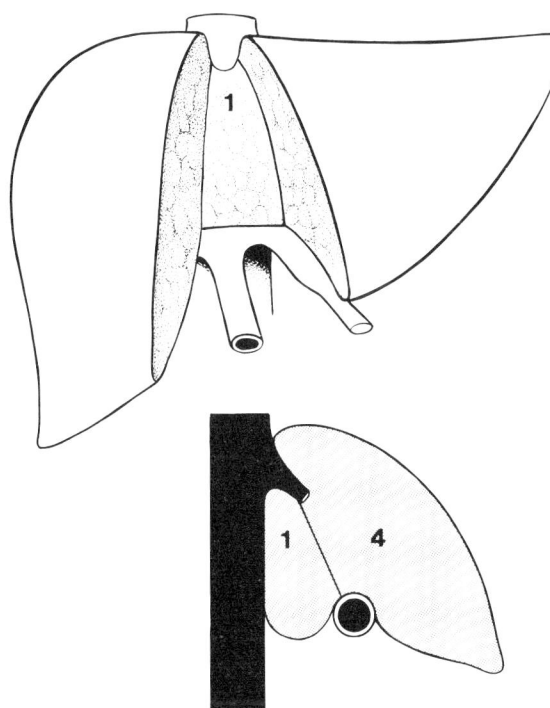

Figure 6.12 *Complete segmentectomy 4: the relationship of segment 4 to segment 1.*

Complete segmentectomy 4

This procedure is equivalent to the complete resection of the medial part of the liver (Figure 6.12). Segment 4 is removed up to the anterior surface of the vena cava.

The first steps are similar to those performed for the resection of the quadrate lobe. However, the two posteriorly directed parenchymatous transections are extended up to the vena cava. The middle hepatic vein, which is usually located posteriorly, close to the vena cava, is not divided during this complete segmentectomy 4. However, when the vein crosses the posterior part of segment 4 transversely to join more anteriorly the left hepatic vein, it may be necessary to ligate it without risk to the remaining parenchyma.

Since segment 4 is just anterior to the spigelian lobe (segment 1), the last step of the resection is to separate these two segments. There is no visible demarcation between the posterior and inferior parts of segment 4 and the anterior and superior parts of segment 1, so, for this reason, this last step can cause bleeding.

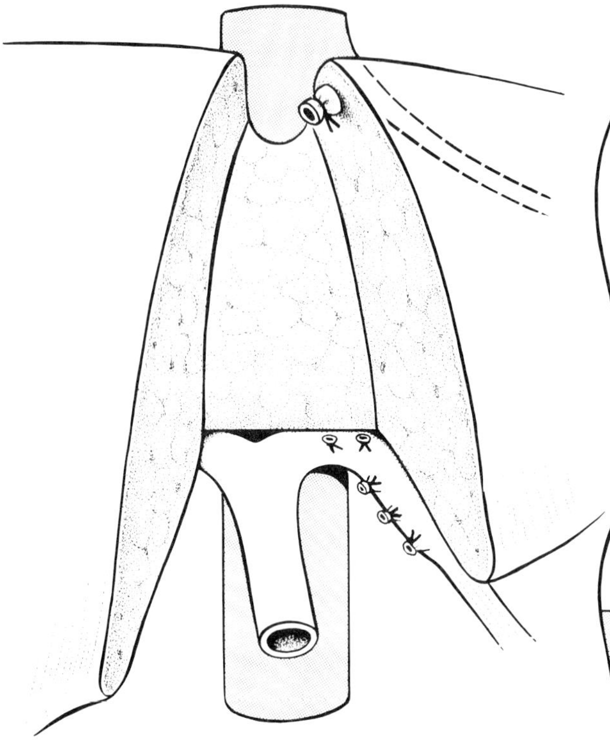

Figure 6.13 *Complete segmentectomy 4.*

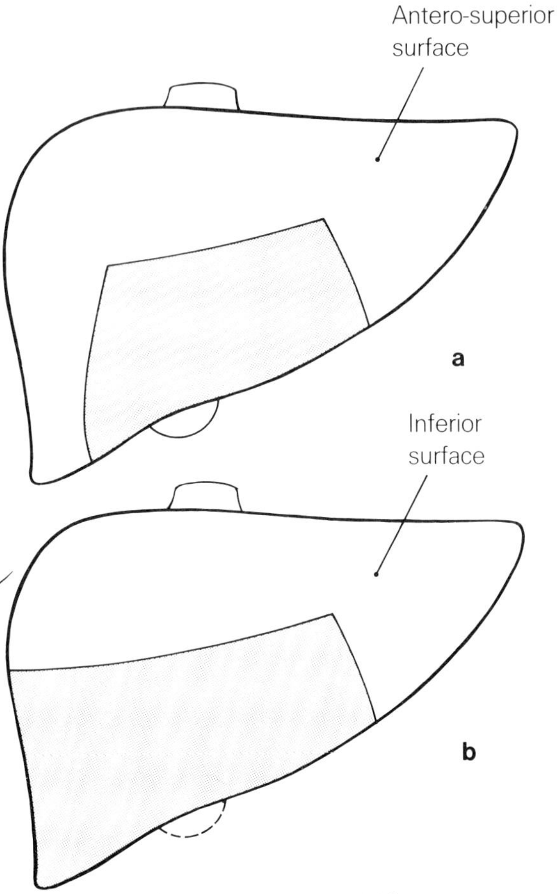

Figure 6.14 *Plurisegmentectomy 4:* **(a)** *bisegmentectomy 4–5;* **(b)** *trisegmentectomy 4–5–6.*

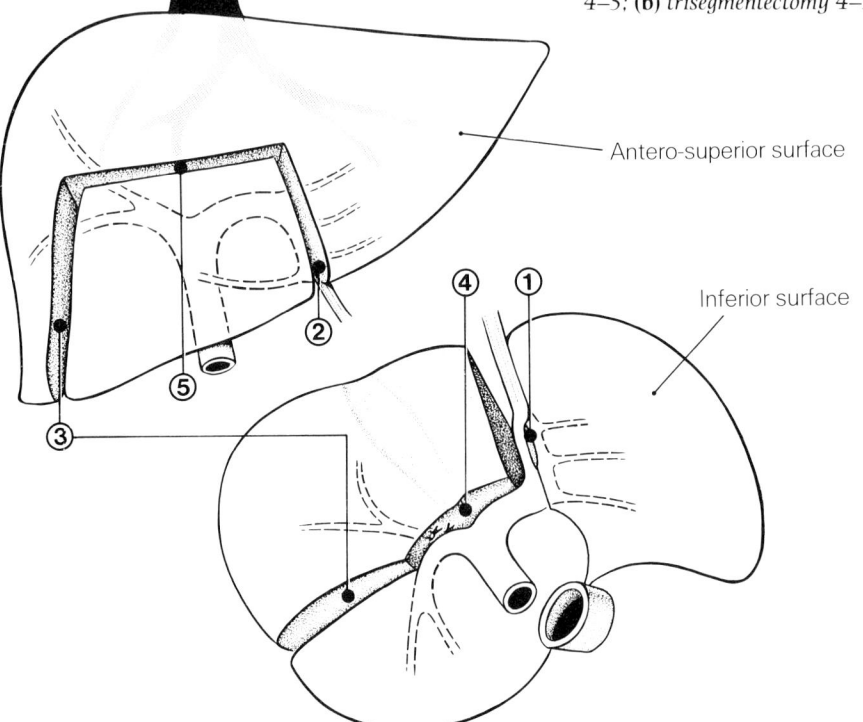

Figure 6.15 *Steps of bisegmentectomy 4–5.*

After complete resection of segment 4 (Figure 6.13), the liver is almost split into two parts and an approximation of the two parts may be necessary to avoid the stomach and duodenum occupying the wide space between the right liver and the left lobe.

PLURISEGMENTECTOMY (Figure 6.14)

Bisegmentectomy 4–5

This operation (Figure 6.15) has an elective indication which is cancer of the gallbladder. Indeed, the gallbladder is located at the level of the main scissura of the liver so a typical resection of the contiguous hepatic parenchyma requires the resection of segments 4 and 5. An extended right hepatectomy (which is necessary when the tumour occupies a large part of the right liver) is, in our opinion,[5] unnecessary when the cancer remains confined to the gallbladder bed or when it is discovered histologically following cholecystectomy for gallstones.

The main technical step in bisegmentectomy 4–5 is the ligation of the portal pedicle of segments 4 and 5. The ligation must be done without impairing the vascularization of the right liver and of the left lobe. The operation is performed through a right subcostal incision. The round ligament and the falciform ligament are divided. The first step of the resection is the ligation of the portal pedicles of segment 4 on the right part of the round ligament, as described for segmentectomy 4.

The second step is the left parenchymatous transection which is conducted along the umbilical fissure. The third step is the right liver transection. This transection must follow the right lateral scissura in which lies the right hepatic vein. However there is no landmark at the surface of the liver for recognizing the scissure. Previously we opened the liver, according to a line parallel to the main hepatic scissura 4 cm on its right. But this is a very approximative way of doing it. Nowadays we use peroperative ultrasound to find the right hepatic vein and the right anterior portal pedicle of segment 5. At the inferior part of the liver, the transection is directed towards the right portal pedicle. During this transection, the large right paramedian portal pedicle is located and only its anterior branch is ligated. The fourth step is the ligation of the portal branches on the posterior part of the quadrate lobe. The fifth step is the posterior parenchymatous transection which joins the left and

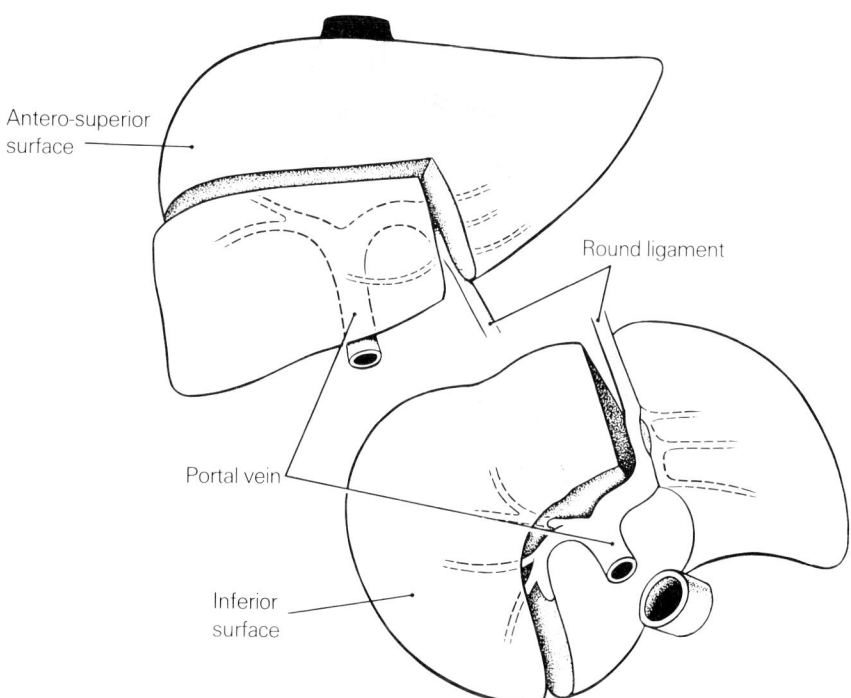

Figure 6.16 *Steps of trisegmentectomy 4–5–6.*

right transections in front of the hilus. During this transverse transection the large middle hepatic vein is ligated and divided.

Trisegmentectomy 4–5–6

Described by Ton That Tung[9] as an extended medial hepatectomy, the resection of segments 4, 5 and 6 was proposed by Couinaud[2] for treatment of carcinoma of the gallbladder because the cystic veins are likely to end in the portal branch of segment 6 (Figure 6.16). The first step of this trisegmentectomy is the same as for the resection of the quadrate lobe: division of the portal pedicles of segment 4 on the right part of the umbilical fissure. Then, the liver is transected along the umbilical fissure up to the level of the hilus. Afterwards, the capsule of Glisson is incised transversely towards the right side of the liver and, from this side, a long transverse transection is performed which leads to division of the portal pedicles of segments 5 and 6, of the origin of the right hepatic and middle hepatic veins.

INDICATIONS FOR SEGMENTECTOMY 4

We have now performed 21 segmentectomies 4 which have been limited to segment 4, or extended to segment 5 or to segments 5 and 6 (Table 6.1).

The indications and results of these liver resections are listed in Tables 6.2, 6.3, 6.4 and 6.5. When a

Table 6.1 *Segmentectomy 4: 21 cases.*

Segmentectomy 4 (anterior, 10; complete, 1)	11
Bisegmentectomy 4–5	6
Trisegmentectomy 4–5–6	4

tumour is located in segment 4, the hepatectomy usually indicated is either a right extended hepatectomy or a left extended hepatectomy (corresponding to what Starzl calls a right or left trisegmentectomy).[10,11] When the tumour is benign or small this resection appears to be very extensive and sometimes disproportionately so, given the objective. In addition, in some patients when the left lobe is small there is a risk of postoperative failure.[12]

The indications for segmentectomy 4 are:

1. Benign tumour
2. Small carcinomas
3. Exposure of the biliary confluence and/or intrahepatic cholangiojejunostomy
4. Carcinomas of the gallbladder

1. When the benign nature of a solid liver tumour is confirmed intraoperatively by frozen section, there is no reason for an extensive resection of the normal surrounding parenchyma. If it appears that

Table 6.2 *Anterior segmentectomy 4.*

	Age and sex	Location and size of the lesions	Postoperative course	Follow up
1 Nodular focal hyperplasia	32 F		Smooth	Alive 4 years
2 Cavernous haemangioma	38 F		Smooth	Alive 4 years
3 Nodular focal hyperplasia	27 F		Smooth	Alive 9 years
4 Nodular focal hyperplasia	17 M		Smooth	Alive 1 year

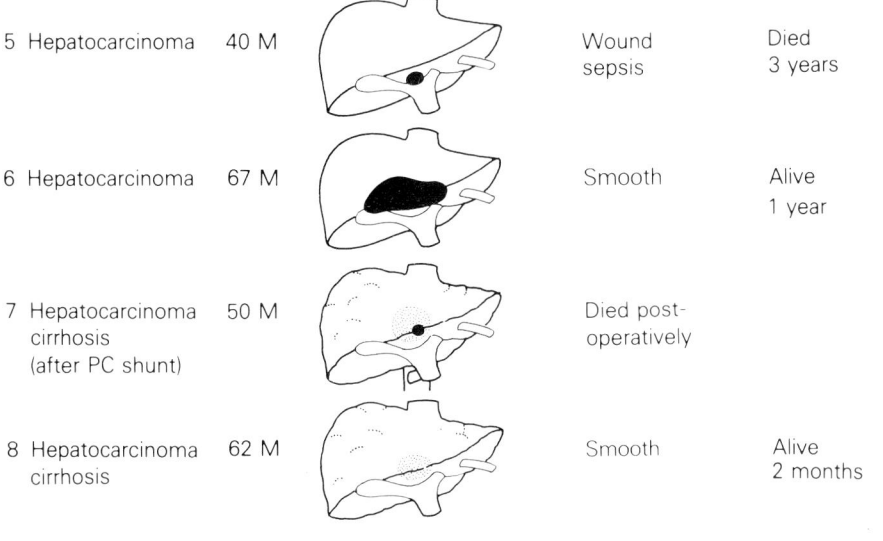

segmental resection could be easily and safely performed in the given case, it is reasonable to choose this type of resection rather than a larger common hepatectomy.

2. Segmental resections in malignant tumours are indicated in some particular conditions. In two cases, the procedure was performed because of associated cirrhosis. In two other cases, the hepatocarcinoma was small and located in the quadrate lobe, equidistant from the main scissura and the umbilical fissure. For these central tumours a right extended hepatectomy or a left hepatectomy has no advantage compared to a segmentectomy 4 which follows the same scissurae.

Table 6.3 *Segmentectomy 4.*

	Age and sex	Location and size of the lesions	Postoperative course	Follow up
1 Hamartoma	10 M		Smooth	Alive 8 years
2 Carcinoma of the hilus	59 M		Smooth	Died 5 years
3 Carcinoma of the hilus	40 M		Smooth	Died 3 years
5 Hepatocarcinoma	40 M		Wound sepsis	Died 3 years
6 Hepatocarcinoma	67 M		Smooth	Alive 1 year
7 Hepatocarcinoma cirrhosis (after PC shunt)	50 M		Died postoperatively	
8 Hepatocarcinoma cirrhosis	62 M		Smooth	Alive 2 months

Table 6.4 *B segmentectomy 4–5.*

	Age and sex	Location and size of the lesions	Postoperative course	Follow up
1 Hepatocarcinoma	42 M		Smooth	Alive 4 years
2 Carcinoma of the gallbladder (reoperation)	39 F		Smooth	Alive 4 years
3 Carcinoma of the gallbladder (reoperation)	57 M		Smooth	Died 2 years
4 Carcinoma of the gallbladder (reoperation)	60 F		Smooth	Alive 5 years
5 Carcinoma of the gallbladder (reoperation)	29 F		Smooth	Alive 5 years
6 Carcinoma of the gallbladder (first operation)	71 M		Smooth	Alive 4 years

Table 6.5 *Trisegmentectomy 4–5–6.*

	Age and sex	Location and size of the lesions	Postoperative course	Follow up
1 Adenoma	29 F		Smooth	Alive 5 years
2 Hepatocarcinoma	65 M		Smooth	Alive 5 years with tumour recurrence
3 Carcinoma of the gallbladder (first operation)	58 M		Smooth	Died 1 year
4 Endocrinoide adenocarcinoma	69 M		Smooth	Alive 6 months

3. The resection of the quadrate lobe can be indicated in the field of biliary surgery when there is the need to gain access to the upper part of the biliary confluence[7] or to perform an intrahepatic cholangioenteric anastomosis.[8]

4. Another indication for segmental liver resection is carcinoma of the gallbladder when malignancy is discovered by histological examination of a gallbladder specimen removed for gallstones. If histology reveals that the carcinoma has extended beyond the wall of the gallbladder, we think that there is an indication for a complementary liver resection. This resection should remove the contiguous liver parenchyma: segments 4 and 5. The right extended hepatectomy, which is often proposed, is in our opinion disproportionate[5] since it removes an almost entirely normal right lobe. Three of our patients operated on by a bisegmentectomy 4–5 after histological discovery of a carcinoma of the gallbladder are at present alive after more than two years with no sign of tumour recurrence.

CONCLUSION

In conclusion, segmentectomies 4 and other hepatic segmentectomies 'réglées' are one of the best illustrations of the anatomical surgery of the liver. They should not be considered as easy and quick surgical options since they are technically demanding. They are interesting alternatives to the common hepatectomies when a more economical resection is permitted by the location and the nature of the lesion, or when a major hepatectomy is likely to expose the patient to the risk of postoperative hepatic failure. Although segmentectomy is not a major resection, a thorough knowledge of the segmental anatomy of the liver is essential for its safe execution.

REFERENCES

1 Bismuth H (1982) Surgical anatomy and anatomical surgery of the liver. *World Journal of Surgery* 6: 3–9.
2 Couinaud C (1957) *Le foie. Etudes Anatomiques et Chirurgicales.* Paris: Masson.
3 Goldsmith NA & Woodbourne RT (1957) The surgical anatomy pertaining to liver resection. *Surgery, Gynecology & Obstetrics* 105: 310–318.
4 Healey JE & Schroy PC (1953) Anatomy of the biliary ducts within the human liver. *Archives of Surgery* 66: 599–616.
5 Bismuth H, Houssin D & Castaing D (1982) Major and minor segmentectomies 'réglées' in liver surgery. *World Journal of Surgery* 6: 10–24.
6 Caprio G (1931) Un caso de extirpacion del lobulo izquierdo del higado. *Bulletin Societad Cirurgia Uruguay (Montevideo)* 2: 159.
7 Champeau M & Pineau P (1964) Voie d'abord élargie transhépatique du canal hépatique gauche. *Mémoires de l'Académie de Chirurgie* (Paris) 90: 602.
8 Bismuth H & Corlette MB (1975) Intrahepatic cholangioenteric anastosis in carcinoma of the hilus of the liver. *Surgery, Gynecology & Obstetrics* 140: 170–178.
9 Ton That Tung (1979) *Les Résections Majeures et Mineures de Foie.* Paris: Masson.
10 Starzl TE, Bell RH, Beart RW & Putnam CW (1975) Hepatic trisegmentectomy and other liver resections. *Surgery, Gynecology & Obstetrics* 141: 429–435.
11 Starzl TE, Iwatsuki S, Shaw, BW, Waterman PM, Vantiez D, Diliz HS, Dekker A & Bron KM (1982) Left hepatic trisegmentectomy. *Surgery, Gynecology & Obstetrics* 155: 21–27.
12 Bismuth H, Houssin D & Mazmanian G (1983) Postoperative liver insufficiency: prevention and management. *World Journal of Surgery* 7: 505–510.

7
Peritoneovenous Shunting for Intractable Ascites

A. Cuschieri

Ascites is detectable clinically when fluid accumulation within the peritoneal cavity exceeds one litre. It may occur with or without evidence of generalized water and salt retention. In some disorders it may be the only or outstanding clinical feature (e.g. cirrhosis, tumours of the peritoneal cavity, tuberculous peritonitis and pancreatic ascites). The protein and cellular content of ascitic fluid carries both diagnostic and therapeutic implications.

The common causes of ascites within the Western hemisphere are cirrhosis and intra-abdominal malignancy. The occurrence of ascites in these conditions signifies severe and advanced disease with a reduced life expectancy. The aim of therapy is therefore essentially palliative.

PATHOGENESIS OF CIRRHOTIC ASCITES

The factors involved in ascites formation are increased hepatic lymph production and leakage, elevated hydrostatic pressure, hypoalbuminaemia and water and salt retention. The enhanced hepatic lymph production results from the post-sinusoidal component of the portal hypertension. It is accompanied by excessive leakage of lymph from the surface of the liver. The elevated hydrostatic pressure induces transudation of fluid from the splanchnic capillaries within the peritoneum. The hypoalbuminaemia is the result of both maldistribution and diminished hepatic synthesis, and leads to a reduced oncotic pressure. There is still some controversy regarding the dominant mechanism responsible for the water and salt retention.[1]

Traditionally the belief has been that renin/aldosterone secretion is induced by a fall in the renal blood flow consequent on fluid sequestration within the splanchnic circulation. However, blood aldosterone levels are often normal in these patients. The alternative hypothesis postulates a primary sodium retention by the renal tubules, leading to an expanded plasma volume.

INTRACTABLE ASCITES

Medical therapy is effective in controlling ascites due to chronic liver disease in the majority of cases. Eventually however some 5% of patients become refractory to medical management. These patients show no response to diuretic therapy (including loop diuretics) and develop pre-renal azotaemia. Patients with malignant ascites do not usually benefit from medical management. By far the most common cause of malignant ascites is secondary peritoneal carcinomatosis. The ascites is usually massive, intractable and the fluid is often haemorrhagic or chylous. The most common site of the primary is the gastrointestinal tract followed by pancreas, breast and ovary.

An increased incidence of peritoneal mesotheliomas has been reported since 1960 and has been attributed to asbestos exposure. Malignant peritoneal mesothelioma is diffuse and unresectable. The majority of cases have been reported in the elderly. The most common presentation is with ascites and/or intestinal obstruction.

Other causes of intractable ascites include the Budd–Chiari syndrome, chylous ascites secondary to lymphoma, and pancreatic ascites. The latter occurs in chronic pancreatitis (usually of alcoholic origin) and in association with pseudocyst or rupture of the pancreatic duct.

Clinical features

The ascites is gross and tense, the elevated intra-abdominal pressure causing venous congestion of the abdominal wall veins and diminished venous return from the lower limbs which aggravates the peripheral oedema. It also causes a tense uncomfortable sensation frequently amounting to abdominal pain and tenderness. Respiratory distress results from splinting of the diaphragm. Mobility is considerably impaired. The umbilicus becomes everted and existing herniae become distended. In patients with chronic liver disease, pre-renal azotaemia is invariably present.

TREATMENT OPTIONS

There are three management options in patients with ascites:

1. Medical therapy
2. Therapeutic paracentesis
3. Peritoneovenous shunting

Medical therapy

This constitutes the first-line approach in patients with cirrhotic ascites and is successful in 95% of cases. The mainstays of medical therapy are dietary salt restriction, spironolactone (anti-aldosterone) and loop diuretics. The objective of medical management is a gradual loss of the fluid overload (3 kg fluid/week) to avoid pre-renal azotaemia. Treatment is stopped if the blood urea rises above 10.0 mmol/l or the creatinine over 120 μmol/l. Dietary salt is restricted to 0.5 g daily and fluid intake to 1500 ml. Initially spironolactone alone is used because this is not attended by K$^+$ loss which is an important consideration since the body K$^+$ store of these patients is depleted. The initial oral dose of spironolactone is 50 mg twice daily with increments of 50–100 mg/day every fourth day up to a maximum dose of 600 mg daily.[2] If spironolactone therapy fails to induce a response, a loop diuretic (frusemide, ethacrynic acid) administered intravenously is used. The initial dose of frusemide is 40 mg/day with increments of 40 mg every 48 hours up to a maximum of 200 mg daily. Ethacrynic acid sometimes succeeds when frusemide has been ineffective but it carries a significant risk of acute ototoxicity especially when administered intravenously. Once reduction of ascites is achieved, maintenance therapy is continued with low salt diet and oral spironolactone with or without oral thiazides, although increasingly K$^+$ sparing diuretics are used in preference to oral thiazides (e.g. amiloride, triamterene).

The complications of medical therapy include volume depletion, hypokalaemia, hyponatraemia and encephalopathy. Furthermore, it is costly and prolonged and does not usually benefit patients with malignant disease.

Therapeutic paracentesis

This is indicated in patients with intractable ascites and prior to the introduction of peritoneovenous shunting was the mainstay of therapy in patients with refractory cirrhotic ascites and patients with malignant disease. Its disadvantages include risk of sepsis, volume depletion, leakage of peritoneal fluid after withdrawal of the cannula and precipitation of encephalopathy in patients wih liver disease.

The procedure is performed under local anaesthesia. A peritoneal dialysis cannula is inserted through a small (1 cm) incision placed in the midline some 2 cm below the umbilicus and then connected to a *closed* system of drainage to minimize the risk of infection. Slow decompression (3–4 litres every 24 hours) is advisable in cirrhotic patients and some advocate intravenous infusion of fresh frozen plasma or salt-poor human albumin solution to prevent volume depletion.

In patients with malignant ascites, instillation of cytotoxic agents into the peritoneal cavity is advocated prior to cannula withdrawal with the objective of preventing recurrence of the ascites, although there is no evidence of any benefit accruing from this approach and it should be stressed that cytotoxic agents administered intraperitoneally are absorbed. This consideration must be borne in mind, especially in patients on systemic chemotherapy, in view of the enhanced risks of bone marrow depression.

Peritoneovenous shunting

This was first reported by Smith in Edinburgh[3] but did not gain widespread use until the introduction of a purpose-designed pressure-activated one-way valve system by LeVeen et al in 1974.[4,5] Since then peritoneovenous shunting has been shown to be effective in the treatment of intractable cirrhotic ascites but incurs a certain morbidity.[6] The problem of clotting of the shunt has been largely overcome with the introduction of systems which incorporate a flushing device. More recently peritoneovenous shunting has been used for malignant ascites.[7]

In cirrhotic ascites, peritoneovenous shunting results in an expansion of the vascular space, enhancement of the effective renal blood flow with a profound diuresis which is sustained for a period of several days. Furthermore, previously refractory patients become responsive to small dose oral diuretic therapy. There is in addition a fall in the plasma aldosterone and renin level, and urinary Na+ excretion is increased.[8]

INDICATIONS AND PATIENT SELECTION FOR PERITONEOVENOUS SHUNTING

Indications

The most common indication has been intractable ascites due to cirrhosis, peritoneovenous shunting being used when diuretic therapy (as previously described) has failed. Others however advocate a trial of 5% of albumin or fresh frozen plasma infusion (500 ml over a period of two hours) followed by intravenous frusemide (50 mg) and 250 ml of 20% mannitol over 20 to 30 minutes, and to resort to peritoneovenous shunting only if the above regimen fails.

Peritoneovenous shunting has also been used in patients with the Budd–Chiari syndrome, although these patients are best served in the long-run by either a side-to-side portacaval or preferably a porta/meso-artrial shunt. Another indication is *chylous ascites* often encountered nowadays in patients with intra-abdominal lymphomas.

Increasingly peritoneovenous shunting is being used to palliate the tense often painful malignant ascites due to peritoneal carcinomatosis, inoperable hepatocellular carcinoma and malignant peritoneal mesothelioma. Good palliation has been experienced by the author in these patients, although it is *rare* for the ascites to disappear completely in this group.

Contraindications

The important contraindications to peritoneovenous shunting are:

Infected ascites. Spontaneous bacterial peritonitis occurs in 8% of cirrhotic ascites. The infection is caused by gram-negative aerobes in 65–70% of cases, with *Staphylococcus albus*, *Streptococcus pneumoniae* and anaerobes being responsible for the remainder.

Encephalopathy. Peritoneovenous shunting is attended by a high mortality from liver failure in these patients.

Bleeding diathesis. The procedure should not be performed in the presence of a grossly prolonged prothrombin and kaolin cephalin time and if the platelet count is below 60 000. The occurrence of disseminated intravascular coagulation (DIC) induced by the shunting may precipitate catastrophic haemorrhage.[9]

Renal failure. This is only a contraindication when it is the result of primary renal disease.

Recent variceal haemorrhage. Obliteration of varices by sclerotherapy should precede peritoneovenous shunting because of the risk of recurrent haemorrhage.

Active liver disease and gross jaundice. Patients with chronic active hepatitis with piecemeal necrosis and those with a bilirubin in excess of 120 μmol/l constitute a high-risk group and peritoneovenous shunting should be postponed until the condition has improved or stabilized with medical therapy.

Other contraindications. These include recent abdominal surgery, cardiac failure and gross pleural effusions.

PREOPERATIVE CARE AND INVESTIGATIONS

Peritoneovenous shunting is carried out as an elective procedure. The patient must be fully investigated and the exact diagnosis established. Absence of any infection must be confirmed before the procedure is performed. The essential preoperative investigations include:

1. Full blood count (including PCV and platelet count).
2. Clotting studies—prothrombin time, kaolin cephalin time, fibrogen and FDP levels.
3. Serum urea, electrolytes and creatinine.
4. Liver function tests.

PERITONEOVENOUS SHUNTING FOR INTRACTABLE ASCITES 109

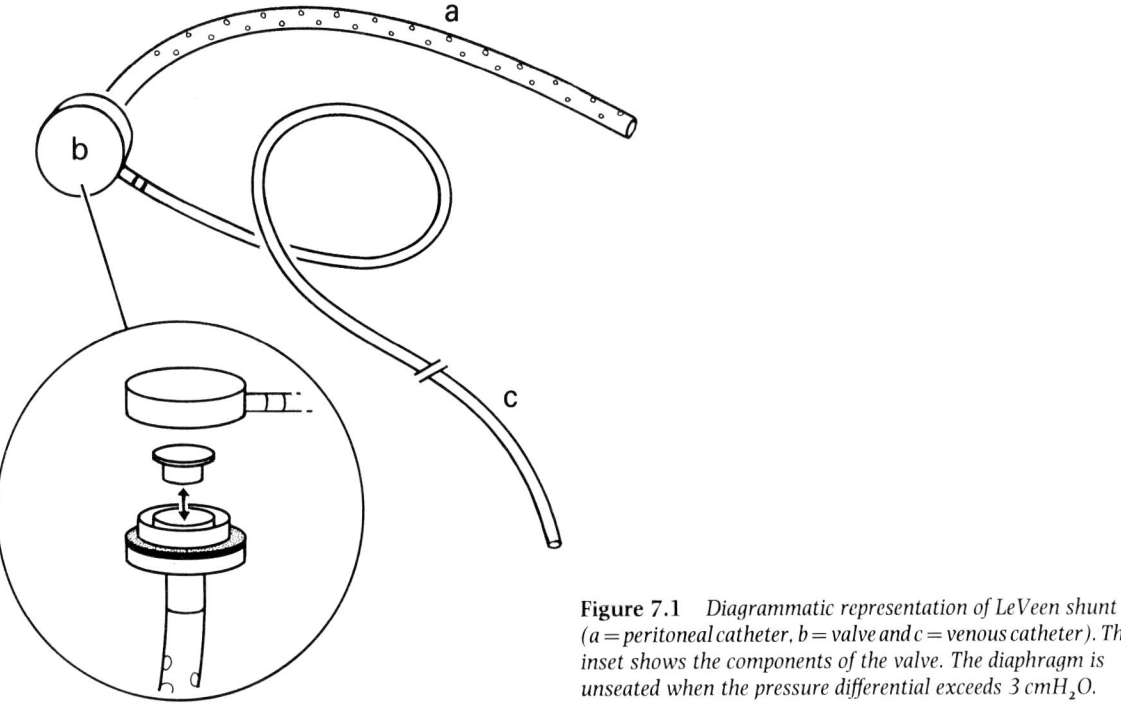

Figure 7.1 *Diagrammatic representation of LeVeen shunt (a = peritoneal catheter, b = valve and c = venous catheter). The inset shows the components of the valve. The diaphragm is unseated when the pressure differential exceeds 3 cmH$_2$O.*

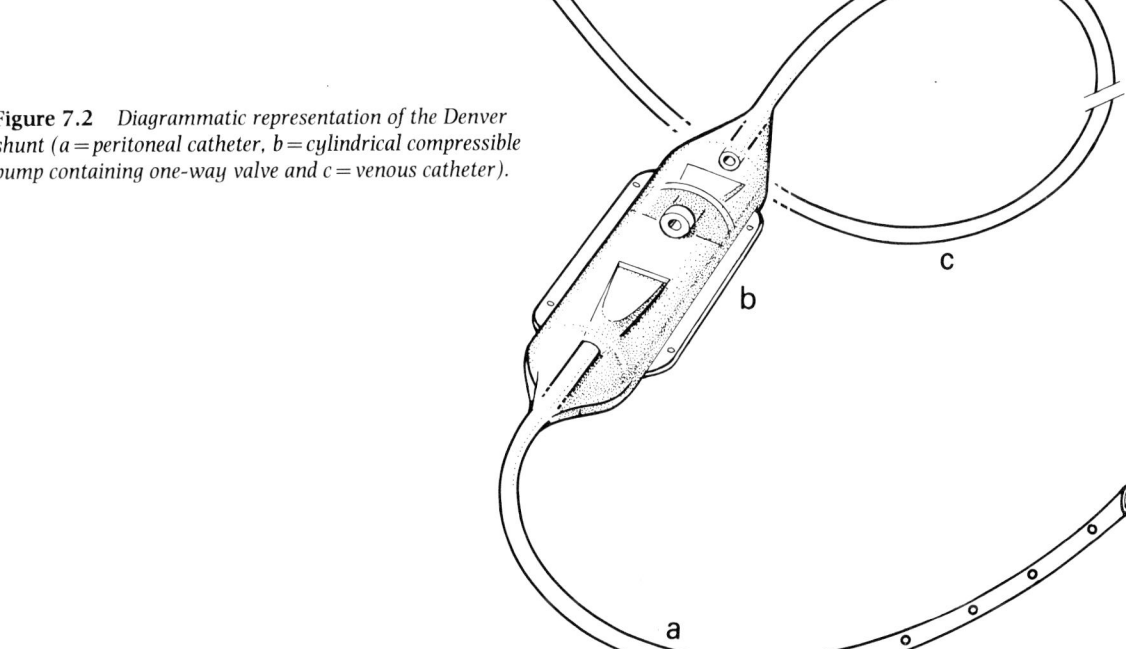

Figure 7.2 *Diagrammatic representation of the Denver shunt (a = peritoneal catheter, b = cylindrical compressible pump containing one-way valve and c = venous catheter).*

5. Diagnostic peritoneal tap. A 20 ml specimen is obtained and sent for biochemical analysis, culture and cytological examination. The protein content of the fluid is an important consideration. If the fluid is an exudate (protein > 2.5 g/l), the risk of shunt blockage is higher than if the fluid has a low protein content and a valve with a flushing mechanism must be used. The cytological examination includes the total cell count in addition to detection of malignant cells.

6. Laparoscopy is an invaluable diagnostic aid in patients with ascites. It is particularly indicated for suspected tuberculous peritonitis, primary mesothelioma and hepatoma complicating cirrhosis. In practice, I use laparoscopy whenever a firm diagnosis has not been established by less invasive methods. It allows biopsy under vision of hepatic lesions and nodules/areas of inflammation of the parietal peritoneum. In patients with previous abdominal surgery, it provides useful information with regard to the intended site of the peritoneal catheter of the shunt.

Antibiotic prophylaxis with cephuroxime is routinely used by the author, 1.5 g being administered intramuscularly with induction.

OPERATIVE DETAILS

Types of shunts

LeVeen shunt (Figure 7.1)

This consists of a diaphragm valve enclosed in a polypropylene casing which connects with the intraperitoneal tubing and the venous line both of which are constructed of silicone tubing. The valve opens only when a positive pressure differential of at least 3 cm H_2O exists between the peritoneal cavity and the central veins. It does not have a flushing mechanism which accounts for the high incidence of shunt obstruction. The valve is placed between the rectus muscle and the posterior rectus sheath.

Denver shunt (Figure 7.2)

This is constructed of medical grade silicone elastomer throughout. The valve mechanism is incorporated within a cylindrical compressible chamber and connects with the venous line proximally and the peritoneal cannula distally. The venous line has tantalum markers for radiological visualization. The pump-valve system is placed over the lower ribs anteriorly to which it is anchored by non-absorbable sutures.

Cordis–Hakim shunt

This is favoured by the author and is shown in Figure 7.3. The valve unit consists of twin Cordis–Hakim valves arranged in parallel. The valve unit is compressible between the two sets of valves and is connected by short tubing to the antechamber, the bottom of which contains a 316 stainless steel needle stop. The chamber is fully compressible and acts as a pump on digital compression. The peritoneal catheter is composed of radio-opaque silicone elastomer and is L-shaped. The peritoneal end has multiple fenestrations and suture grooves,

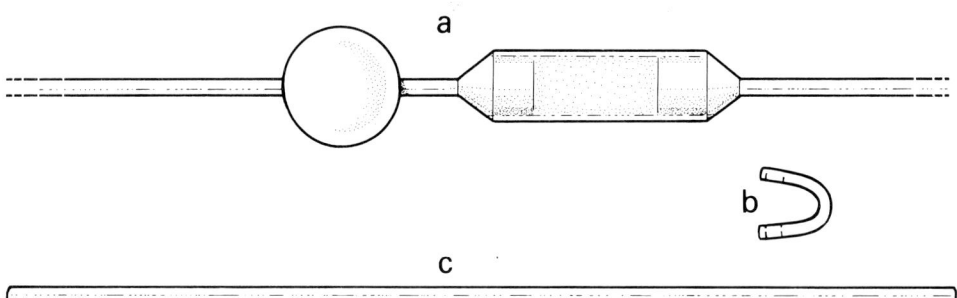

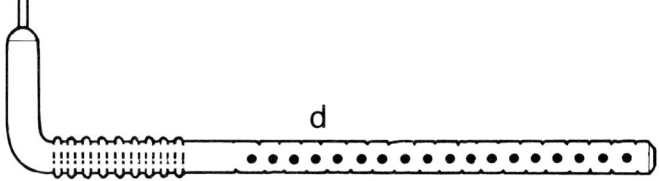

Figure 7.3 *Diagrammatic representation of Cordis – Hakim shunt (a = valve unit– antechamber assembly, b = metal U-shaped connector, c = venous catheter and d = peritoneal catheter with straight integral connector).*

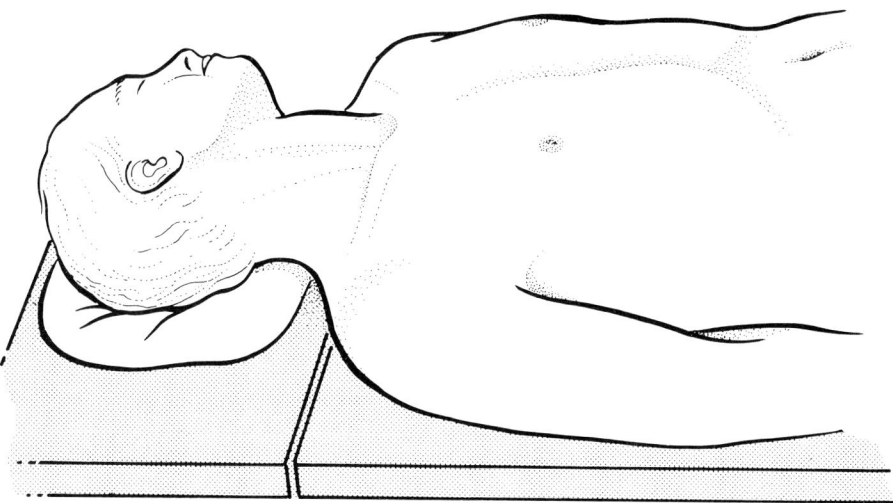

Figure 7.4 *Positioning of the patient on the operating table. The neck is extended and rotated away from the operative side.*

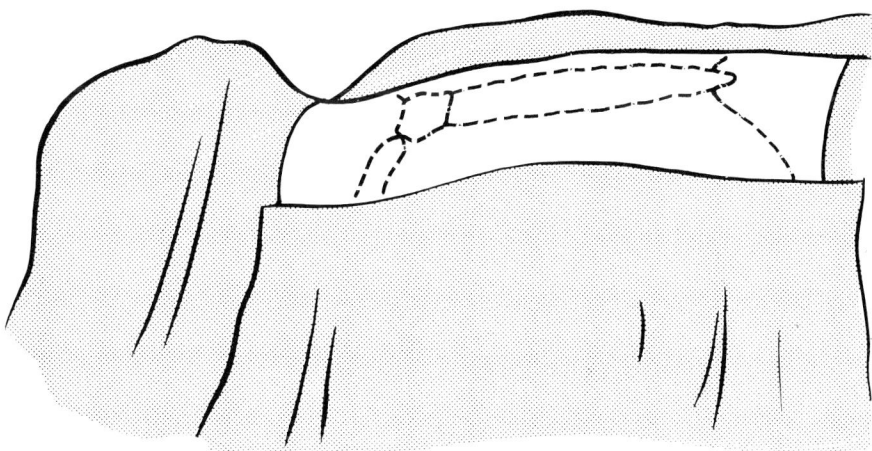

Figure 7.5 *Towelling of operative area.*

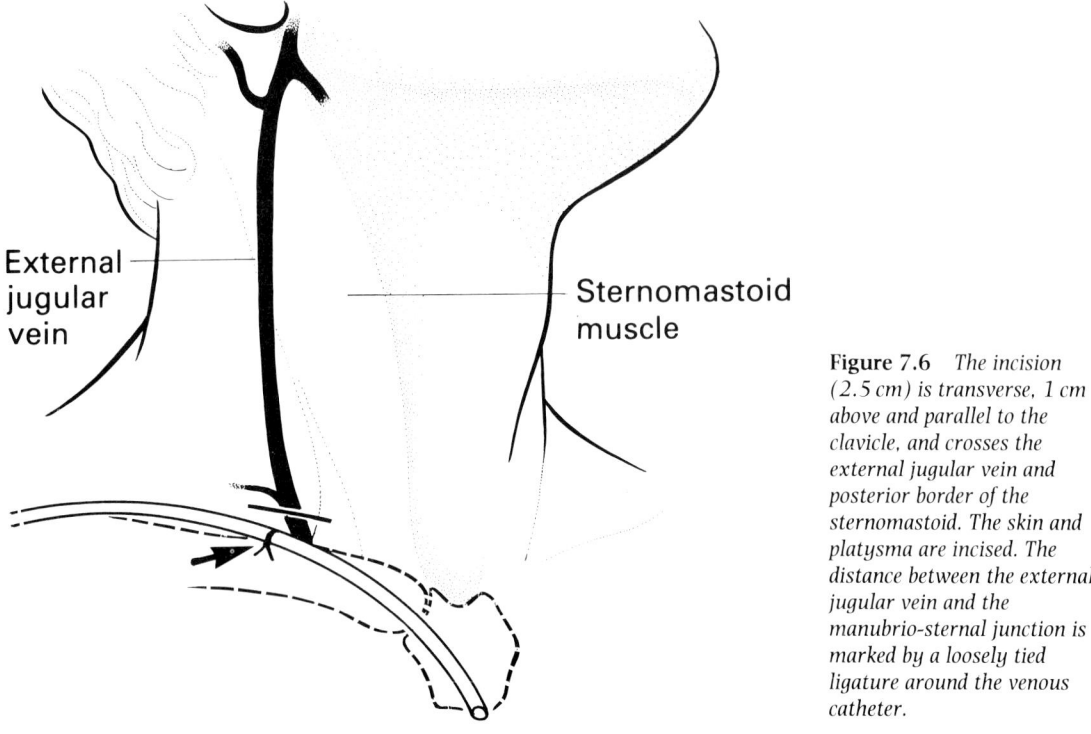

Figure 7.6 *The incision (2.5 cm) is transverse, 1 cm above and parallel to the clavicle, and crosses the external jugular vein and posterior border of the sternomastoid. The skin and platysma are incised. The distance between the external jugular vein and the manubrio-sternal junction is marked by a loosely tied ligature around the venous catheter.*

Figure 7.7 *The external jugular has been exposed by incision of skin and platysma and the vein tied proximally in continuity. The venous catheter fitted with a three-way tap and filled with heparinized saline has been inserted into the vein up to the marking suture. It is important to check the position of the atrial catheter by injecting contrast while viewing with the image intensifier.*

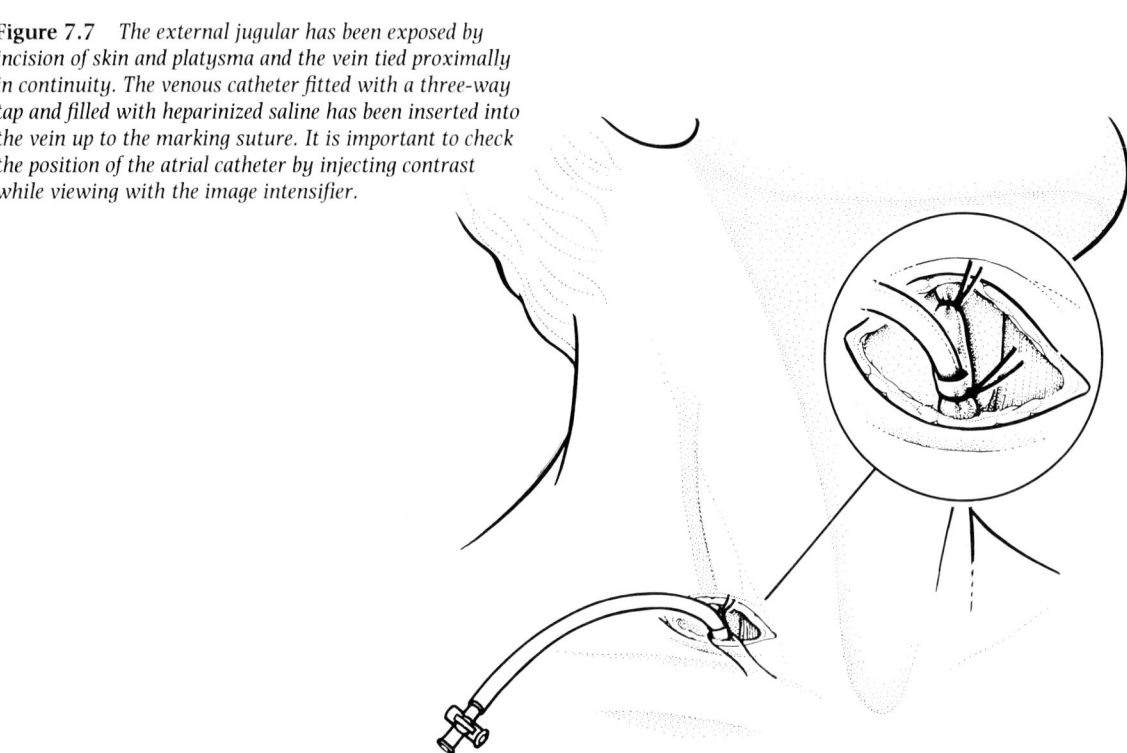

and the proximal end has an integral stainless steel connector for the tubing leading to the antechamber-valve unit. The atrial catheter is also made of radio-opaque silicone tubing and a U-shaped or straight connector of stainless steel is used to join the atrial catheter to the tubing leading to the valve unit. The entire system has an opening pressure of 1–3 cm H_2O. The flow capacity of the system is pressure-dependent and varies from 90–110 ml/h at a pressure differential of 4.2 cm H_2O to 200–300 ml/h at a pressure head of 6 cm H_2O.

Operative insertion of shunt (Cordis–Hakim)

The operation can be performed under local anaesthesia but where the patient's general condition permits, general anaesthesia facilitates the procedure and is preferred by the author.

Patient positioning

The patient is kept in the supine position with the neck extended and the head rotated away from the intended operative site (Figure 7.4). The area from the chin down to the umbilicus is prepared with Hibitane soap followed by an antiseptic lotion of choice and towelling is applied such that the side of the neck, sternal region and upper quadrant are left exposed (Figure 7.5).

Insertion of venous (atrial) catheter

The best approach is through the external jugular vein. Availability of image intensification for exact positioning of the atrial catheter is essential. Initially the distance between the intended entry point in the external jugular vein and the manubriosternal angle is measured and the catheter is marked accordingly by a loosely tied ligature round it. This step provides a rough but reliable guide to the depth of insertion of the venous catheter (Figure 7.6).

The external jugular vein is exposed through a 2.5 cm transverse incision along the upper border of the clavicle, crossing the external jugular vein. The vein is exposed after division of the platysma and is then dissected over a distance of 1 cm. Any small tributaries are ligated. Non-absorbable ligatures are inserted round the mobilized vein and the cephalad one is tied. At this stage the table should be tilted (30°) to the Trendelenburg position as a prophylaxis against air embolism. A three-way tap is fitted to the venous catheter which is filled with heparinized saline. The external jugular vein is opened transversely and the cannula is introduced as far as the marking tie which is then removed. The distal vein ligature is tied loosely (one throw) around the vein and catheter (Figure 7.7). Sodium diatrizoate (Hypaque) is injected through the three-way tap to check the position of the tip of the venous catheter by screening with the image intensifier. The ideal position of the catheter is such that its tip lies at the junction of the superior vena cava with the right atrium. *In practice, exact positioning of the atrial catheter constitutes the most crucial part of the operation.* Having achieved this, the catheter is securely tied to the external jugular vein, is then flushed with heparinized saline and the three-way tap closed. It is unwise to trim off the excess catheter length at this stage.

Insertion of the peritoneal catheter

To avoid leakage of peritoneal fluid the metal connector of the peritoneal catheter is closed. This is achieved by fitting a small segment of collapsible tubing over the metal segment and then tying the tubing tightly beyond the segment (Figure 7.8).

A 4 cm transverse skin incision is made 2.5 cm from the linea alba and 6 cm below the xyphoid process (Figure 7.9). The incision is deepened to expose the anterior rectus sheath which is divided, together with the underlying rectus muscle, using the cutting diathermy knife. Careful attention to haemostasis is essential. Large high-pressure venous collaterals are often encountered in cirrhotic patients and require individual ligation. Extreme care must be taken when dividing the rectus muscle not to damage the posterior rectus sheath which is exposed further by blunt mobilization of the cut rectus muscle. An area, 2 cm square, of exposed posterior rectus sheath is required for in-

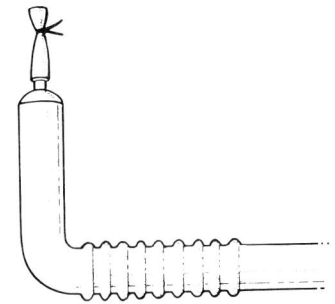

Figure 7.8 *Temporary closure of integral metal connector of the peritoneal catheter by tubing which is tied beyond the metal end.*

114 GENERAL SURGERY

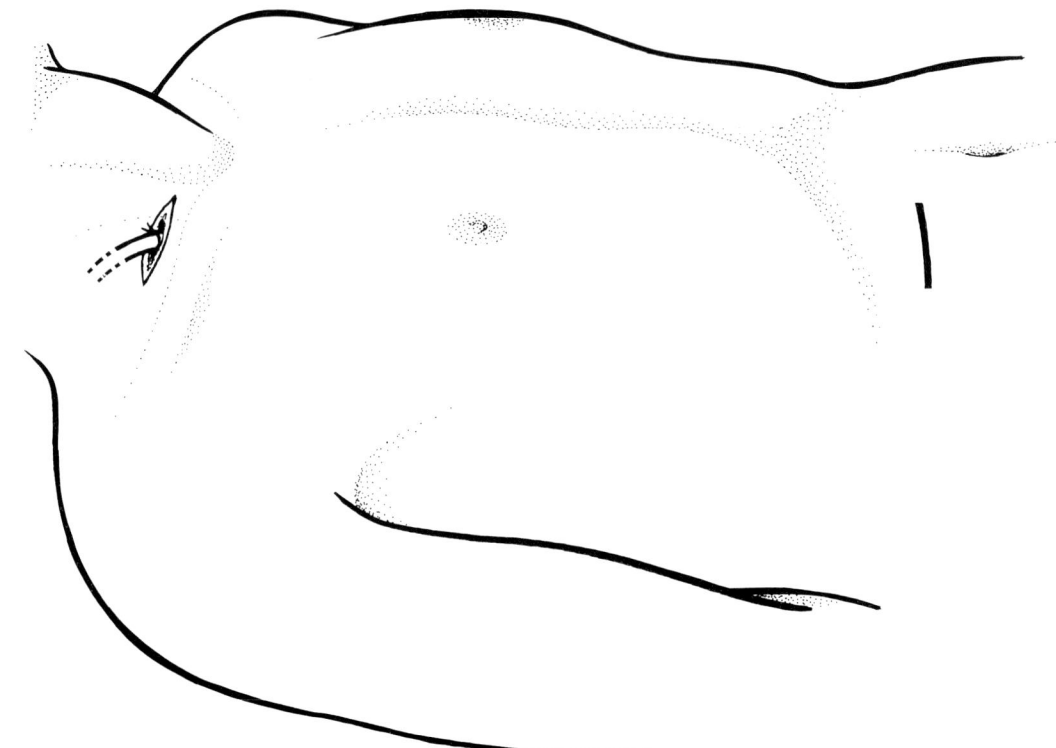

Figure 7.9 *Abdominal transverse skin incision which is situated one inch from the linea alba and 6 cm below the xiphoid process.*

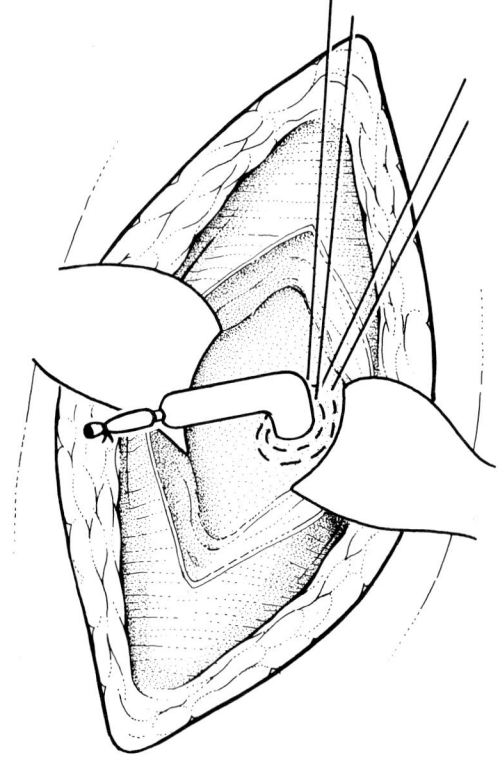

Figure 7.10 *Insertion of peritoneal catheter. Two purse-string sutures are used to prevent leakage of ascitic fluid around the catheter.*

PERITONEOVENOUS SHUNTING FOR INTRACTABLE ASCITES 115

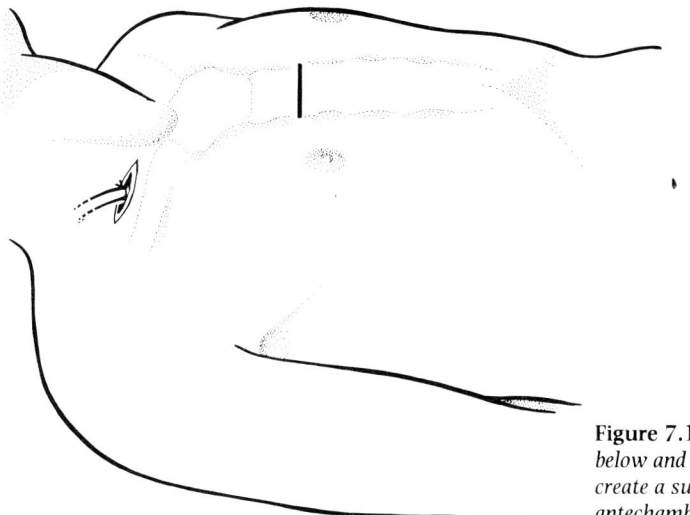

Figure 7.11 *Transverse incision over the sternum 4 cm below and parallel to the manubriosternal angle is used to create a subcutaneous pocket for the insertion of the antechamber–valve unit.*

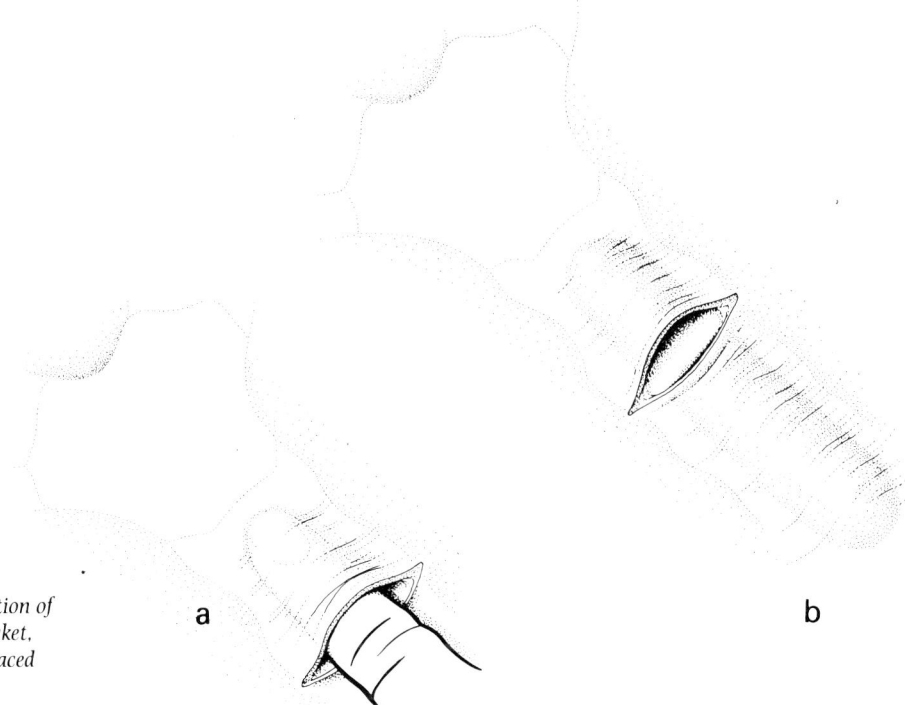

Figure 7.12 *Construction of subcutaneous sternal pocket, two-thirds of which is placed distal to the transverse sternal wound.*

a

b

116 GENERAL SURGERY

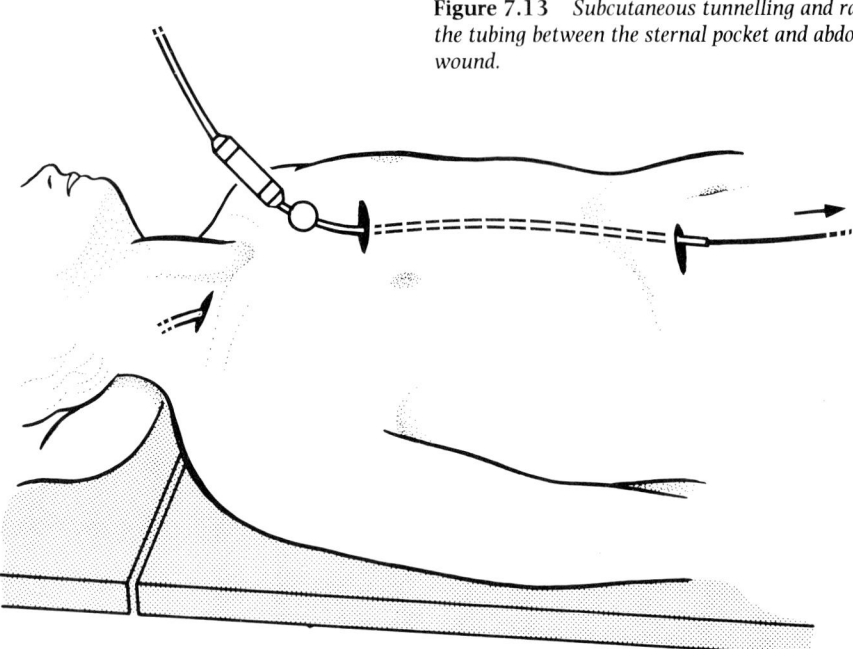

Figure 7.13 *Subcutaneous tunnelling and railroading of the tubing between the sternal pocket and abdominal wound.*

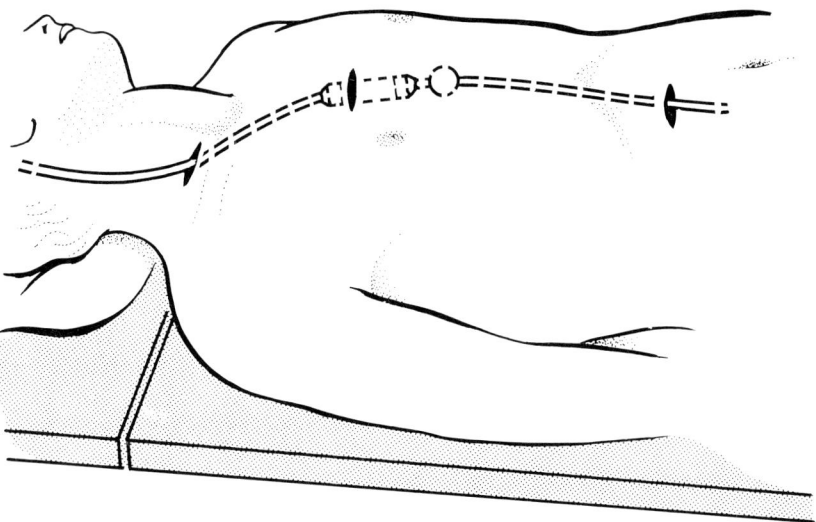

Figure 7.14 *Subcutaneous tunnelling and railroading of tubing between upper end of valve unit and cervical wound.*

sertion and fixation of the peritoneal catheter. A self-retaining mastoid-type retractor is inserted. An atraumatic purse-string suture (1/0 non-absorbable) is inserted around the proposed entry site and encircling an area of approximately 1.5 cm diameter. A second purse-string suture of the same material is then inserted 0.5 cm outside the first one (Figure 7.10). A stab incision with a pointed scalpel is made in the posterior rectus sheath. Ascitic fluid leaks through, confirming complete penetration of the sheath and peritoneum. The peritoneal catheter is then inserted up to the grooved segment and the inner purse string suture tied securely round it using a surgeon's knot. The second purse-string suture is next tied. The purpose of the second purse-string suture is to bunch the rectus sheath around the catheter, thereby ensuring a water-tight seal around the emergent peritoneal catheter.

Fashioning the bed for the valve–antechamber unit

A transverse incision, 2 cm long, is made 4 cm distal and parallel to the manubriosternal angle (Figure 7.11). By a combination of scissor and finger dissection the skin is elevated from the underlying sternum to create a subcutaneous pocket, two-thirds of which lies below the incision (Figure 7.12). The pocket must be of the right size such that when the valve and antechamber assembly are inserted, the intervening tube between them assumes a straight line.

A narrow subcutaneous tunnel is effected between the abdominal wound and the sternal pocket using a metal probe or fine long artery forceps. The tubing attached to the antechamber is fixed to the probe (or grasped by the artery forceps) and railroaded down to the abdominal wound (Figure 7.13). A second subcutaneous tunnel is next made between the sternal pouch and the cervical wound and the tubing attached to the valve railroaded to the neck (Figure 7.14). The valve and antechamber unit is then inserted in the subcutaneous sternal pocket and mild traction is applied to the tubing at both the cervical and abdominal wounds. After ensuring an adequate lie of the valve–antechamber unit, the distal tubing is inserted through a stab in the rectus sheath, excess length is cut off and then fitted to the metal end of the peritoneal catheter being secured to this by a non-absorbable ligature (Figure 7.15).

The antechamber is then compressed six to 10 times until the whole system is filled with ascitic fluid and a steady stream emerges from the cervical tubing. The cervical tubing connecting with the valve is trimmed to size and fittted to the U-shaped metal connector to which it is secured by a non-absorbable ligature. The excess length of the caval catheter is then cut off, after which the cannula is fitted to the other end of the U-shaped metal connector and secured to it by an encircling ligature. Accurate placing of the metal connection by means of a non-absorbable suture around its apex to the underlying muscle ensures against angulation or kinking (Figure 7.16).

Wound closure

The wounds are sprayed with povidone-iodine spray and closed in layers. Suture of the anterior rectus sheath covers the peritoneal catheter completely and likewise suture of the platysma, the metal connection between the valve tubing and the atrial catheter. Dressings are applied to the wounds. The position of the antechamber is marked on the overlying skin to facilitate pump compression by the nursing staff and patient in the postoperative period. An elastic abdominal corset is applied.

POSTOPERATIVE CARE AND EARLY COMPLICATIONS

Postoperative care

The patient is nursed in the semi-recumbent position. Essential monitoring include CVP, urine output, urea and electrolytes, PCV and platelet count, fibrogen and FDP levels in addition to prothrombin and kaolin-cephalin times. Some elevation of the CVP occurs in about 15% of cirrhotic patients and if marked, heralds the onset of circulatory overload and cardiac failure. A marked diuresis at times amounting to 5 litres/24 hours is observed during the first three to four days. A daily weight and fluid balance chart is continued for seven to 10 days after surgery.

The antechamber is compressed six to 10 times every six hours for the first few days. The abdominal corset is worn indefinitely. The patient is instructed how to exhale through a straw for periods of 10 minutes three times daily. This procedure increases the differential between the intra-abdominal pressure and the cervical venous pressure.

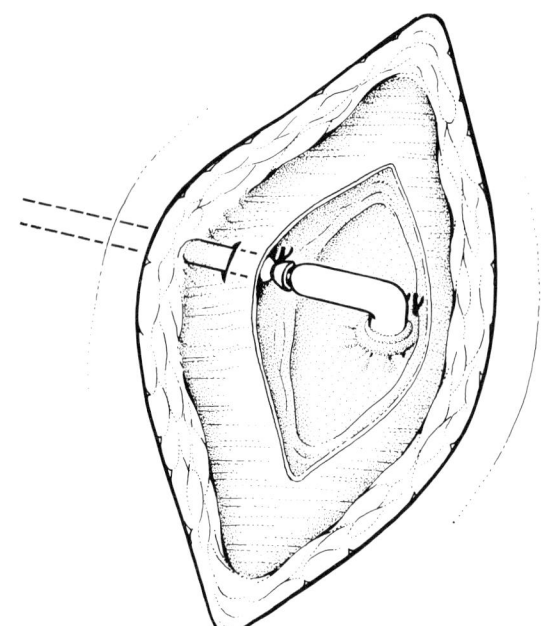

Figure 7.15 *The tubing is passed through a stab wound under the anterior rectus sheath, the excess trimmed off and then fitted to the integral metal connector of the peritoneal catheter to which it is anchored by an encircling non-absorbable suture.*

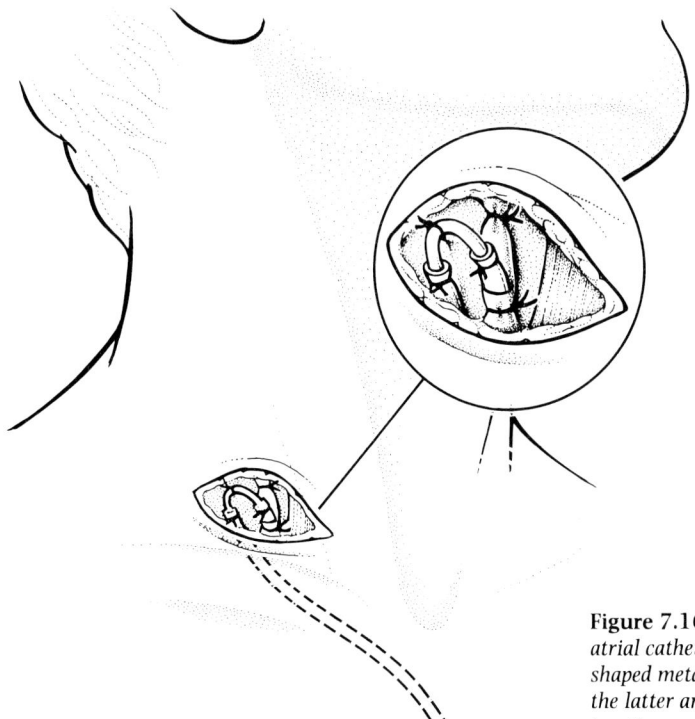

Figure 7.16 *The excess length of the cervical tubing and atrial catheter is cut off and the two connected by a U-shaped metal connector. A suture surrounding the apex of the latter and including the subjacent muscle fixes the junction and avoids kinking.*

PERITONEOVENOUS SHUNTING FOR INTRACTABLE ASCITES 119

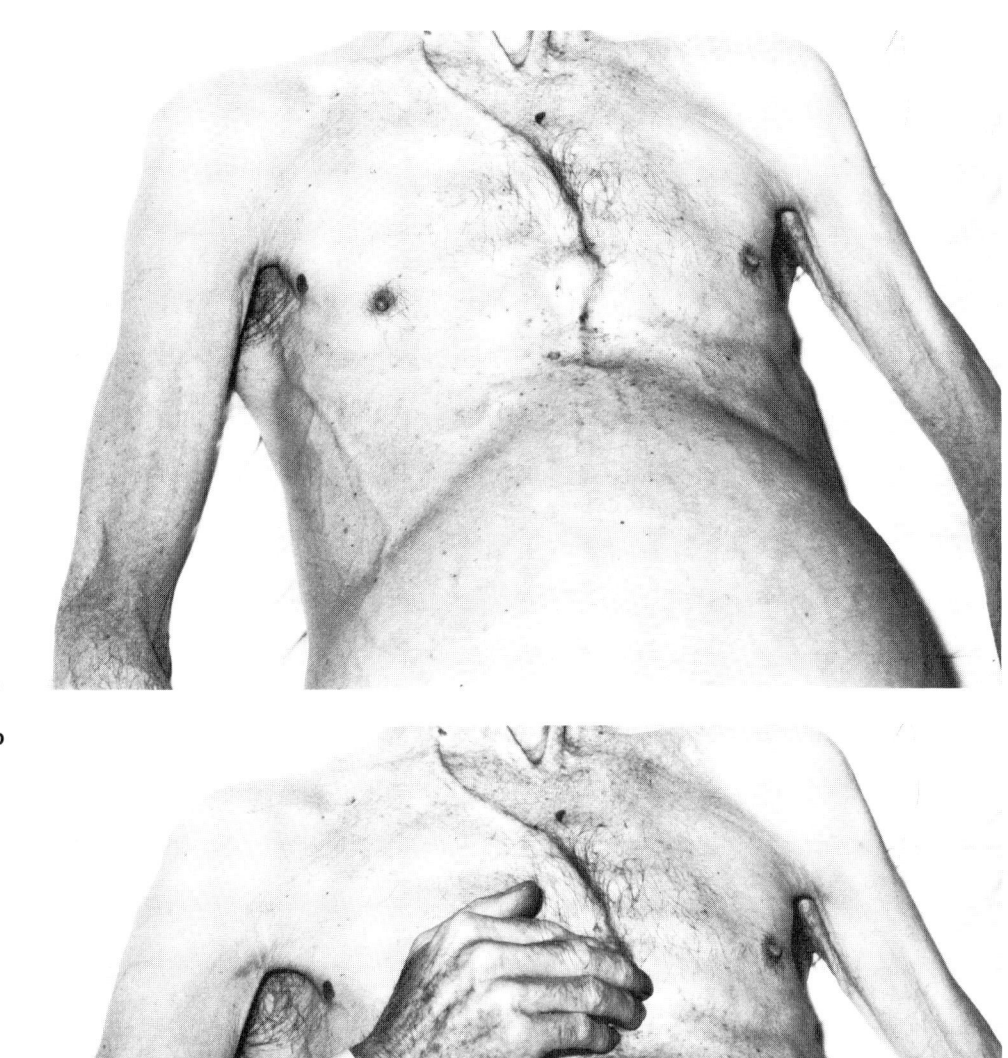

a

b

Figure 7.17 *Cordis – Hakim shunt in situ. Manual compression of the pump antechamber by the patient.*

Early complications

Disseminated intravascular coagulation is reported to occur in some of these patients with death from widespread haemorrhage in 25% of those who develop it. The condition is diagnosed by a marked lowering of the platelet count and fibrinogen level together with a high titre of fibrinogen degradation products. In the author's experience haematological evidence of subclinical DIC occurs in 30% but the full-blown condition is rare and has not been encountered in the author's series. The cause of the DIC is unknown and has been variously ascribed to the presence of a procoagulant in the ascitic fluid, infection or endotoxin. The occurrence of severe DIC is an indication for immediate shunt removal followed by heparin therapy using an infusion pump.

Cardiac complications include arrhythmias and congestive cardiac failure. Arrhythmias are usually due to malposition of the atrial catheter such that it lies against the myocardium. Congestive cardiac failure as a result of volume overload occurs in patients with diminished cardiac reserve and is treated conservatively. It is usually self-limiting since the marked diuresis rapidly reduces the expanded plasma volume.

OUTCOME AND LONG-TERM COMPLICATIONS

Cirrhotic ascites

In the absence of complications, an effective decompression of the ascites is obtained in all the patients but complete abolition of the ascites is rare. The maximal diuretic response is obtained during the first seven to 10 days. Thereafter the daily urine output levels off since the pressure differential between the peritoneal cavity and the central venous pressure drops and when it equalizes, flow through the shunt does not occur spontaneously. At this stage flow is maintained by external compression of the antechamber by the patient who is instructed to compress it intermittently during the waking hours (10 compressions) over a period of five minutes three or four times per day (Figure 7.17). The patient is also instructed to continue to wear an elastic corset since this helps to maintain the pressure differential.

Most of these patients need to be maintained on a low salt diet and on low oral doses of spironolactone and/or a K^+ sparing loop diuretic (amiloride).

Malignant effusions

The results obtained in patients with peritoneal carcinomatosis can be gratifying with abolition of the distressing symptoms of the tense ascites, although complete disappearance of the latter does not occur. In the author's experience these patients do not seem to benefit from additional therapy with spironolactone or loop diuretics. Cytological examination of samples of the fluid from the antechamber in these patients has demonstrated a constant flow of malignant cells into the circulation (Figure 7.18) but this does not appear to be associated with widespread dissemination of the tumour or any adverse reactions. By contrast the clinical impression has been that these patients survive for long periods in the absence of any chemotherapy and despite their extensive disease. The average survival in this group has been eight months with a range of two to 23 months.

Long-term complications

Infection

This is perhaps the most serious complication and in the author's experience occurs usually after discharge and is generally a late complication. The problem is linked with the risk of spontaneous bacterial peritonitis which is a known complication of cirrhotic ascites. Evidence for introduction of sepsis at the time of surgery is usually lacking. The symptoms, which are mild and easily missed, are rigors, a low-grade pyrexia and abdominal pain. Often abdominal tenderness and rebound are absent and it is rare to encounter the classical picture of bacterial peritonitis. A diagnostic tap from the peritoneal cavity or the antechamber reveals turbid fluid

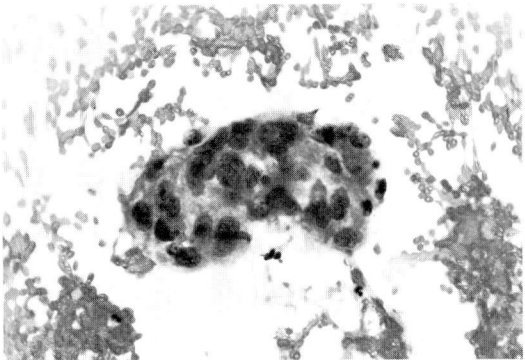

Figure 7.18 *Cytology of aspirate from antechamber obtained from a patient with malignant ascites, showing malignant cells in the fluid.*

and culture usually grows gram-negative aerobes, pneumococcus or *Staphylococcus albus*. Shunt infection often precipitates encephalopathy in these patients and is attended by a high mortality. Treatment entails shunt removal and appropriate antibiotic therapy.

Shunt blockage

Obstruction of the shunt is a common complication of the LeVeen shunt, and surgical revision and replacement was necessary in 70% of patients within four months of insertion of this shunt. Obstruction still occurs with the Cordis–Hakim shunt but is far less common and is usually reversible by conservative measures.

The signs of shunt occlusion include an increase in the abdominal girth and tenderness, a decrease in the urine output and a rise in the haematocrit. When the peritoneal catheter is occluded, the pump antechamber refills very slowly after compression. The obstruction is usually cleared by allowing the antechamber to refill. The tubing between the valve unit and antechamber is then occluded by external finger compression and the antechamber pressed firmly. This procedure which forces fluid back through the peritoneal catheter is repeated two to three times. If the antechamber does not refill adequately after compression or the above measures fail, sterile saline is injected with a fine needle into the antechamber while occluding the tubing between it and the valve unit.

Obstruction can also occur between the antechamber and the valve unit. This is characterized by failure of the valve unit to refill after compression despite a functioning antechamber. This obstruction is remedied by occlusion of the tubing between the antechamber and the peritoneal catheter. Thereafter the antechamber is pressed firmly thereby forcing ascitic fluid through the valve unit and venous line. The procedure is repeated two to three times. If unsuccessful, sterile saline is injected into the antechamber while occluding the tubing between it and the peritoneal catheter.

Obstruction of the venous (atrial) catheter is characterized by a functioning antechamber but the valve unit resists compression. Remedial action consists of forceful compression of the valve unit. If this fails saline is injected through the antechamber after occlusion of the tubing between it and the peritoneal catheter. If patency is not restored by this measure, the system, or more usually the atrial catheter, is replaced surgically.

Leakage of peritoneal fluid

This results from loosening of the purse-string suture around the peritoneal catheter or stretching of the rectus sheath. It causes leakage of peritoneal fluid along the tract surrounding the tubing and the antechamber–valve unit (Figure 7.19). Untreated it leads to occlusion of the shunt. The treatment consists of exploration of the abdominal wound and insertion of a new purse-string suture round the peritoneal catheter. This complication is prevented by the insertion of two purse-string sutures around the emergent peritoneal catheter at the time of insertion of the shunt.

Other late complications

The author has encountered one instance of skin necrosis over the pump antechamber with exposure of the latter and infection. This was due to

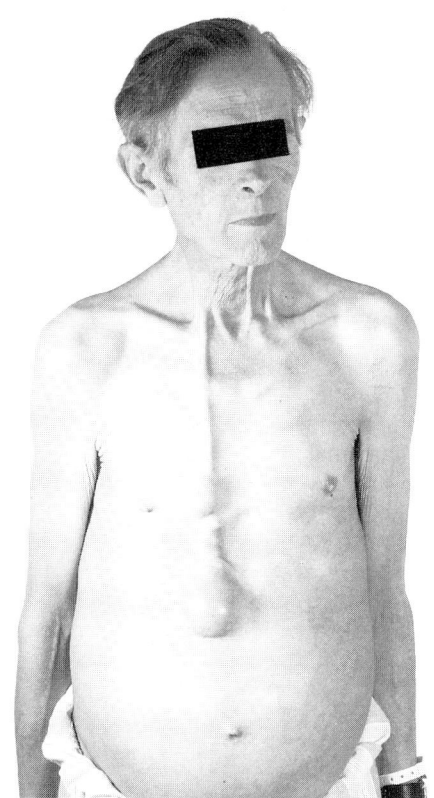

Figure 7.19 *Leakage of peritoneal fluid around peritoneal catheter. This complication is caused by loosening of the purse-string suture or stretching of the posterior rectus sheath. The complication is prevented by the insertion of two purse-string sutures around the emergent peritoneal catheter at the time of insertion of the shunt.*

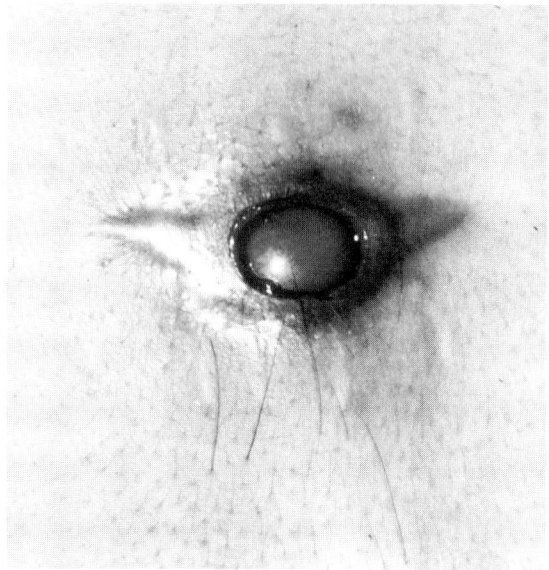

Figure 7.20 *Necrosis of scar with exposure of the antechamber and infection.*

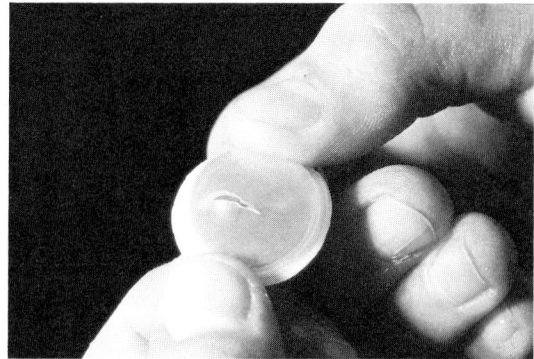

Figure 7.21 *Mechanical failure with fracture of the antechamber.*

faulty positioning of the antechamber such that it was sited beneath the transverse sternal wound used to fashion the pocket to accommodate the antechamber–valve unit assembly (Figure 7.20). The placement of the antechamber distal to the sternal wound is an important practical step since the repeated compression by the patient of the antechamber will induce pressure necrosis of the relatively avascular scar.

Mechanical failure of the pump antechamber due to fracture, causing accumulation of fluid surrounding the shunt system, was encountered in one patient (Figure 7.21). This may have been due to obsessive and vigorous compression of the chamber by a rather anxious patient or to a defective unit in the first instance.

REFERENCES

1. Wilkinson SP & Williams R (1980) Renin–angiotensin–aldosterone system in cirrhosis. *Gut* **21**: 545–554.
2. Campra JL & Reynolds TB (1978) Effectiveness of high-dose spironolactone therapy in patients with chronic liver disease and relatively refractory ascites. *Digestive Diseases* **23**: 1025–1030.
3. Smith AN (1962) Peritoneocaval shunt with a Holter valve in the treatment of ascites. *Lancet* **i**: 671–672.
4. LeVeen HH, Christondeas G, Moon IP et al (1974) Peritoneovenous shunting for ascites. *Annals of Surgery* **180**: 580–591.
5. LeVeen HH, Wapnick S & Grosberg S (1976) Further experience with peritoneovenous shunting for ascites. *Annals of Surgery* **174**: 574–581.
6. Greenlee HB, Stanley MM & Reinhardt GF (1981) Intractable ascites treated with peritoneovenous shunt (LeVeen). *Archives of Surgery* **116**: 518–524.
7. Oosterlee J (1980) Peritoneovenous shunting for ascites in cancer patients. *British Journal of Surgery* **67**: 667–668.
8. Greig PD, Blendis LM, Langer B et al (1981) Renal and haemodynamic effects of the peritoneovenous shunt. *Gastroenterology* **80**: 119–125.
9. Matseshe JW, Beart RW, Bartholomew LG et al (1978) Fatal disseminated intravascular coagulation after peritoneovenous shunt for intractable ascites. *Mayo Clinic Proceedings* **53**: 526–528.

8

Surgery for Morbid Obesity

Robert J. Freeark

Morbid Obesity is commonly defined as a body weight of 100 lbs (45 kg) or more above the ideal for a person of that height, age and sex, and which has existed for at least five years in spite of conscientious efforts to control it. While there are many limitations to this definition, for the most part it describes a group of patients who are predominantly female and whose weight gain began early in life and has continued in a largely uninterrupted fashion throughout their 20s in spite of a myriad of therapies, diets and drugs which are usually administered under medical direction. Many of these patients deny excessive intake of food and few of them eat three meals per day, almost always eschewing breakfast but acknowledging a propensity to compulsive eating at times of stress. They have often responded to diet programmes with as much as 30–50 lb weight loss only to regain the weight rapidly once they have abandoned the particular diet or programme. They are commonly depressed, have low self-esteem and severely restrict their physical and social activities.

Surgical considerations

In the USA, severe obesity exists in an estimated 5% of the male and 7% of the female population. The rationale behind a surgical treatment of this problem rests with the assumption that persistence of this morbid condition will lead to a host of medical problems and will significantly shorten the patient's life expectancy. It is similarly assumed that these effects can be prevented by returning to and maintaining their weight at near normal levels. While this rationale is as yet unproven, the failure of alternative methods of weight control and a growing awareness of the medical, psychological and social consequences of excessive body weight has, over the past two decades, led to a large-scale effort to find a safe and effective surgical treatment.

In spite of two decades of experimental and clinical investigation, there is at present no agreement as to the role of surgery in the management of severe obesity. Surgeons who are engaged in this endeavour have a clear obligation to familiarize themselves and their patients with the important lessons gleaned from past experiences, as well as the many uncertainties which still exist.

Historical perspective

From 1964 to 1975, the operation of choice for the surgical management of morbid obesity was the jejunoileal bypass.[1]

Morbidly obese patients were assumed to be incapable of long-term control of their caloric intake so it was thought that weight reduction could best be achieved by the early diversion of ingested food into the large intestine. Although considerable controversy surrounded issues of technique and the prevention and management of serious side-effects, the operation was performed on a large number of patients in major medical centres and small hospitals around the world. Important lessons learned from this clinical experience were:

1. In the proper setting major surgery could be performed on morbidly obese patients with a low operative morbidity and mortality.

2. Surgically induced rapid weight loss over a period of 12 to 18 months was generally well tolerated, and that many of the undesirable side-effects were self-limited, easily controlled or reversible.

3. Both serious and life-endangering complications from this procedure occurred in a small (10%) but significant group of patients and would ultimately lead to the virtual abandonment of this method as a definitive form of treatment.[2]

4. Seemingly small details of operative technique, e.g. measurement of the length of intestinal segments, could have a profound influence on the results of surgery.

5. Few patients achieved their ideal weight by bypass alone.

6. Early and impressive weight loss was not consistently maintained.

7. While some morbidly obese patients could learn to modify their eating habits, a significant few persisted in their excessive intake of readily absorbable high-calorie food which effectively undid the anticipated effects of the procedure.

8. When it was found necessary or advisable to take down an intestinal bypass, virtually all patients regained their lost weight unless other surgical procedures to control obesity were performed simultaneously.

The years from 1975 to the present have reflected a growing emphasis on operations which limit the amount of food entering the small intestine and have been characterized by a bewildering variety of minor technical modifications designed to overcome the early or late complications of these procedures and to assure their long-term success. As in the earlier experience with intestinal bypass, it has become increasingly apparent that early weight loss is not always maintained, and that late and unanticipated sequelae occur, requiring constant long-term surveillance of patients undergoing these procedures.

PATIENT SELECTION

With few exceptions, obesity surgery should be confined to good-risk patients who have weighed in excess of 100 lbs (45 kg) over their ideal weight for a period of more than five years in spite of medically supervised efforts to control their obesity.

'Good risk' refers to both the physical and emotional capacity of the patient to withstand the operation and its medical as well as psychosocial consequences. A distinction should be made between prophylactic and therapeutic obesity surgery. The former is generally confined to younger patients of 20–40 years of age who have experienced none of the recognized medical consequences of morbid obesity, but whose persistent excessive weight clearly poses a threat to their future health and well being. 'Therapeutic surgery' is undertaken in those patients who have sustained one or more of the sequelae of morbid obesity and are being operated on in an effort to control or reverse its medical effects. Such patients may have cardiovascular disease, hypertension, arthritis, diabetes, hyperlipidaemia, metabolic disturbances or gout, all of which contribute to the hazards of the anaesthetic and the operation, and can impede postoperative recovery. This increased risk must be balanced against the likelihood of significant benefit in these complicating medical problems.

In both prophylactic and therapeutic obesity surgery, great emphasis should be placed on the emotional health of the candidates and their ability to adjust to the rigours of the procedure and its consequences. Psychological disorders commonly accompany morbid obesity, and both psychiatric and psychological problems may arise as a consequence of treatment. While a number of psychological tests have been advocated to assist in the evaluation process, we have found a personal assessment by the responsible team members to be sufficient for the evaluation of most patients. Experience suggests that patients with a history of inpatient psychiatric treatment, as well as those addicted to alcohol or cola drinks, are more likely to experience medical complications, while those with a strong oral dependency may be unable to tolerate a gastric restrictive procedure. Of the utmost importance is an assessment of the patients' ability to modify their eating habits during the period of restricted intake and to sustain these modifications once the restrictive aspects of the procedure have begun to disappear. Gentry et al found that patients who understood before surgery that the success of the operation depended on changing their eating behaviour lost more weight.[3] They emphasized the need for patients to have a realistic attitude towards the impact of weight loss on their life, as well as the importance of consistent postoperative reinforcement of dietary principles for optimal results.

Criteria

As with other elective procedures, operations for morbid obesity are recommended only after a thorough assessment of the risks and benefits for the patient in question. The following are generally accepted criteria.

1. Severe exogenous obesity: Variously defined as weight twice that of the normal for similar age, sex and height; 100% over ideal weight; or 100 lbs (45 kg) in excess of ideal weight. The excess weight developed in the absence of any demonstrable endocrinological or metabolic disorder.
2. Intractable: The excess weight has persisted for longer than five years in spite of documented medically supervised attempts at weight reduction.
3. Satisfactory health: Defined as medically and emotionally capable of tolerating the proposed procedure and its immediate and long-term consequences.

Within these criteria, considerable latitude exists for determining the need and wisdom of operative treatment. Patient selection is, however, the single most important factor in achieving a satisfactory result in obesity surgery. The following are offered as guidelines.

Age. Limited experience with the results of obesity surgery in patients under the age of 20 years, as well as uncertainty as regards the long-term consequences of these procedures, suggest that great caution should be exercised in recommending operative treatment for patients who are less than 20 years of age.

Morbidly obese patients over the age of 50 years are more likely to have experienced the late sequelae of long-term excess weight and face a higher risk/benefit ratio from operative intervention. They should seldom be considered for surgery unless there are compelling medical problems which are likely to be benefited by profound weight reduction, i.e. a 'therapeutic' procedure. In contrast, patients in the 20–50 years age range who fulfil the criteria listed above and who have no known medical disorder as a result of obesity are candidates for 'prophylactic' surgery.

Sex. While severe or morbid obesity is more common in females and they constitute the largest number of patients undergoing obesity surgery, the health risk and reduced longevity resulting from severe obesity is not as well documented in females as in males. In the author's experience, male patients accepted the undesirable side-effects of both the intestinal and gastric procedures better and lost more weight in the early follow-up period. Lack of compliance of male patients in long-term follow up precludes a definitive statement with regard to the degree of long-term benefits.

Severity of excess weight. Most studies have confirmed a greater degree of weight loss in patients with the most to lose. The more severe cases of morbid obesity are less likely to return to or near their ideal weight.

Associated medical illness. Medical problems such as adult onset diabetes, hypertension, cardiovascular disease, hyperlipidaemia, hyperuricaemia, Pickwickian syndrome, arthritis, and sleep apnoea syndrome are likely to benefit from successful surgery. On occasion, obesity surgery will be required to effect weight loss prior to the undertaking of another operative procedure, e.g. spinal stenosis, joint replacement, repair of giant hernia, etc. In contrast, patients with severe liver disease or those with medical problems of sufficient severity to preclude general anaesthesia or major abdominal surgery are clearly ineligible for obesity surgery. Particular attention should be paid to the presence of endocrine disturbances, such as hypothyroidism and conditions which impair pulmonary and cardiovascular function.

Psychological disturbances. While severe obesity is associated with several known organic diseases and may be a manifestation of a severe psychological disorder, successful operative treatment may provide significant benefit to a wide range of emotional and psychosocial problems. Strict guidelines for patient selection are not possible but the following deserve emphasis.[3]

1. There was no correlation between weight loss and psychologic status in patients undergoing gastric bypass who were studied by Saltzstein and Guttman.[4]
2. Psychiatric inpatient treatment correlated with a high incidence of medical complications following surgery, but outpatient psychiatric history did not.
3. Obesity patients have more depressive traits and lower self-esteem than a normal population, and these remain unchanged after successful weight-reduction surgery.
4. Patients who are addicted to alcohol or cola drugs and those with severe oral dependency are unsuitable candidates for gastric obesity surgery.
5. An MMPI (Minnesota Multiphasic Personality Inventory) score that is greater than two standard deviations above the mean (indicates psychopathology) correlates with a higher incidence of medical and psychological complications.

Compliance. Since postoperative dietary compliance is the single most important determinant of successful obesity surgery, it is unfortunate that no reliable method exists to measure this in preoperative evaluations. Clearly, a willingness to accept the severe intake restrictions imposed by the gastric operations, as well as the commitment to permanent modification of eating patterns, maintenance of recommended vitamin and dietary supplements, and returning for periodic evaluations are essential to long-term success.

PREOPERATIVE CARE AND INVESTIGATIONS

In addition to the usual history, physical examination and routine laboratory tests employed on all patients undergoing major abdominal surgery, the following are of special importance in operative procedures in obese patients.

Prior to admission

1. Patients should be seen by an attending anaesthesiologist for evaluation of any special problems relating to identified medical conditions, e.g. hypertension, current or proposed medications, past anaesthetic history of patient or family, anatomical problems related to airway and its maintenance, and difficulties of intraoperative monitoring techniques.

2. Patients should stop smoking for at least two weeks prior to operation and begin a liquid diet two days prior to surgery to facilitate an empty colon.

3. Cutaneous infection anywhere on the body surface should be eradicated, and areas of skin irritation commonly seen in the depths of skin folds of the obese patient should be controlled by twice daily showering with an antiseptic soap and careful drying of intertriginous areas.

4. The use of aspirin containing medications should cease at least 10 days prior to surgery.

5. When indicated (see below) special radiological, haematological, metabolic or endocrinological studies should be completed in time for any remedial action.

6. All the criteria for a truly informed consent to operation should have been fulfilled prior to admission following a lengthy discussion of the operation, risks, benefits and alternatives with the patient and nearest relative.

On admission

1. The high incidence of cholelithiasis in morbidly obese patients has led many surgeons to obtain gallbladder studies (ultrasound, oral cholecystography) prior to surgery. Our preference is to rely on palpation of the gallbladder at the time of surgery and to recommend removal only if stones are identified. Cholecystectomy is listed as one of the procedures on the patient's consent form. It is seldom performed prophylactically.

2. Except under circumstances suggesting an abnormality of structure or function, we do not perform routine radiological examinations of the gastrointestinal or genitourinary systems.

3. Patients are given a laxative on the day of admission and receive cleansing enemas the night prior to surgery. Except in the case of intestinal bypass surgery, antibiotic bowel preparation is not employed.

4. The need for and method of prophylaxis for venous thromboembolism is evaluated on admission. Specific measures are undertaken only in patients with a past history or clinical evidence of deep venous thrombosis.

Day of surgery

All gastric operations receive a systemic broad-spectrum antibiotic, currently cephalosporin, one hour prior to operation and every four hours during and following the operative procedure for a period of 24 hours.

AVAILABLE OPTIONS

Jejunoileal bypass

Although largely abandoned as the sole surgical treatment of morbid obesity, we share with a minority of bariatric surgeons the conviction that, under special circumstances, intestinal bypass is an acceptable procedure for selected patients. When currently employed by us, it constitutes the first stage of a two-stage operative approach. The jejunoileal bypass is performed with the clear understanding that it will be taken down after a period of maximal weight loss, and the patient will undergo a gastric restrictive procedure at that time. This two-stage approach is preferred for patients with 'super obesity' (usually in excess of 400 lbs), patients whose morbid obesity is associated with severe hyperlipidaemia or diabetes and patients who are emotionally incapable of accepting the restricted intake of the gastric procedures. On occasion, it is employed when, for technical, medical or anaesthetic considerations an upper abdominal (gastric) procedure is inadvisable until some weight loss has been achieved.

In our experience, weight loss in excess of 200 lb is rarely accomplished by a gastric procedure alone, although such losses were not uncommon with jejunoileal bypass. Careful surveillance during the 12–24 months following jejunoileal bypass will usually permit the early detection of electrolyte imbalance, or liver or kidney disturbances before irreversible damage has occurred. Liberal use of antibiotics during this period has also tended to eliminate the various intestinal complications of this procedure. The intestinal bypass patients usually learn to modify their intake over a period of time in an effort to control their surgically induced diarrhoea. This reduced intake of calories, in addition to the impaired absorption of ingested calories, usually leads to marked weight loss which can subsequently be enhanced by the safer long-term procedure of gastric bypass. While subjecting the patients to the risks, costs and discomfort of two major operations, the efficacy of the two-step approach has been confirmed by a number of patients who required takedown of what was originally intended to be a definitive intestinal bypass and by a smaller number of patients in whom the intestinal operation was a temporary first step in preparation for a definitive gastric procedure.

Jejunoileal bypass as the first stage of a two-step approach to morbid obesity is always performed end to side to simplify the procedure and to facilitate subsequent takedown. We prefer a transverse incision just above the level of the umbilicus and transect the jejunum 12 inches below the ligament of Treitz as measured on the mesenteric side of a tightly stretched first jejunal segment. The distal jejunum is closed and turned back on itself to discourage intussusception. The proximal jejunum is anastomosed end to side of the distal ileum 4 inches from the ileocolic junction after first removing the ileocaecal fat pad and appendix.

Following discharge from the hospital, jejunoileal bypass patients are seen at weekly intervals in the outpatient centre until the initial diarrhoea and accompanying fluid and electrolyte disturbance begins to subside. Careful assessment of the patient is then carried out at one- to three-month intervals for signs of the recognized nutritional and metabolic complications of this procedure. At the first sign of significant hepatomegaly, hepatic dysfunction, renal impairment, urinary calculi formation, severe electrolyte disturbance or profound protein caloric malnutrition, the patient is hospitalized for corrective measures, and plans are made for early takedown of the intestinal bypass. In the absence of significant side-effects, the bypass is left intact until the patient is no longer experiencing significant weight loss. At this time, usually after 12–18 months, the patient is scheduled for take-

Table 8.1 *Gastric restrictive procedures.*

	Gastroplasty	Gastric bypass
Essential components		
Small pouch	50 ml capacity or less	50 ml capacity or less
Small stoma	<12 mm diameter	<12 mm diameter
Gastric partition	Permanent, leak free	Permanent, leak free
Special requirements		
Stoma	Requires reinforcement	Reinforcement advisable?
Early complications		
Leak	Infrequent (stoma, partition, pouch)	2–10% anastomotic
Stomal stenosis	Common (10–15%)	Rare
Late complications		
Inadequate weight loss (<25% excess weight)	20%*	10%*
Oesophagitis	Rare	10%*
Intolerance requiring takedown	5%	Rare
Anaemia (Fe deficiency, B_{12})	Rare	15%?
Afferent loop syndrome	None	Varies with technique

*Percentage occurrence varies considerably with techniques employed and individual reports.

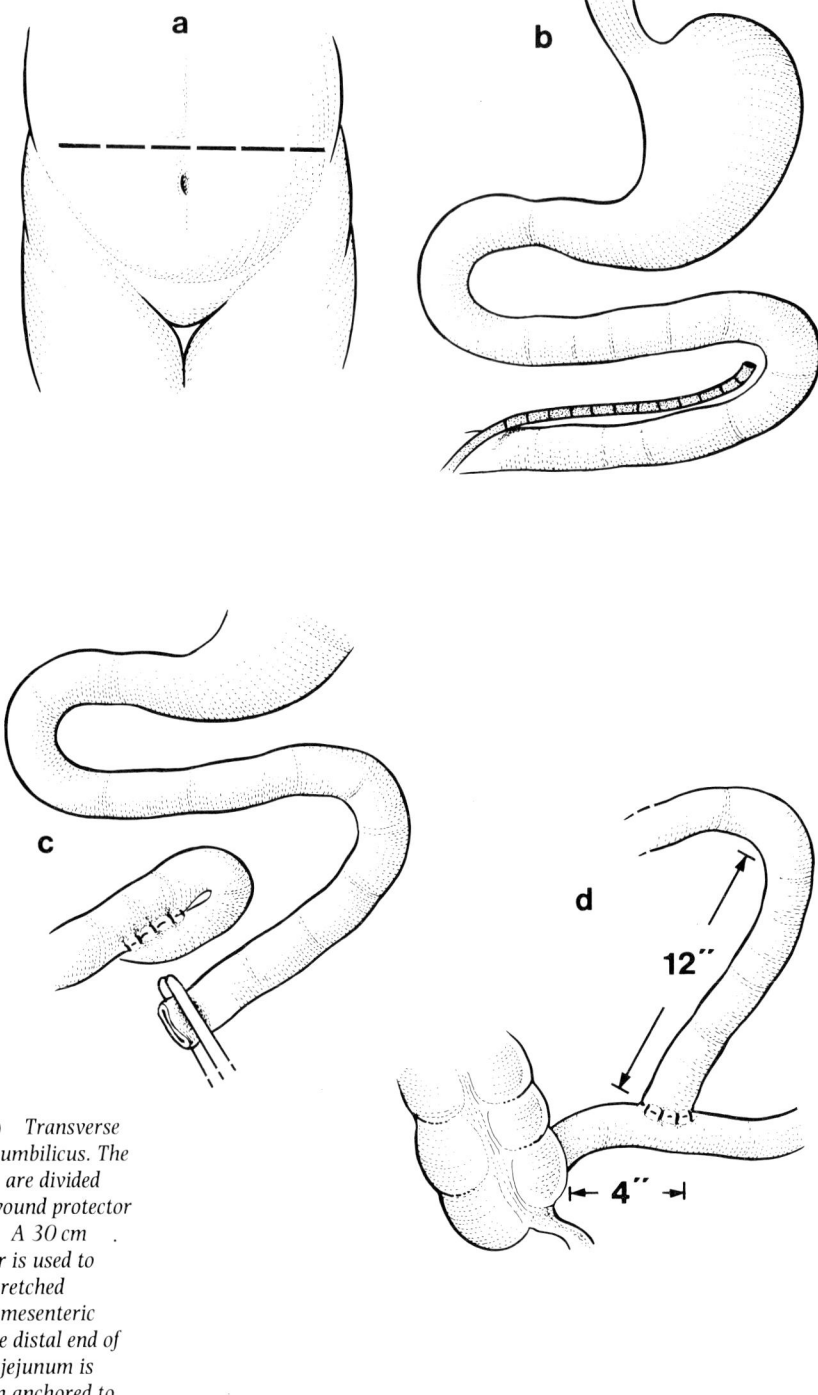

Figure 8.1 (a) *Transverse incision above umbilicus. The rectus muscles are divided and a plastic wound protector is inserted.* (b) *A 30 cm rubber catheter is used to measure the stretched jejunum at its mesenteric border.* (c) *The distal end of the transected jejunum is closed and then anchored to itself to discourage intussusception.* (d) *The proximal cut end of the jejunum is anastomosed end to side to the distal ileum 10 cm from the ileocaecal junction.*

down and gastric restrictive procedure on an elective basis.

Gastric restrictive procedures (Table 8.1)

Current surgical management of morbid obesity relies largely on procedures which limit the intake of calories by controlling the size of the gastric reservoir and the opening which allows food to continue down the alimentary tract. In gastroplasty (GP), a proximal gastric pouch of less than 50 ml capacity is created by partitioning the stomach with surgical staples. This pouch communicates with the distal stomach through a stoma of 10 mm or less that is surgically created through one of several techniques. The procedure as currently employed is relatively easy to perform with few of the risks or hazards of gastrointestinal anastomoses. Reoperation for stenosis or dilatation of the stoma, or disruption or marked enlargement of the gastric reservoir is fairly common. Weight loss is less than in procedures which bypass the distal stomach,[5] but gastroplasty patients are relatively free from the long-term hazards of iron and vitamin B_{12} deficiency.

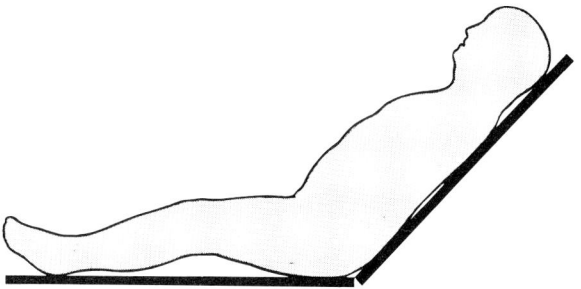

Figure 8.2 *Patient position for gastric restrictive procedures. The semi-recumbent posture is used with chest and abdomen up to 45° from the horizontal plane in order to facilitate downward displacement of the stomach and upper abdominal viscera.*

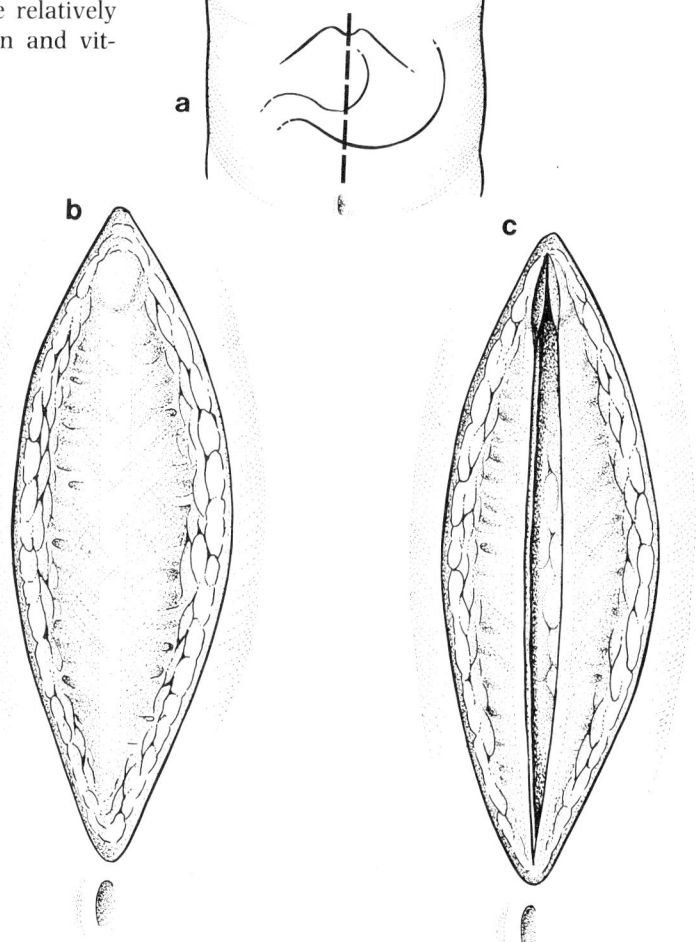

Figure 8.3 (a) *A high upper abdominal midline incision extending over the xiphoid process facilitates excision of xiphoid and identification of linea alba.* **(b)** *The abundant subcutaneous fat is separated by firm lateral traction after first incising the skin. A 1 cm strip of linea alba is cleared of overlying fat precisely along the midline (tip of xiphoid).* **(c)** *The linea alba is incised exposing the fat of the falciform ligament. The incision extends from the umbilicus to include all of the xiphoid process which is cleared of its attachments and excised using heavy scissors. The peritoneal cavity is then entered through the lateral leaf of the falciform ligament.*

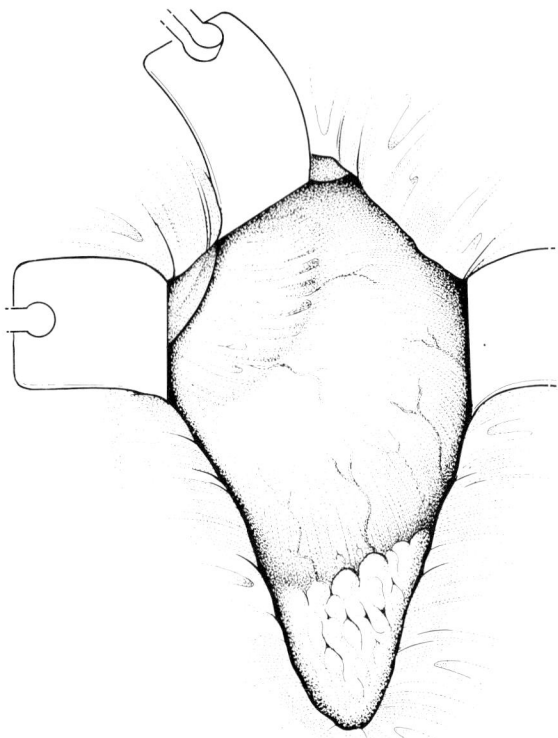

Figure 8.3 (d) *The falciform ligament is detached from the under-surface of the abdominal wall and a plastic wound protector is inserted. Table-anchored wound retractors are positioned to provide upward and lateral traction on both costal margins and under-surface of the left lobe of the liver.*

In gastric bypass (GBP), a proximal gastric pouch of 50 ml capacity or less is completely separated from the distal stomach by two rows of staples or, in our hands, by transection and suture closure. A gastrojejunal anastomosis is then carried out using either a loop or Roux-en-Y technique. The stoma of the gastric pouch is constructed at a diameter of 12 mm or less, usually without external banding or restrictive suture. The longer operative procedure and increased risk of suture line disruption is in part compensated for by a more predictable degree of weight reduction and the rarity of stomal stenosis or closure. Late dilatation of both the pouch and/or the stoma remains a problem in this procedure as it does in gastroplasty. The use of the loop gastrojejunostomy increases the risk of reflux oesophagitis but avoids the necessity for a vent in the bypassed gastric pouch. If Roux-en-Y reconstruction is employed, it should usually be accompanied by a temporary decompressive tube gastrostomy in the distal gastric pouch.

OPERATIVE PROCEDURES

Jejunoileal bypass end to side (Figure 8.1)

Through a transverse skin incision both rectus muscles are completely divided and the peritoneal cavity is entered. A plastic wound protector is inserted and limited abdominal exploration is carried out. A needle biopsy of the liver is performed. Using a rubber catheter 30 cm in length, the mesenteric border of tightly stretched proximal jejunum is measured and the bowel transected. The distal end is closed and sutured distally to discourage intussusception. The proximal end is anastomosed end to side to the distal ileum at a distance of 10 cm from the ileocaecal valve. The mesentery is closed. Wall closure is carried out in layers using non absorbable suture and the skin is closed with nylon and Steristrips.

Gastric restrictive procedures (Figures 8.2 and 8.3)

A high upper abdominal midline incision is made over the xiphoid process to allow for accurate identification of linea alba and complete excision of xiphoid process.

Abundant subcutaneous fat is separated by firm traction rather than cut to expose midline fascia.

A 1 cm strip of linea alba is cleared of overlying fat precisely in the midline (tip of xiphoid) and incised sharply in the centre to expose the underlying falciform ligament. The linea alba is incised down to the umbilicus or farther as required.

The xiphoid process is totally excised by first clearing its anterior and posterior surfaces of fat and musculofascial attachments, and heavy scissors and cautery are used to effect removal.

The free peritoneal cavity is entered through the lateral leaf of the falciform ligament where it joins the parietal peritoneum. The ligament is then detached from the upper surface of the anterior abdominal wall throughout its length and remains attached to the anterior surface of the liver.

A disposable plastic wound protector (9–11 inches in diameter) is inserted to cover the entire abdominal wound throughout the procedure.

Table-anchored wound retractors are positioned to provide upward and lateral traction on both costal margins as well as the upper surface of the left lobe of the liver.

Abdominal exploration is carried out with emphasis on the presence of gallstones, splenic adhesions and pelvic viscera in the female. The generally good health in the age group usually undergoing obesity surgery and the difficulties of abdominal exploration in obese patients make palpation of all abdominal viscera unnecessary.

Procedure for loop gastric bypass (Figure 8.4)

The following is the author's technique:

1. Mobilization of greater curvature is begun at the bare area between vas breva and uppermost point of gastroepiploic arcade. The vessel on the gastric side is ligated in continuity with 2/0 silk, while the splenic side vessels are doubly clipped prior to section.

2. The entire greater curvature is dissected free to the level of the oesophagogastric junction, both laterally and posteriorly. The anterior fat pad is preserved proximally.

3. The mobilized proximal stomach is retracted laterally and posteriorly, and the upper portion of the lesser curvature is skeletonized for a distance of 5 cm up to 1 cm of the oesophagogastric junction. The many small branches of both the vagus nerve and left gastric artery are sectioned between 3/0 silk ligatures (gastric side) and clips. Great care is taken to preserve the entire length of the ascending branch of the left gastric artery as well as maintaining its entry into the stomach at the level of the oesophagogastric junction.

4. A point 4 cm from the oesophagogastric junction on the greater curvature is selected as the anastomotic site, and a Kocher clamp is applied at a right angle to the curvature, incorporating 1.5 cm of gastric wall. A second Kocher clamp is applied parallel to and 1 cm distal to the first clamp and incorporates 2.5 cm of stomach wall. The

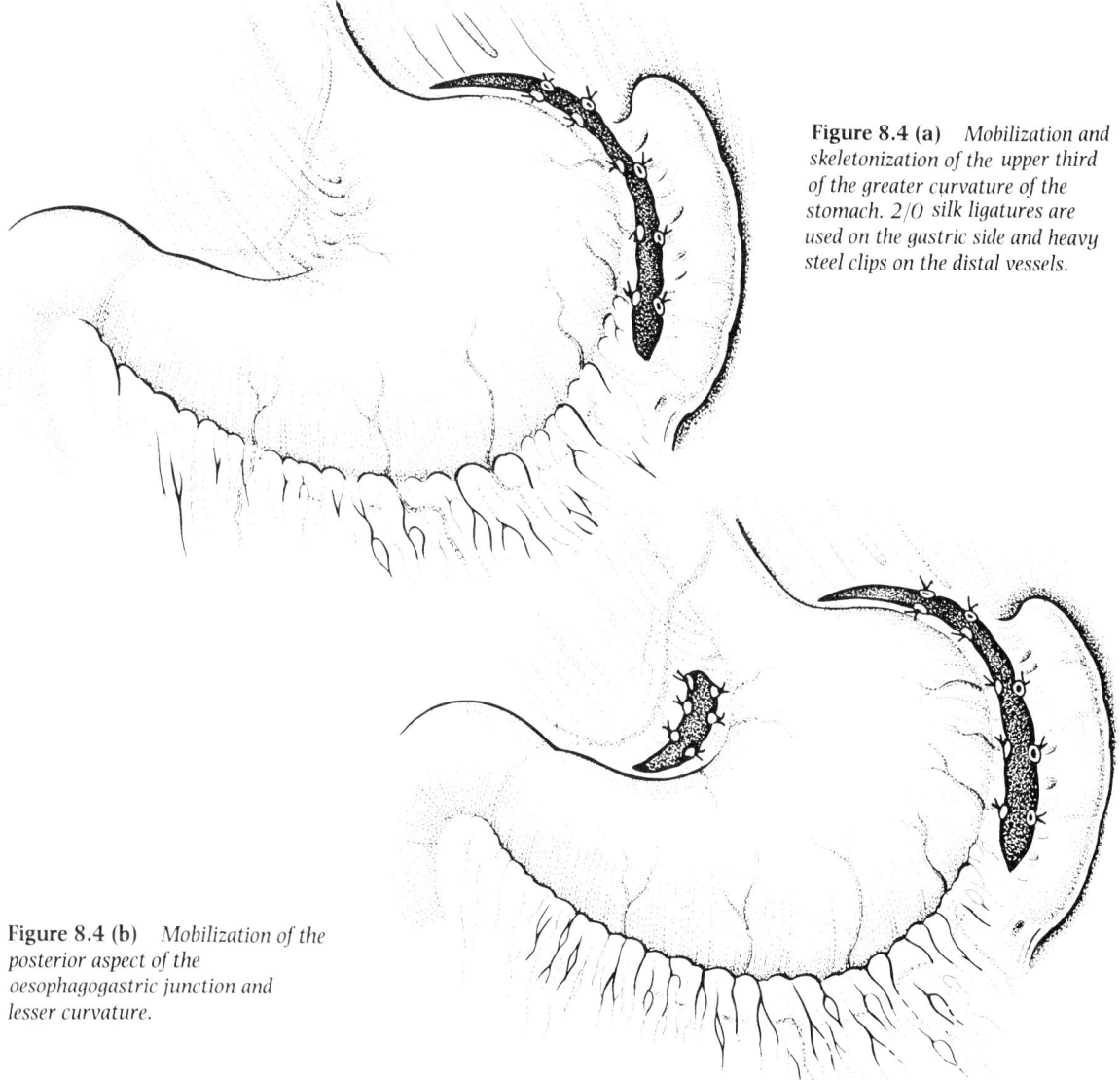

Figure 8.4 (a) *Mobilization and skeletonization of the upper third of the greater curvature of the stomach. 2/0 silk ligatures are used on the gastric side and heavy steel clips on the distal vessels.*

Figure 8.4 (b) *Mobilization of the posterior aspect of the oesophagogastric junction and lesser curvature.*

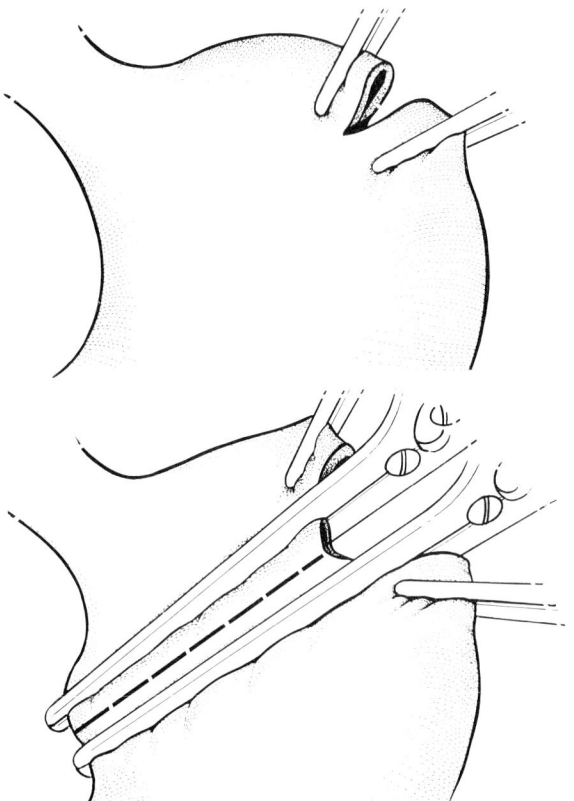

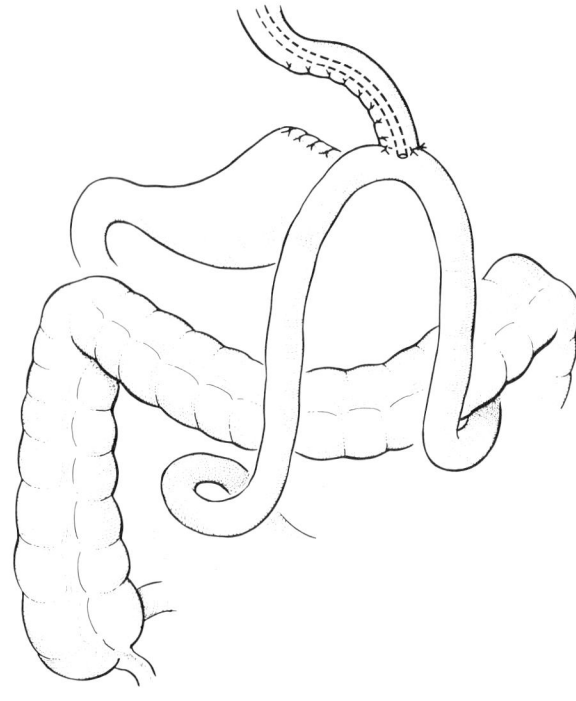

Figure 8.4 (e) *Antecolic loop gastrojejunostomy is performed between the lateral extremity of the pouch and a loop of upper jejunum. This anastomosis should be approximately 1 cm in diameter.*

Figure 8.4 (c) *Anastomotic clamps are applied to the greater curvature 5 cm below the oesophagogastric junction, and the stomach is divided between them. Payr clamps are then applied across the remainder of the stomach which is then completely transected.*

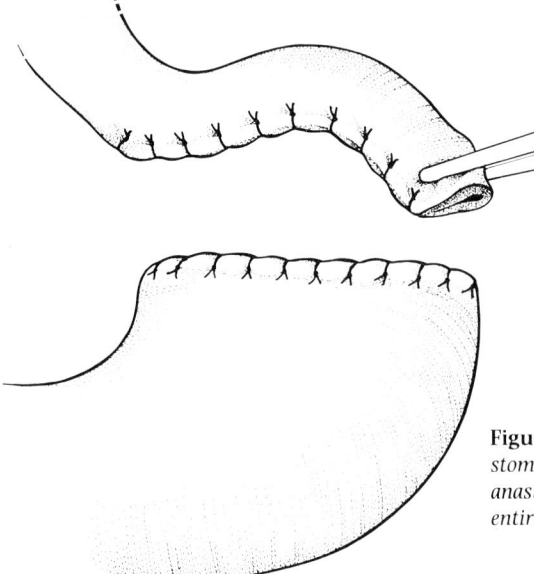

stomach between the two clamps is sectioned to the tip of the more proximal clamp.

5. The space between the two clamps is then used to insert additional clamps between the remaining stomach and the window along the lesser curvature (because of their security and haemostatic effects, the author prefers to use two Payr clamps for this purpose).

6. The stomach is then transected between these final clamps, and the proximal portion is closed to the level of the proximal anastomotic clamp, using a running 2/0 catgut beneath the proximal clamp with a returning running lock stitch of the same suture once the clamp is removed. This lesser curvature side of the proximal gastric pouch is then closed further with interrupted seromuscular sutures of 3/0 silk.

7. The distal gastric pouch is then closed in a

Figure 8.4 (d) *The lesser curvature and proximal stomach are closed with three layers down to the first anastomotic clamp. The distal stomach is closed along its entire length.*

similar fashion throughout its cut edge with emphasis on careful hemostasis of the transected stomach.

8. An antecolic (preferred) loop gastrojejunostomy is then carried out between the tiny proximal gastric pouch (estimated volume 25 cc) and the side of the proximal jejunum approximately 1 cm from its mesenteric border.

   (a) The author prefers to employ a layer of interrupted 3/0 seromuscular sutures posteriorly which are tied, held and cut sequentially to facilitate a second layer of running 3/0 chromic catgut which traverses the full thickness of both walls posteriorly.

   (b) The anterior portion of this small (1.0 cm) anastomosis is closed by a running 3/0 catgut on mucosa only followed by a similar suture approximating, but not inverting, the cut edge of seromuscular tissue. A final layer of interrupted 3/0 silk seromuscular sutures is then added anteriorly.

9. On completion, the small gastric remnant (less than 2% of stomach, or 25 ml capacity) is anastomosed to the proximal jejunum with an estimated stomal diameter of 1.0 cm. The 18 F Salem sump nasogastric tube is then advanced, usually with some difficulty, through the anastomosis and anchored at the nose to make sure that tube openings allow for decompression of both the oesophagogastric remnant and jejunum.

ALTERNATIVE APPROACHES TO GASTRIC BYPASS

The author recognizes that the procedure described above departs from those employed by other authors. As described, the author's technique is lengthy (on average: 4.0 hours) and technically demanding, requiring adequate exposure, good assistants and precise suture technique. It is similar to that used in near total gastrectomy for tumour. This technique has been performed in over 100 patients by a large number of resident surgeons with the author often serving as first assistant. Thus far, it has proved to be safe with no deaths attributable to the method and with only a single instance of anastomotic leak when employed primarily in the treatment of morbid obesity. Two other anastomotic leaks occurred in patients in whom a jejunoileal bypass was taken down, and the atrophic limb of bypassed jejunum was anastomosed to the remnant in a Roux-en-Y manner, a method that is no longer employed.

There were no instances of anastomotic stenosis or stricture requiring treatment of any kind.

More popular and for many surgeons more practical alternatives to the above method of gastric bypass are listed below along with the author's reasons for not employing the modification.

Staple partitioning of the stomach

The application of one or two rows of surgical staples to establish the proximal gastric pouch greatly shortens operating time and is employed by most surgeons performing gastric bypass.

Comment. Though largely overcome by the use of a double row of staples 0.5 cm apart, the author prefers to avoid the risk of partition breakthrough that continues to occur in staple closure of the stomach and cannot arise when the stomach is transected and closed. In addition, the use of the Hofmeister modification of the Polya method for closing the cut ends of the gastric pouch permits construction of a smaller pouch that empties at its distal portion without difficulties and facilitates endoscopic cannulation if required.

Roux-en-Y gastrojejunostomy

A Roux-en-Y limb of jejunum, at least 45 cm in length, is commonly used for anastomosis to the gastric pouch. In most instances, it is passed through the transverse mesocolon (retrocolic) and can facilitate a tension-free anastomosis when excessive colonic size or mesenteric fat makes either an antecolic or retrocolic loop jejunostomy difficult. Many authorities feel that reflux of biliary and pancreatic juice from a loop jejunostomy gives rise to a significant incidence of oesophagitis in bypassed patients and prefer the Roux-en-Y limb technique for this reason.

Comment. The author has not been impressed with the frequency of symptomatic oesophagitis or gastritis in patients with loop bypass, probably because of the extremely small stoma employed. Moreover, there are a number of reports which suggest significant delays in the emptying of the Roux-en-Y limb and disagreement as to the proper length to prevent reflux. The author's long experience and general satisfaction with loop jejunostomy, and one fatal complication occurring in a Roux-en-Y limb reconstruction (severe afferent loop syndrome) has discouraged a change. If the Roux-en-Y limb gastric bypass is used, a temporary gastrostomy tube should be placed in the distal gastric pouch to assure its decompression in the immediate postoperative period.

Suture line reinforcement

Almost all patients undergoing gastric bypass begin to stabilize their weight after a period of 12–24 months. In addition, they usually report an increased capacity for ingested food and a tolerance for more solid food that was initially not present. In some 25% of patients, this increased capacity is associated with a regaining of some of the lost weight.

Radiological or endoscopic investigation of these late failures usually reveals an increase in the size of the gastric pouch (or partitioned upper stomach) or an increase in the size of the gastrojejunal stoma. Both of these changes, to some extent, seem inevitable and are the principal reason for encouraging patients to modify their eating habits during the period of limited capacity and rapid weight loss. This often occurs and is bolstered by the positive influence and satisfaction of significant weight reduction (often for the first time after years of failed obesity therapy). This prospect of an increased capacity and greater variety of food intake is important for some patients who cannot accept a lifetime of marked dietary restriction.

For those patients who do not learn to modify their intake and eating habits, and continue to engage in compulsive eating or drinking of high caloric foods, the gastric bypass, as described, offers little except the nutritional impairment of a near total gastrectomy. The inevitability of some degree of dilatation of the gastrojejunal stoma has led to the use of a variety of techniques to restrict the size of the stoma permanently. Such techniques are now employed routinely in patients undergoing gastroplasty (see later). The use of Marlex mesh or Prolene or similar non-absorbable suture materials to restrict the size of the gastrojejunostomy permanently is also employed by some surgeons. With the exception of the report of Flickinger,[6] none of these authors have provided sufficient follow-up data to determine its benefit or its rate of complications (erosion, stenosis or disruption). We have had occasion to encircle a dilated gastrojejunal stoma with Prolene on a failed gastric bypass and were pleased with its ease and efficacy on a short period of follow up. It is possible that it should be a routine part of both gastric restrictive procedures.

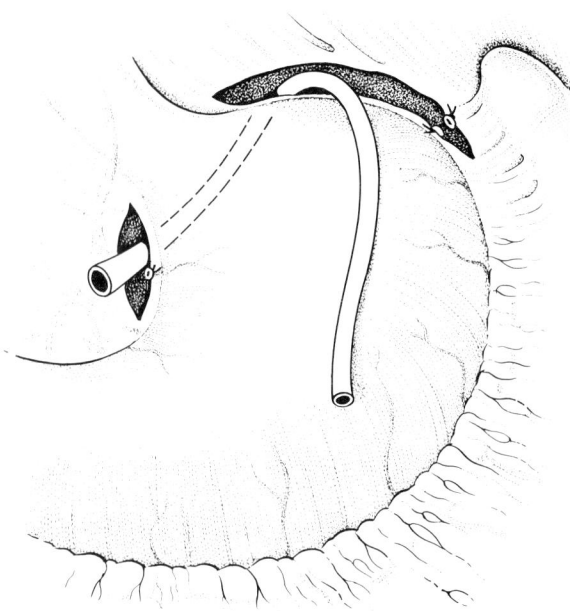

Figure 8.5 (a) *The lesser curvature is cleared for 5 cm near the hiatus and inside the nerve and vascular pedicle. A bare area on the fundus near the hiatus is entered and the greater curvature of the stomach is cleared for 6–8 cm. One or two vasa brevia may require ligation and division. A rubber catheter is then passed around the stomach to facilitate insertion of the TA 90 stapler.*

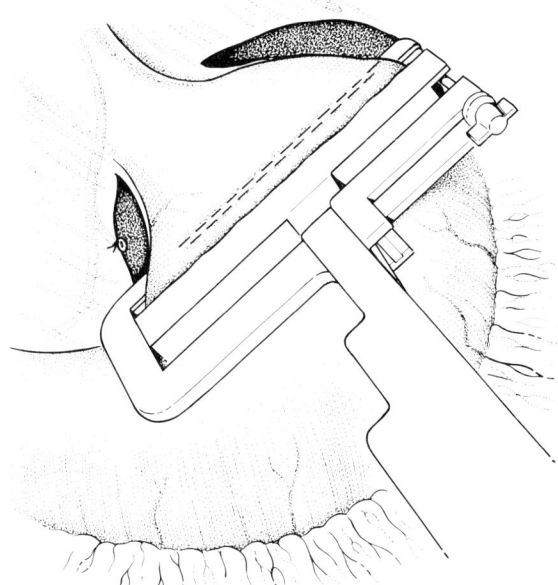

Figure 8.5 (b) *The TA-90 stapler with four staples removed at the medial end is inserted from the lesser curvature side using the rubber catheter (which is fitted over the anvil) to facilitate insertion and positioning of the stapler across the stomach.*

SURGERY FOR MORBID OBESITY 135

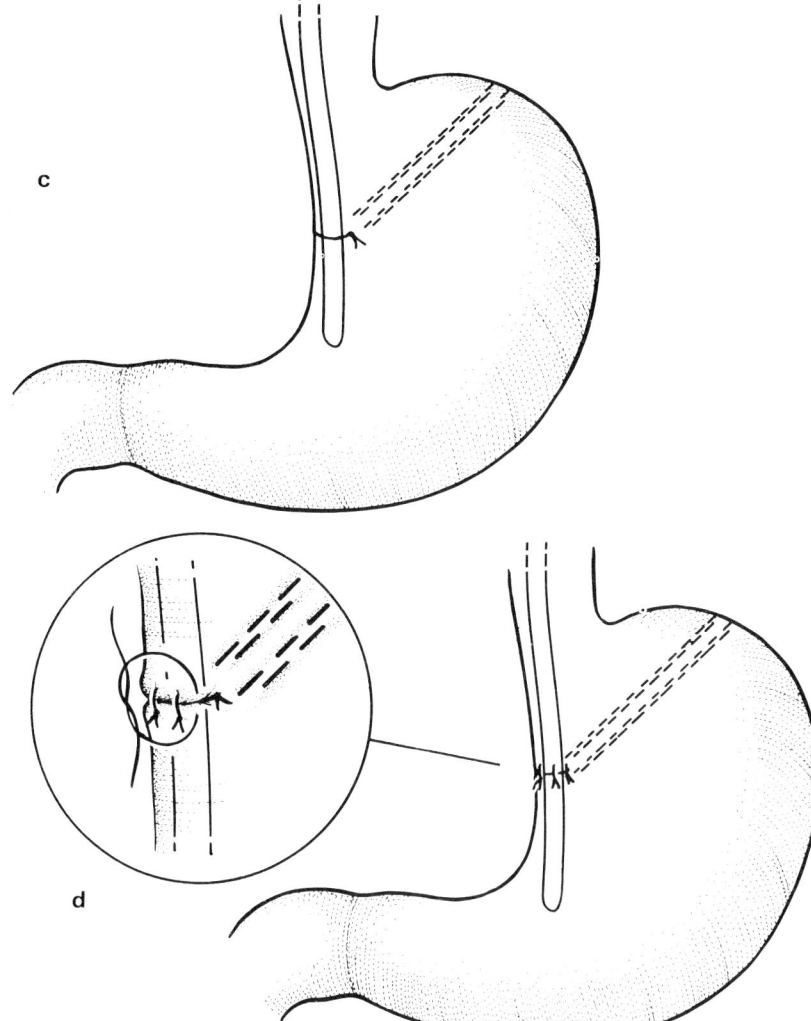

Figure 8.5 (c) *Two rows of staples divide the stomach except near the lesser curvature. A 32 Hurst bougie has been passed alongside the lesser curvature into the distal stomach. An encircling 2/0 Dexon suture is passed through both walls of the stomach and tied round the lesser curvature and the dilator.* **(d)** *Seromuscular sutures are used to cover the encircling Dexon ligature. The Hurst bougie is replaced by a nasogastric tube located to ensure decompression of proximal and distal stomach.*

Tube decompression of the distal gastric pouch

As discussed above, this is performed routinely in patients with Roux-en-Y limb gastric bypass, but is not felt to be necessary in loop bypass. Some authors feel it should be employed in all patients.

Use of the distal gastric pouch to reinforce the gastrojejunal stoma

This additional protection against suture line disruption is theoretically attractive but has not been found necessary in our experience. We return the closed distal gastric pouch to the upper abdomen adjacent to the stoma but take no steps to affix it to the area of the anastomosis.

GASTROPLASTY (VERTICAL, REINFORCED)
(Figure 8.5)

1. The preoperative and early operative management is similar to that described under gastric bypass. Once the upper stomach has been exposed and any splenic adhesions noted and appropriately managed, the lesser bursa is entered through the avascular area in the gastrohepatic ligament and the upper stomach is elevated digitally from the posterior peritoneum.

2. An avascular area between the oesophagogastric junction and the uppermost vasa brevia on the greater curvature at the top of fundus is bluntly developed, and the entire stomach and lesser curvature vessels are encircled with a No. 14 round rubber catheter.

3. A 2.0 cm area on the lesser curvature beginning 5 cm below the oesophagogastric junction is cleared of all penetrating vessels and nerves. A tunnel is created retrogastrically between the two openings and the rubber catheter is rerouted to exit through this window inside the ascending vessels on the lesser curvature. The encircled pouch of upper stomach is estimated to be no larger than a 50 ml capacity.

4. The jaws of the TA-90 stapler are directed from below upwards by means of the catheter to encompass the previously encircled upper stomach. The cartridge is prepared by removing four of the staples that are closest to the handle of the stapler.

5. Two rows of staples are then inserted 0.5 cm apart and in a vertically directed manner in such a way as to encroach medially on the lesser curvature (Figure 8.5b).

6. The two rows of staples that serve as a partition between the upper and lower stomach are then reinforced by a series of interrupted through and through silk sutures to discourage late disruption of the stapled partition. A no. 32 Hurst dilator is inserted by the anaesthetist after withdrawal of the nasogastric tube. It is passed into the upper pouch and directed through the opening along the lesser curvature (unstapled section) into the distal stomach.

7. A 0/0 Dexon suture is then passed through the stomach at the lower end of the partition and is tied snugly round the Hurst dilator and remaining lesser curvature of the stomach to form the reinforced channel by which liquid and food leaves the upper pouch to continue down the gastrointestinal canal (Figure 8.5c).

8. The dilator is then removed. This encircling Dexon suture is then 'covered' by a series of interrupted 4/0 Prolene seromuscular sutures in the gastric wall. The absorbable Dexon suture is believed to result in a ring of scar tissue which limits stomal size without the hazards of late erosion seen with permanent suture material.

9. The 'stoma' is calibrated by attempts to pass the dilator through the opening, and once deemed sufficiently snug, is replaced by a nasogastric tube which is positioned to decompress both the upper and lower stomach.

POSTOPERATIVE COMPLICATIONS

Obesity surgery in general

Surgery in morbidly obese patients carries with it a high incidence of complications and a risk of mortality. Both of these concerns can be greatly minimized by surgical experience, attention to detail, patient selection and good quality support services, in particular, anaesthesiology and nursing care. Three areas deserve particular attention.

Pulmonary

The often massive amounts of extra- and intra-abdominal fat combine with the usual splinting which follows abdominal surgery to impair respiration and increase the risk of postoperative atelectasis, impaired gas exchange and pneumonia. Careful monitoring of blood gases pre-, per- and postoperatively is essential. The decision to wean from respirators and/or extubate, or transfer from the recovery unit should be a thoughtful one based on standard criteria and a knowledge of the degree of surveillance and care available in alternative areas.

Medical and nursing staff must be sufficient in number and fully aware of the correct management of nasogastric tubes, the need for early ambulation, effective pulmonary toilet, anti-atelectasis measures, fluid management and careful monitoring of vital signs. Elevation of the head of the bed helps coughing and effective ventilation, but often discourages changes in position and impairs nasogastric decompression.

Wound care

Systemic antibiotics are administered prior to incision and for 24 hours thereafter. All layers of the abdominal wall are isolated from external or endogenous contamination throughout the procedure by the immediate insertion of a disposable plastic wound protector which is removed only after the operative team has changed gloves and removed potential contaminants prior to closure. The muscular and fascial layers of the abdominal wall are closed with interrupted sutures, preferably using a double-stranded 3/0 stainless steel wire with the strands placed 1.5 cm apart and 1.5 cm from the cut edge. Experience of tying wire is essential if this suture material is to be employed effectively in these patients. The often massive subcutaneous layer is irrigated copiously after careful haemostasis and the skin is approximated with staples, suture or Steristrips, without the use of drains or subcutaneous sutures. We avoid retention sutures but do not hesitate to delay skin wound closure if contamination has occurred. External garments or binders to 'support' the wound are occasionally employed when a giant pannus exists.

Unexplained fever, particularly arising after the nasogastric tube has been removed, suggests the possibility of wound infection—an infrequent complication in our experience. Personnel should be reminded of the frequent absence of any external signs of such infection in these patients. If fever is not otherwise accounted for it is our practice to paint the abdominal incision with Betadine solutions and probe the wound. This is carried out with minimal discomfort to the patient by inserting sterile cotton swabs between intact sutures using a twisting motion. The swab is advanced to the level of the deep external fascia. Early identification and drainage of a deep subcutaneous pocket of pus is important to prevent impairment of fascial healing and the development of incisional hernia.

In a personal series of over 250 operations for morbid obesity, there were no instances of evisceration, the wound infection rate is less than 5% and late incisional hernias are rarely seen.

Thromboembolism

In spite of the time-honoured concept of an increased risk of thromboembolism in obese patients undergoing surgery, we are not impressed with this problem. As a consequence, for most patients under 40 years of age, we have relied on early and frequent ambulation to prevent serious thromboembolic problems. Patients with a history of deep venous thrombosis or evidence of severe varicosities are given 5000 units of subcutaneous Heparin (minidose) preoperatively and twice daily until fully ambulatory. For elderly patients, we frequently employ the intraoperative intermittent compression device on the lower extremities.

POSTOPERATIVE COMPLICATIONS IN THE VARIOUS OPERATIVE PROCEDURES

Complications of intestinal bypass

Early complications

Complications in the immediate postoperative period, including those noted above, are infrequent and this is one of the reasons which have led us to continue to use this procedure as a first-stage measure in selected patients, including those who are poor anaesthetic risks due to extreme obesity.

Diarrhoea. From 10 to 20 liquid stools per day is an anticipated consequence of the short circuiting of upper gastrointestinal secretions into the colon. Careful monitoring of fluid and electrolyte balance is essential to avoid serious problems and rectal irritation is common. Antidiarrhoeal medications are not often required and six to eight semi solid stools are usually achieved spontaneously within a three-month period. The severity and discomfort of the frequent stools are influenced by diet and are a major factor in the patient's reduced caloric intake.

Fluid and electrolyte disorders. Dehydration, hypocalcaemia, hypokalaemia and hypomagnesaemia are particularly common but they usually respond to routine measures.

Late complications

Renal. A 10–15% incidence of urinary calculi and the less frequent interstitial nephropathy are one of the principal reasons why the operation has fallen into disfavour. All patients must be monitored for impairment of renal function which results from the increased oxalate absorption in the colon and hyperoxaluria. Several authors believe the incidence of oxalate urolithiasis can be reduced by the administration of oral calcium to the diet which additionally protects against the problems of hypocalcaemia. Significant changes in the serum creatinine should be followed by clearance studies and will usually respond promptly to takedown of the bypass.

Hepatic. An increase in fatty infiltration of the liver regularly occurs in association with weight loss secondary to ileojejunal bypass. Of greatest concern is an estimated 20% of patients who will develop varying degrees of centrilobular fibrosis and portal cell infiltrates. Irreversible hepatic failure and cirrhosis may occur and all patients must be regularly evaluated for excessive hepatomegaly, serious deterioration of liver function tests and significant histological changes on serial liver biopsies. Post-bypass hepatopathy usually occurs in the first year following surgery and is manifested by nausea, vomiting, asthenia and excessive weight loss. Treatment requires prompt intensive and hypercaloric therapy and most patients will require reversal of the bypass procedure.

Gastrointestinal. The chronic diarrhoea is usually well tolerated but acute exacerbations with fluid and electrolyte disorders may require hospitalization and dietary measures. Additional problems include excessive and foul-smelling flatus, fever, pain and abdominal distension. Bowel obstruction secondary to adhesions, hernia or intussusception must be considered as well as bypass enteropathy, pseudo-obstruction, pneumatosis cystoides intestinalis, transmural ileocolitis and megacolon. Most of these side-effects can be managed by dietary measures such as avoidance of fat and/or the use of broad-spectrum antibiotics aimed at reducing the overgrowth of anaerobic bacteria in the bypassed small bowel. Severe or technical problems require revision or takedown.

The incidence of cholelithiasis following intestinal bypass is variously reported as 10–40%, prompting some to recommend routine cholecystectomy at the time of weight reduction surgery. Symptomatic gall stone disease is treated surgically after assuring an adequate nutritional state.

Musculoskeletal. Severe demineralization of the bony skeleton and specific forms of arthromyalgias are encountered in some patients. Malabsorption, deficiency of fat-soluble vitamins, circulating cryoproteins and immune complexes have all been implicated. Vitamin supplements are advisable in all patients and anti-inflammatory agents are useful in controlling arthritic symptoms.

Alopecia. Thinning of hair occurs in a significant number of patients probably as a result of protein deficiency. It uniformly improves once weight loss has been achieved.

Anaemia. Anaemia is an infrequent complication of intestinal bypass but may arise as a result of ileocolitis or impaired vitamin B_{12} absorption due to the exclusion of receptor sites in the terminal ileum. Parenteral administration of vitamin B_{12} is advisable in patients with reduced B_{12} levels and significant anaemia of any type should be thoroughly evaluated.

Complications of gastric reduction procedures

Common to both types of gastric reduction procedures is an increased risk of pulmonary problems secondary to the upper abdominal incision.

Early complications

Leak. Leakage of gastrointestinal contents from an anastomosis, staple suture line, or proximal or distal pouch is the most feared complication of this surgery. The site, frequency and cause vary with the procedure employed and the experience of the surgeon. Some element of ischaemia, nasogastric tube pressure or technical error is usually implicated. Symptoms are often very subtle and may consist only of unexplained tachycardia, leukocytosis and back or shoulder pain. The presence or absence of free air is seldom helpful. Suspicion of perforation should be studied immediately by instillation of water-soluble contrast material down the nasogastric tube and careful radiological evaluation. The prognosis varies with the age of the patient, size and site of leak, and the experience of the surgeon. In most instances, reoperation to establish adequate drainage, antibiotics, intake restriction and total parenteral nutrition will be followed by spontaneous closure and a satisfactory result.

Stomal stenosis. See late complications.

Late complications

Failure to lose the anticipated amount of excess weight. Failure of patients to lose more than 50% of excess weight is the most common and disturbing of the late complications. This is usually the result of one or more of the following: (a) stomal dilatation, (b) pouch dilatation, (c) partition disruption and (d) high intake of liquid calories. Prevention and treatment of these problems is a matter of intense debate and study, and is the principal reason for familiarizing oneself with the collective experience of others before undertaking obesity surgery.

Stomal stenosis. This occurs more commonly in gastroplasty procedures and is characterized by vomiting of ingested food and even pooled saliva. Early and milder cases respond to a period of nasogastric suction, return to liquid diet and the use of cimetidine and Regulan. Endoscopic study should be carried out and many cases will respond to balloon dilatation using the Gruntzig balloon technique. Severe cases require reoperation, usually with conversion to a gastric bypass procedure.

Episodic vomiting. Some emesis is encountered in all gastric restrictive procedures and its causes vary widely from specific food intolerances (e.g. to red meat) to stomal obliteration (see above). Its occurrence should be noted since it may lead to dehydration, oesophagitis and severe malnutrition. Fortunately, in most instances it responds to a return to the simpler diets of the early postoperative period. Some patients will be emotionally incapable of tolerating the restrictions of oral intake and, if identifiable, may be better candidates for intestinal bypass as a first-stage procedure. When vomiting is accompanied by abdominal pain the possibility of gallbladder disease, bowel obstruction or peptic ulcer should be investigated.

Anaemia and malnutrition. These are the principal non-life endangering side-effects of the gastric reductive procedures. Anaemia is much more common after gastric bypass and is due primarily to reduced absorption of vitamin B_{12}, folic acid and iron from the bypassed segments. Lassitude and easy fatigue are common symptoms accompanying marked weight loss, but the protein calorie depletion is seldom so severe as to discredit the reason for the procedure in properly selected patients. The rate of weight loss should be monitored. Routine assessment of blood counts, serum albumin, and vitamin B_{12} and folic acid levels are part of the long-term follow up of these patients. The use of iron and vitamin supplements is appropriate prophylaxis. Parenteral administration may be required once significant anaemia occurs.

Bleeding. Blood loss secondary to erosions or inflammatory changes within both the proximal and distal gastric pouch has been described. Rarely it occurs secondary to peptic ulcers. Endoscopic diagnosis is essential and bleeding from a variety of causes has responded to the use of cimetidine. As with other causes of gastrointestinal bleeding, surgery may be required but preoperative localization is essential.

Non-compliance. Non-compliance is frequent and contributes significantly to most of the other complications. While inability to control their intake and appetite is a fundamental problem of the morbidly obese it is not clear why some patients fail to take their vitamin and mineral supplements or refuse to return for long-term follow up. Unless this problem is corrected, existing uncertainties regarding the benefits of obesity surgery will continue.

Reflux gastritis, oesophagitis. Both of these problems have been documented in some patients following gastric restrictive procedures. The usual symptoms are those of heart burn, nausea and dyspepsia, but respiratory difficulties including asthma-like attacks may occur. Mild cases of oesophagitis will respond to dietary measures, antacids, H_2 blockers and avoidance of recumbency after meals. More severe cases should be studied by 24-hour pH monitoring and may require surgical intervention. Since the problem is encountered primarily in patients with loop gastric bypass or gastroplasty, conversion to Roux-en-Y bypass can be employed.

Bile reflux into the bypassed gastric remnant with metaplasia of the gastric mucosa has been described as early as three months following gastric bypass.[6]

Dumping syndrome. Variations on the dumping syndrome have been noted after gastric bypass and are usually encountered early in the postoperative period when a liquid diet is employed. Most patients respond to dietary measures.

OUTCOME: OVERALL RESULTS

At the present time, it is impossible to state with any degree of accuracy the final results of the surgery for morbid obesity. Our own experience with over 500 patients operated on during the past 10 years lacks statistical validity and defies analysis because of three factors common to most reports on obesity surgery.

These are:

1. **Variation in procedures employed.** Early in our experience, the majority of patients underwent intestinal bypass by either the end-to-side or end-to-end technique. More recently, we have performed one of the two gastric restrictive procedures. Many early patients had their intestinal bypass taken down at a time when they were no longer morbidly obese—the precise contribution of the gastric bypass or gastroplasty to the final result is therefore difficult to assess.

2. **Variations in technique for a given procedure.** During the early experience with intestinal bypass, it became obvious that individual surgeons would vary greatly in their measurement of the length of jejunum or ileum employed, and that the same surgeon would change measurement technique as their experience and confidence in the procedure increased. Similarly, in the gastric restrictive procedures, such important variables as pouch size, stomal diameter, methods of partition, gastroenterostomy technique and use of suture line reinforcement varied between surgeons and often changed from one patient to the next with individual surgeons.

3. **Lack of consistent follow-up information on operated patients.** In spite of the fact that all obesity surgery in our medical centre was per-

formed by two senior surgeons in a single hospital located in a stable and affluent suburban area, over one-third of our patients were lost to follow up within two years of the operation. This occurred in spite of the employment of a full-time clinical nurse specialist who conscientiously pursued by telephone and letter the whereabouts and status of non-compliant patients. Other authors have expressed similar concerns, and most believe that patients lost to follow up probably constitute treatment failures and should be so classified.

Recent reports of 100% follow up of patients undergoing carefully standardized operations are only now becoming available.[5,6] For meaningful data, the patients should be selected according to strict criteria, and results expressed in terms of percentage excess weight lost. Such studies should continue for a period of at least five years to allow for a reasonably accurate prediction of the ultimate benefits of this type of surgery for individual patients.

In spite of uncertainty in regard to the consistency or permanence of weight loss, as well as the late consequences of obesity surgery, there is clear evidence of significant improvement in health and life-style for many patients who have undergone these procedures. While various authors employ different criteria to define a satisfactory result, a loss of greater than 25% of weight occurs in the majority of patients treated in established centres. Successful weight reduction is regularly associated with improvement in blood pressure, diabetic control, cardiac and pulmonary function, and relief of the various related syndromes (e.g. Pickwickian, sleep apnoea). Relief of arthritis and back problems is common and hyperlipidaemia may be ameliorated. Most surveys reflect a high degree of patient satisfaction, improved work capacity and social adjustment. The principal source of referral for obesity surgery is from patients and family of those who have undergone the procedure.

CONCLUSIONS

The indications for and ideal surgical treatment of morbid obesity have not been established. At the present time, gastric restrictive procedures which limit caloric intake and provide early satiety appear to offer a more physiological method of weight reduction than intestinal bypass. The ease and relative safety of various forms of gastroplasty are accompanied by an increased likelihood of inadequate or unsustained weight loss. In contrast, gastric bypass procedures pose a greater risk of serious postoperative complications and chronic anaemia, but appear to be better tolerated by most patients and to be capable of more consistent and sustained weight loss. The failure of many patients to comply with recommended medications and dietary measures, and to return for periodic evaluations greatly compromise the success, safety and certainty on which operative treatment is based. Under proper circumstances, surgery can offer significant relief from the medical, social and economic consequences of severe obesity to a large number of those afflicted.

REFERENCES

1. Payne H & DeWind LF (1963) Surgical treatment of obesity. *American Journal of Surgery* 106: 273.
2. Griffen WO Jr, Bevins BA & Bell M (1983) The decline and fall of the jejuno-ileal bypass. *Surgery, Gynecology & Obstetrics* 157 (4): 301–307.
3. Gentry K, Halverson JD & Huster S (1984) Psychologic assessment of mordibly obese patients undergoing gastric bypass: a comparison of preoperative and postoperative adjustment. *Surgery* 95 (2): 215–220.
4. Saltzstein F & Guttman M (1980) Gastric bypass for morbid obesity. Preoperative and postoperative psychological evaluation of patients. *Archives of Surgery* 115: 21–28.
5. Pories WJ, Flickinger EG, Meelheim D et al (1982) The effectiveness of gastric bypass over gastric partition in morbid obesity. *Annals of Surgery* 196: 389–399.
6. Flickinger EG, Pories WJ, Meelheim D, Sinor DR, Blase IL & Thomas FT (1984) The Greenville gastric bypass: progress report after three years. *Annals of Surgery* 199 (5): 555–563.

9

Injection Sclerotherapy for Oesophageal Varices

T. P. J. Hennessy

Injection sclerotherapy has been shown to be effective in the treatment of acute bleeding from oesophageal varices. Evidence has also been presented demonstrating its value in reducing the incidence of bleeding and prolonging the life of patients with varices when used electively. Its use has also been advocated in the prophylactic treatment of oesophageal varices.

The technique was first described by Crafoord and Frenckner[1] in 1939 and introduced into Britain in 1943 by McBeth.[2] The early success and rising popularity of portal systemic shunting hindered its general acceptance and much is owed to the work of Johnston and Rodgers[3] in reestablishing the technique in 1973. This, coupled with the increasing awareness of the limitations and complications of portosystemic shunts, has led to a renewed appreciation of injection sclerotherapy as a valuable technique in the treatment of oesophageal varices.

Controversy continues on the merits of different methods of injection. The original technique consisted of direct intravariceal injection via the rigid oesophagoscope. Modern variations include the use of (a) the flexible fibreoptic oesophagoscope with or without a sheath, (b) multiple perivariceal injections to provide a thickened fibrotic mucosa, leaving the varices themselves intact, and (c) a variety of sclerosants, the most popular of which are ethanolamine oleate for intravariceal injections and polidocanol for perivariceal injection. Modifications have also been made in the original endoscopic technique. Bailey and Dawson[4] recommended the provision of a window or slot opposite the beak of the Negus oesophagoscope through which the varix presents for injection. Rotation of the scope allows the injected varix to be compressed while the next varix projects into the slot for injection. Proximal fibreoptic lighting and distal

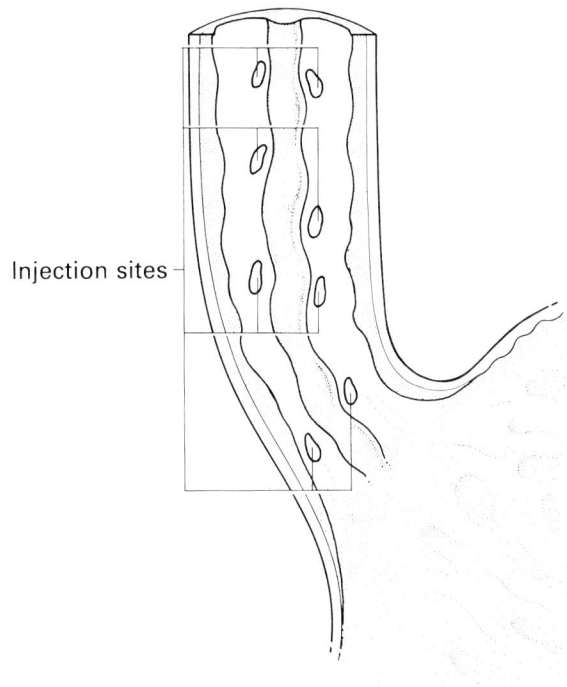

Figure 9.1 *On either side of the column of varices a series of parallel sites show where the multiple perivariceal or extravariceal injections should be made to produce fibrosis, thus obliterating the varices.*

suction are of great value in providing adequate vision for the injection of bleeding varices. The Stortz rigid oesophagoscope with built-in needle and telescope and with distal suction greatly facilitates injection in the emergency situation. Other means of controlling bleeding during injection are the attachment of a balloon to the flexible scope and the use of the Linton-Nachlas[5] balloon to compress the varices at the oesophagogastric junction, thus controlling bleeding during injection.

CONTROL OF ACUTE BLEEDING

Commonly, a period of variceal compression with the Sengstaken tube is employed initially in bleeding varices during the period of admission and assessment. Continuous infusion of intravenous vasopressin is also employed (0.2–0.4 u/min). Our own practice is to limit this period to between 12 and 24 hours. If bleeding has stopped on decompression of the balloon, injection is deferred to a convenient time within the succeeeding few days. If bleeding resumes on decompression, the balloon is repositioned temporarily and the patient is scheduled for immediate sclerotherapy via the rigid oesophagoscope.

The original sclerosant used was quinine. Sodium morrhuate was used in the USA. The most frequently used sclerosant in Great Britain is ethanolamine oleate which seems to produce fewer complications and is non-toxic. Polidocanol is used extensively in Europe. Systemic toxicity has been reported and its use is confined to perivariceal injection. Sodium tetradecyl sulphate has also been used, and so has 50% dextrose, though not widely.

TECHNIQUE OF INJECTION SCLEROTHERAPY USING THE RIGID OESOPHAGOSCOPE

Anaesthesia

Anaesthesia is induced with sodium thiopentone and suxamethonium, and is maintained with nitrous oxide/oxygen and intermittent thiopentone and suxamethonium. If there is active bleeding the Sengstaken tube is maintained in situ until intubation has been achieved.

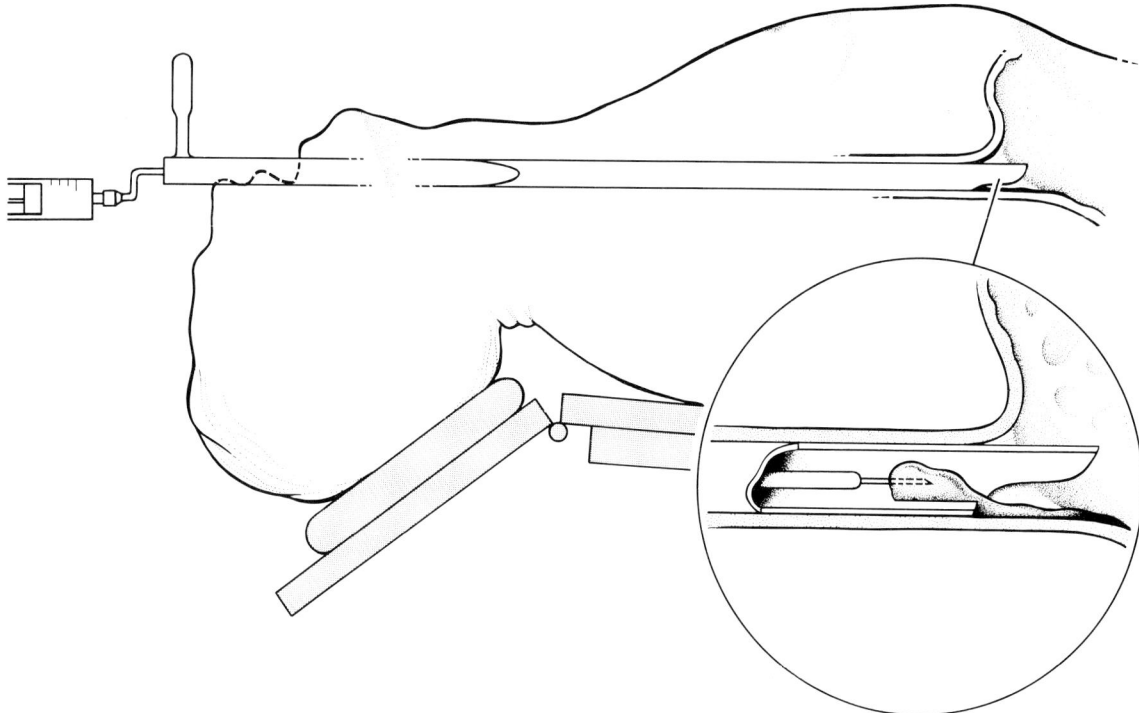

Figure 9.2 *The rigid Negus oesophagoscope is passed down the oesophagus to its lower end. There is a slot at the lower end of the oesophagoscope through which a varix presents. The tip of the needle has been inserted into the varix prior to injecting sclerosant from the syringe attached to the hub of the needle.*

Sclerotherapy

A 50 cm Negus oesophagoscope (with a slot as described by Bailey and Dawson) is passed to the oesophagogastric junction. Suction is employed to remove blood and clots. The bleeding varix is identified and injected first. A McBeth or Roberts needle is passed down the scope and the tip inserted into the varix. Five millilitres of ethanolamine oleate are injected. The scope is immediately rotated to compress the injected varix and allow the next varix to present either into the slot if the modified scope is in use or into the lumen of the standard scope. A total of 15–25 ml may be given at one sitting. The scope is kept in place for five minutes after injection. If the injections have been given for active bleeding it is wise to reintroduce the Sengstaken tube for a further six-hour period of compression. It is not our custom to do this, however, if the injections have been part of an elective course of sclerotherapy and in these circumstances we have not found post-injection bleeding to be a problem.

SCLEROTHERAPY USING THE FLEXIBLE OESOPHAGOSCOPE

This may be done in adults without general anaesthesia using Diazepam sedation in the elective situation. If there is active bleeding it is safer to anaesthetize and intubate the patient. The preferred instrument is the Olympus GIF-K oblique-viewing scope.

The Williams tube or sheath is passed down the oesophagus over the oesophagoscope until the slot in the tube reaches the gastro-oesophageal junction. The sheath is then positioned to allow a varix to protrude through the slot at its distal end. Injection is achieved via the flexible Olympus NM-3 needle which is passed down the biopsy channel of the scope. The sheath is then rotated to allow the next varix to be injected. Each varix is injected with 3–6 ml of 5% ethanolamine oleate to a total of 20–25 ml.

CHILDREN

Injections in children are preferably done via the flexible oesophagoscope under general anaesthesia and without using the sheath. An injection of 2 or 3 ml of 5% ethanolamine oleate is made into each varix to a maximum of 10 ml. Very occasionally compression with the Sengstaken tube may be required after elective injection.

PERIVARICEAL INJECTION

This technique has been used extensively by Paquet[6] and others using the rigid oesophagoscope for acute bleeding and the flexible oesophagoscope for elective injection.

The sclerosant used is polidocanol 0.5% or 1% depending on the response of the mucosa to injection. If there is little ulceration the higher concentration may be used. There is some evidence that the use of this sclerosant intravascularly could lead to systemic reactions, e.g. pulmonary oedema and pulmonary fibrosis.

The lower 6 cm of oesophagus is chosen for perivariceal injection. The injections are placed submucosally on either side of the columns of varices. About 40 individual injections of 0.5 ml are given at one sitting and the procedure is repeated for two or four sessions at five- to eight-day intervals.

COMPLICATIONS OF INJECTION SCLEROTHERAPY

A common complaint after injection sclerotherapy is chest pain located retrosternally and often accompanied by transient dysphagia. This usually clears up after a day or two and does not seem to be of any ominous significance.

Ulceration of the oesophageal mucosa can be a serious complication and if it overlies a varix can lead to severe re-bleeding. Severe ulceration may be responsible for subsequent stricture formation. Mucosal ulceration has followed both perivariceal and intravariceal injection. The frequency and number of injections and the amount of sclerosant used may be significant factors. Westaby et al[7] found that mucosal ulceration was more frequent in patients receiving weekly intravariceal injections than in those receiving injections at three-weekly intervals, but the increased frequency of ulceration was not associated with a higher incidence of stricture formation. Sorensen et al[8] found a correlation between more frequent injections using greater amounts of sclerosant for perivariceal injection and the development of mucosal ulceration and subsequent stricture formation. Treatment of the ulcer depends on its severity. The majority respond to cimetidine. Sometimes the Linton tube is required to control bleeding. Occasionally, resection of the oesophagus has had to be carried out.

The incidence of stricture formation in Sorensen's series was 59%. However, many studies have reported a much lower incidence.[3,9] Reilly et al[10] suggest that post-sclerotherapy strictures are the result of acid reflux and delayed oesophageal clearance due to the adverse effect of sclerotherapy on oesophageal motility. They advocate antacids and other antireflux measures for these patients. Strictures generally respond to simple dilatation.

Small perioesophageal leaks have been demonstrated but do not present a serious problem. Chest infection is a common hazard and the risk of perforating the oesophagus, particularly with rigid instruments, must be borne in mind.

FREQUENCY OF INJECTIONS

No defined policy on the frequency of injection has been determined. Some patients require only a few injections at three- to four-week intervals, after which the varices appear to be thrombosed or eradicated. Other patients require many more injections before a satisfactory result is obtained. Some workers recommend more frequent injections at one- or two-week intervals. All patients should be followed up by endoscopy at six-monthly intervals so that new variceal channels, if they appear, may be injected.

GASTRIC VARICES

At present it is generally agreed that gastric varices are not a major problem from the point of view of bleeding and it is not usual to attempt to inject them. It may be that the thrombosis induced at the oesophagogastric junction extends distally to include gastric varices.

RESULTS OF SCLEROTHERAPY

The ability of injection sclerotherapy to control acute variceal haemorrhage,[3] obliterate varices[7] and increase long-term survival[9] has been demonstrated. Re-bleeding may occur during treatment. Large varices and poor liver function increase the risk of re-bleeding[11] but re-bleeding from varices undergoing sclerotherapy tends to be relatively mild. The number of injections required for eradication of varices is very variable and may be any number from one to eight or 10. Varices, once obliterated, may remain so for long periods. In Terblanche's trial,[12] the average period of obliteration was 21.5 months. However, most varices eventually recur and repeated endoscopy and re-injection of new variceal channels must be continued for the patient's lifetime.

REFERENCES

1. Crafoord C & Frenckner P (1939) New surgical treatment of varicose veins of the oesophagus. *Acta Otolaryngologica* **27**, 422–429.
2. Macbeth R (1955) Treatment of oesophageal varices in portal hypertension by means of sclerosing injections. *British Medical Journal* **ii**: 877–880.
3. Johnston GW & Rodgers HW (1973) A review of 15 years' experience in the use of sclerotherapy in the control of acute haemorrhage from oesophageal varices. *British Journal of Surgery* **60**: 797.
4. Bailey ME & Dawson JL (1975) Modified oesophagoscope for injection oesophageal varices. *British Medical Journal* **ii**: 540–541.
5. Nachlas MM (1955) A new triple lumen tube for the diagnosis and treatment of upper gastrointestinal haemorrhage. *New England Journal of Medicine* **252**: 820–821.
6. Paquet KJ (1982) In Westaby D, MacDougall BRD & Williams R (eds) *Variceal Bleeding*, pp 148–156. London: Pitman.
7. Westaby D, Melia WM, Macdougall BRD, Hegarty JE & Williams R (1984) Injection sclerotherapy for oesophageal varices: a prospective randomized trial of different treatment schedules. *Gut* **25**: 129–132.
8. Sorensen T, Burcharth F, Pedersen ML & Findahl F (1984) Oesophageal stricture and dysphagia after endoscopic sclerotherapy for bleeding varices. *Gut* **25**: 473–477.
9. Macdougall BRD, Westaby D, Theodossi A, Dawson JL & Williams R (1982) Increased long-term survival in variceal haemorrhage using injection sclerotherapy. Results of a controlled trial. *Lancet* **i**: 124–127.
10. Reilly JG, Sclade RR & Van Thiel DS (1984) Esophageal function after injection sclerotherapy: pathogenesis of esophageal stricture. *American Journal of Surgery* **147**: 85–88.
11. Rose JDR, Crane MD & Smith PM (1983) Factors affecting successful endoscopic sclerotherapy for oesophageal varices. *Gut* **24**: 946–949.
12. Terblanche, J, Bornman PC, Delawir K, Jonker MAT, Campbell, JAH, Wright J & Kirsch R (1983) Failure of repeated injection sclerotherapy to improve long-term survival after oesophageal variceal bleeding. *Lancet* **ii**: 1328–1332.

Index

Adhesion division during pyloric reconstruction, 46–8
Age limits for obesity surgery, 125
Alcohol abuse causing oesophageal bleeding, 29
Alopecia following gastric bypass, 138
Anaemia following obesity surgery, 138, 139
Anaesthesia, for injection sclerotherapy, 142
    for pyloric reconstruction, 45
Analgesics for breast pain, 4–5
Anastomotic leakage, following gastric reservoir reconstruction, 72
    following oesophageal transection, 38
    from gastric reduction procedures, 138
    stenosis, 73
Antibiotics following pyloric reconstruction, 59
Ascites
    following peritoneovenous shunt, 120
    infected, 108
    intractable, 106–7
    medical therapy for, 107
    paracentesis for, 107
    pathogenesis of cirrhotic, 106
    peritoneovenous shunting for, 107–8
Aspiration cytology, 2, 5–6
Axillary clearance, lower, 8–10

Biliary anastomosis, intrahepatic, 98
Biopsy, breast, 2, 5–7
Bisegmentectomy, 100–2, 104
Bleeding *see* Haemorrhage
Bleeding diathesis as contraindication to shunting, 108
Breast, attitude of patient to surgery of, 1
    carcinoma, diagnosis of, 5–7
        surgery for, 7–19
    conservation, 7–8
    conservative surgery, 1–20
    deformity, 1
    disease, premalignant, 10–11
    implants, 12
    lower axillary clearance, 8–10
    lump, 2
    lumpiness, 2
    pain, 4–5, 10
    reconstruction following total mastectomy, 20–25
    smears, cytological grading of, 7
    subcutaneous mastectomy of, 10–19
    surgery, complications of, 19–20
        postoperative care, 19
        wide local excision, 7
        wound closure, 18
    see also Nipple
Bromocriptine for breast pain, 4
Budd–Chiari syndrome, 108

Capsule formation following breast surgery, 19–20
Capsulotomy, 19
Carcinoma, breast, diagnosis of, 5–7
    surgery for, 7–19
    epidermotrophic, of nipple ducts, 3
    hepatic, segmentectomy for, 102–5
Cardiac complications following peritoneovenous shunting, 120
Catheter insertion for peritoneovenous shunting, 113–17
Cherry red spots in oesophagus, 28
^{14}C-Cholate breath test, 63–4
Cholelithiasis following gastric bypass, 138
Chylous ascites, 108
Cirrhosis, surgery and, 32
Cirrhotic ascites, pathogenesis of, 106
Collagen, microcrystalline, for splenic haemostasis, 78–9
Cone excision of nipple, 4
Cordis–Hakim shunt, 110–13
    blockage, 121

Cordis–Hakim shunt—*cont.*
  insertion, 113–17
Cysts, breast, 2
  splenic, 75, 76–7

Danazol for breast pain, 4
Denver shunt, 109–10
Diarrhoea following gastric bypass, 137
Disseminated intravascular coagulation following peritoneovenous shunt, 120
Drains following splenic surgery, 87, 90
Dumping syndrome, 42
  diagnosis, 43
  following gastric reduction, 139
  following pyloric reconstruction, 59
  provocation test, 43
  severity, 43–4
  symptoms, causes, 44–5
Duodenojejunal anastomosis, 71
Dysphagia following oesophageal transection, 38

Encapsulation following breast surgery, 19–20
Encephalopathy, as contraindication to shunting, 108
  following oesophageal transection, 38
Endoscopy, for diagnosing peptic ulcer recurrence, 45
  in oesophageal bleeding, 30
Entero-enteric anastomosis, 62, 68
Enterolysis, 67
Epithelial hyperplasia, 10–11
Ethacrynic acid for ascites, 107
Evening primrose oil for breast pain, 4
Excision biopsy for breast lump, 2, 7

Fibrocystic disease, 11
Fine needle aspiration cytology, 5–6
Fluid accumulation following breast surgery, 19
Frusemide for ascites, 107

Gallbladder carcinoma, 105
Gastric bypass, 130, 131–3
    complications of, 137
    emptying rate following dumping provocation, 44
    pouch decompression, 135
    use for reinforcing gastrojejunal stoma, 135
  reduction procedures complications, 138–9
  reservoir reconstruction, 62–73
    operative technique, 64–71
    outcome, 73
    patient selection and preoperative preparation, 63–4
    postoperative care and complications, 72–3
  restrictive procedures, 127, 129–31
  stasis following pyloric reconstruction, 58–9
  varices, 145
Gastrointestinal complications following gastric bypass, 137–8
Gastrojejunal anastomosis separation, 67

Gastrojejunostomy, Roux-en-Y, 133–4
Gastroplasty, 129, 134, 135–6
Grafts, nipple–areola, 25

Haemorrhage, acute, control of, 31
  following obesity surgery, 139
  from oesophageal varices, as contraindication to shunting, 108
    clinical features, 28–30
    early management of patient, 30–31
    injection sclerotherapy for, 32, 141–4
    pathophysiology, 27–8
    preoperative assessment and patient selection, 31–2
    postoperative, following oesophageal transection, 38–9
Heartburn following oesophageal transection, 38
Henley's operation, 62–3
Hepatic complications following gastric bypass, 137
Hypersplenism, 75–6

Iatrogenic splenic injury, 74, 92
Immunization, preoperative, 77
Implants, breast, 12–18
  splenic, 90–91
Infection following breast surgery, 19
  following peritoneovenous shunt, 120–21
Injection sclerotherapy for variceal bleeding, 32, 141–4
Insulin for dumping syndrome, 45
Interposed isoperistaltic loop technique, 62
Intraepithelial channels in oesophagus, 28

Jaundice as contraindication to shunting, 108
Jejunal interposition, reservoir, 64–71
  loop reservoirs, 62
Jejunogastric–oesophageal anastomosis, 62
Jejunoileal bypass, 126–9, 130

Kehr incision, 79
  sign, 76

Laparoscopy for ascites, 110
Latissimus dorsi myocutaneous flap, 21–5
LaVeen shunt, 109–10
Liver
  bisegmentectomy, 100–2, 104
  disease, as contraindication to shunting, 108
    physical examination for, 30
  plurisegmentectomy, 100–102
  segmentectomy, 94–9, 102–5
  segments, 93
  tests for preoperative assessment, 32
  trisegmentectomy, 102, 104
Loop jejunostomy, 65
Lump, breast, 2

Lumpectomy, 8
Lumpiness, breast, 2
Lung physiotherapy following pyloric reconstruction, 59

Malignant effusions following peritoneovenous shunt, 120
Malnutrition following obesity surgery, 139
Mammography, 2, 3, 7
Marker biopsy for breast cancer, 7
Mastalgia, 4–5
Mastectomy, reconstruction following, 20–5
   subcutaneous, 10–19
      for breast pain, 5
Microdochectomy for nipple discharge, 3
Mortality following oesophageal transection, 39
Musculoskeletal complications following gastric bypass, 138

Necrosis of gastric reservoir, 73
   of shunt scar, 121–2
Needle aspiration cytology, 2, 5–7
Negus oesophagoscope, 142
Nipple–areola grafting, 25
      reconstruction, 25
   cone excision, 4
   disc, demarcation and preservation, 11
   discharge, 2–3
   excoriation, 3–4
Nutritional management in malnutrition, 64

Obesity, surgery
   available options, 126–30
   historical perspective, 123–4
   patient selection, 124–5
   postoperative complications, 136–40
   preoperative care and investigations, 126
   surgical considerations, 123
   techniques, 130–36
Oesophageal anastomosis, 69–71
   leak following transection, 38
   mucosa ulceration, 143
   reflux following transection, 38
   stricture following sclerotherapy, 143–4
   tamponade, 31
   transection–devascularization, complications of, 38–9
      mortality following, 39
      preoperative problems, 37
      results of, 37–9
      survival following, 39
      technique, 32–7
   varices, bleeding, as contraindication to shunting, 108
      clinical features of, 28–30
      early management of patient, 30–31
      injection sclerotherapy for, 32, 141–4
      pathophysiology of, 27–8
      preoperative assessment and patient selection, 31–2
      rebleeding, 144
Oesophagitis following gastric reduction, 139
Oesophagogastric junction, vessel pattern at, 28
Oesophagoscope, flexible, 143
   rigid, 142

Paget's disease of nipple, 3–4
Pain, breast, 4–5, 10
Paracentesis for ascites, 107
Pectoralis minor exposure, 8
Peritoneal catheter insertion, 113–17
   fluid leakage, 121
   mesothelioma, 106
   tap, diagnostic, 110
Peritoneovenous shunting, blockage, 121
   failure, 122
   indications and patient selection, 108
   outcome, 120–22
   postoperative care and complications, 117–20
   preoperative care and investigations, 108–10
   technique, 110–17
Perivariceal injection, 144
Plasma volume following dumping provocation, 44
   following pyloric reconstruction, 59
Plurisegmentectomy, 100–102
Polya restoration, 65, 67
Portal hypertension causing oesophageal varices, 27–8
Psychiatric problems and obesity, 124, 125
Pulmonary complications following obesity surgery, 136
Pyloric ring identification, 49, 52
   repair, 50, 53
   reconstruction, patient selection for, 43–5
      postoperative care, 58–9
      results, 59–60
      technique, 45–8
Pyloroduodenal channel examination, 48, 49, 52
Pyloroplasty, excision of scar, 47, 48
   Finney, reversal of, 53–8
   Heinecke–Mikulicz, anatomy of, 47, 48
   reversal of, 45, 48–53

Quadrantectomy, 8

Reflux gastritis following gastric reduction, 139
Renal complications following gastric bypass, 137
Reservoir jejunal interposition, 64–71
Roux-en-Y gastrojejunostomy, 133–4
   reconstruction, 62, 65–7
Resuscitation of haemorrhaging patient, 30

Sclerosants, 143
Sclerotherapy for variceal bleeding, 32, 141–4
Segmentectomy, breast, 8
Segmentectomy 4, of liver, 93, 103
   anterior, 94–5, 102–3

Segmentectomy 4—*cont.*
  anterior—*cont.*
    for intrahepatic biliary anastomosis, 98
    for resection of quadrate lobe, 95–8
  complete, 99–101
  indications, 102–5
Serous fluid accumulation, 19
Sex parameters of obesity surgery, 125
Shunt surgery for variceal bleeding, 32
Silicone implants, 12–18
Skin incision, circumareolar/lateral, 12
  for gastric restrictive procedures, 129
  for jejunoileal bypass, 128
  for oesophageal transection, 34
  for peritoneovenous shunt, 112, 113
  for pyloric reconstruction, 46, 48
  for reservoir jejunal interposition, 64–5
  for shunt insertion, 114–15
  for splenic surgery, 79
  latissimus dorsi muscle/ellipse, 20–21
  lower axillary, 8
  necrosis, following breast surgery, 18, 24
Spironolactone for ascites, 107
Splenectomy, partial, 85–9
Splenic artery control, 79
  cysts, 75, 76–7
  non-malignant hypersplenic states, 75–6
  surgery
    implants, 90–91
    mobilization, 79–80
    outcome, 91–2
    patient selection, 74–6
    postoperative care, 91
    preoperative care and investigations, 76–7
    selective devascularization, 80–81
    techniques, 77–91
  trauma, 74–5, 76, 77–9
Splenomegaly, physical examination for, 30

Splenorrhaphy, 79–84
Stapling guns, 34
Stenosis of anastomosis, 73
  of stoma, 138
Sternal pocket construction, subcutaneous, 115
Stomach, staple partitioning of, 133
Stomal stenosis, 138
Subcutaneous mastectomy, 10–20
Subpectoral pouch extension, 16–18
Sutures, for breast surgery, 18
  for obesity surgery, 136
  for peritoneovenous shunting, 117
  for splenectomy, 87
  for splenorrhaphy, 82–4
  reinforcement in gastric restrictive procedures, 134

Tamponade, oesophageal, 31
Thromboembolism following obesity surgery, 137
Transection–devascularization technique for oesophageal varices, 32–7
Trisegmentectomy, 102, 104
Tylectomy, 8

Urolithiasis reduction, 137

Varices *see* Oesophageal varices
Vascular pedicle construction, 68
Vasopressin for variceal bleeding, 31, 142
Venous catheter insertion, 113
Vomiting, episodic, following gastric reduction, 138–9

Weight loss following gastric reduction, 138
Wound care following obesity surgery, 136–7